Critical Pathways for Collaborative Nursing Care

Suzanne C. Beyea, RN, CS, PhD

Department of Nursing
Saint Anselm College
Manchester, New Hampshire

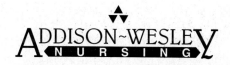
ADDISON~WESLEY
NURSING

A Division of the Benjamin/Cummings Publishing Company, Inc.
Menlo Park, California • Reading, Massachusetts • New York
Don Mills, Ontario • Wokingham, UK • Amsterdam • Bonn • Paris
Milan • Madrid • Sydney • Singapore • Tokyo • Seoul • Taipei
Mexico City • San Juan

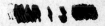

Executive Editor: Patricia L. Cleary
Managing Editor: Wendy Earl
Production Editor: Eleanor Renner Brown
Text Designer: Brad Greene
Cover Designer: Yvo Riezebos
Copyeditor: Kristin Barendsen
Proofreader: Eleanor Renner Brown
Compositor: London Road Design
Indexer: Nancy Kopper
Printer: Courier, Kendallville

The quilt pictured on the cover, "Postmodern XX" was designed by Jane Reeves of Canton, Ohio.

Library of Congress Cataloging-in Publication Data

Beyea, Suzanne C.
    Critical pathways for collaborative nursing care / Suzanne C. Beyea.
        p.   cm.
    Includes index.
    ISBN 0–8053–7230–X
    1. Nursing--Planning.   2. Critical path analysis.   3. Patient education.
I. Title.
    [DNLM: 1. Patient Care Planning.   2. Nursing Care.   WY 100 B573c
1996]
RT49.B49 1996
610.73--dc20
DNLM/DLC   95-41649
for Library of Congress   CIP

ISBN 0–8053–7230–x
1 2 3 4 5 6 7 8 9 10—CRK—99 98 97 96 95

Addison-Wesley Nursing
A Division of the Benjamin/Cummings Publishing Company, Inc.
2725 Sand Hill Road
Menlo Park, California 94025

Reviewers

Ann K. Beaver, RN, BS
William Beaumont Hospital
Royal Oak, Michigan

Joea E. Bierchen, RN, EdD, Emeritus
St. Petersburg Jr. College
St. Petersburg, Florida

B.J. Bockenhauer, MSN, RN
Nurse Educator
New Hampshire Hospital
Concord, New Hampshire

Liz Byrne-Rodzik, RN, BSN
Adjunct Faculty
Oakland Community College
Highland Lakes Campus, Michigan

Suzann J. Caldon, RN, CARN
Detox Program Coordinator
Lakes Region General Hospital
Laconia, New Hampshire

Karen Groth
RN, CS, MN, PhDc
Gonzaga University
Spokane, Washington

Carla Hronek, RN, MSN, CDE, OCN
Overland Park Regional Medical Center
Overland Park, Kansas

Karen Lavallee, BSN, RN
Assistant Nurse Manager
Catholic Medical Center
Manchester, New Hampshire

Nancy Tisdale, MS, RN, C, CNA
Assistant Director of Nursing Standards, Education, and Research
New Hampshire Hospital
Concord, New Hampshire

Christine Williams-Burgess, DNSc, RN
Associate Professor
University of Miami
Miami, Florida

Preface

This book presents examples of critical pathways for a number of health conditions. Critical pathways are one approach to deliver collaborative outcome-driven health care. Fast replacing traditional nursing care plans in many settings, critical pathways specify progressive interventions and predetermined outcomes.

Within this text, the user will see how health care interventions and outcomes may progress within a critical pathway. There is no such thing as a "perfect" critical pathway. Each agency and health care team must consider clinical resources, the population served, the setting, and community resources when developing a pathway. The critical pathways within this book present examples that have been based on a consensus process of practice patterns across the United States.

However, each client is unique and a given pathway may not be appropriate to a specific client situation. Each client must be individually assessed and a plan of care implemented based on those needs. If the critical pathway is utilized, the nurse must carefully assess the client's needs and responses to therapies on a regular and ongoing basis. Specific care should only be implemented if it is appropriate to the client's condition and situation. For example, most pathways provide medication recommendations. However, if the client is allergic to that medication, it should not be given.

The typical nursing textbook discusses nursing interventions and client outcomes in a somewhat broad fashion. It is only infrequently that a length of stay is discussed or progressive interventions are described. The beginning practitioner can view the complexities of care, but may not understand how to provide care in an incremental fashion. This book of critical pathways provides examples of how care may be provided to achieve outcomes across a timeline. An effort has been made to be holistic and address the complexity of care.

No pathway in this book should be considered a standard of care. In fact, the pathways presented are only one example of how to provide care for a certain client population. Nurses using these pathways may have suggestions or ideas to improve them, and I welcome comments and thoughts. It is my hope that these pathways will assist students and faculty in the teaching/learning process and provide examples of how pathways can be developed.

This book is organized according to specialty areas: medical, surgical, obstetric, pediatric, and psychiatric. For each pathway, potential client variances have been identified. For each specialty area, discharge teaching plans have been included.

Potential Client Variances

Potential client variances identify situations that may affect a client's progress on a particular pathway. These potential variances alert the caregiver to risks for complications, health situations, or nursing diagnoses that may affect the client's progress on a critical pathway.

Discharge Teaching Forms

Diagnosis-specific sample discharge teaching forms have been developed for the medical/surgical and pediatric critical pathways. These discharge teaching forms can be individualized to a client-specific situation. Models for assessing discharge needs for psychiatric and obstetrical patients are also included.

Dedication

This book is dedicated to my husband George, my sons Nate and Matt, my friends, and my students. These individuals have truly taught me about life, learning, love, and peace.

Acknowledgements

This book could never have been completed without the efforts and dedication of many others and I am grateful for those many contributions. I would like to offer a most sincere thank you to those individuals:

- Barbara Kozier and Glenora Erb whose vision for nursing started me on this pathway.

- Patti Cleary, for her untiring support, encouragement, and patience.

- Dorothy Zinky, for without her I would never have survived the struggle of compiling the materials. Her kind, encouraging words helped along the way.

- Dr. Joanne Farley, who has backed my efforts with words of encouragement and ongoing support.

- The reviewers, for their helpful comments and suggestions and their feedback that advanced my thinking and writing.

- Eleanor Renner Brown, whose dedication and thoroughness has made this book possible. She tutored me through the process of copyediting and processing pages. Her helpfulness has been beyond belief.

- Erin Mulligan for help and support at various stages.

- Wendy Earl, whose design and production efforts have made this book a reality.
- Kristin Barendsen for careful checking, helpful style suggestions, and making the printed word more readable.
- Emilie Dasch, RN, BSN, Nursing Director, Medical College Hospitals, Toledo, Ohio, who graciously discussed and shared a critical pathway for clients with sickle cell anemia. Her comments and suggestions were most helpful.
- Susan Smith, RN, BSN, Director of Women's and Children's Health Services, Lakes Region General Hospital, Laconia, New Hampshire, who provided helpful assistance by sharing a teaching needs assessment for maternity clients.
- Nancy Tisdale, RN, MSN, whose friendship and professionalism has guided me more than once. My thanks for discussion time and encouragement and sharing her knowledge of psychiatric clients and their needs. I am also grateful for her sharing the teaching protocol for inclusion as a guide in addressing knowledge deficits of psychiatric clients.
- B. J. Bockenhauer, RN, MSN, for valuable discussions about critical pathways for psychiatric populations and sharing her knowledge of the nursing process. Her assistance was instrumental in the development of the pathways for psychiatric clients.
- Norma Phillips at Lakes Region General Hospital who has endlessly provided materials that have supported this and many other projects.
- Brad Greene, for his clear and readable text design.
- Yvo Riezebos, whose vision and careful layout make the cover compliment the title.
- Nancy Kopper, whose attention to detail on the index will help others find their way to the information within these pages.

Finally, I thank my family and friends who have provided me with the support and love to make this possible.

"They are people who, in some mysterious way, are there when my need is greatest and help me to save my own life and the lives of those I love." (Tim Dayton)

Suzanne C. Beyea

Contents

Part 1

Introduction

Part 2

Critical Pathways

Medical Pathways 17

Burns, Severe Thermal 19
Cerebral Vascular Accident (CVA) 22
Congestive Heart Failure (CHF) 28
Chronic Obstructive Pulmonary Disease (COPD) 33
Deep Vein Thrombosis 38
Diabetes (Type II), New Onset 43
Diarrhea and Dehydration 48
Diverticulitis and Constipation 53
Gastrointestinal Bleeding (Upper) 58
Myocardial Infarction (Uncomplicated) 63
Osteomyelitis 68
Pneumonia 73
Sickle Cell Crisis 78
Weight Loss Program 83
Wound Management at Home 85

Surgical Pathways 87

Abdominal Aortic Aneurysm Repair 89
Appendectomy 95
Arm Fracture (Upper), with Open Reduction 99
Carotid Endarterectomy 103
Cataract Surgery 108
Cholecystectomy (Laparoscopic) 111
Colon Resection 114
Coronary Angioplasty, Percutaneous Transluminal 120
Coronary Artery Bypass Surgery 123
Craniotomy for Brain Tumor 131
Cystectomy with Ileal Conduit 135
Femoral Popliteal Bypass Graft 141
Gastrectomy (Partial) 146
Hernia Repair (Laparoscopic) 152
Hip Pinning (Fractured Hip with Prosthesis or Internal Fixation) 155
Hip Replacement (Total) 163
Hysterectomy (Abdominal) 168
Hysterectomy (Vaginal) 172

Knee Replacement (Total) 176
Laminectomy (Lumbar) 182
Laryngectomy 186
Lower Leg Fracture (Open Reduction and Internal Fixation) 194
Mastectomy 198
Microdiskectomy 202
Nephrectomy 205
Permanent Pacemaker Insertion 211
Proctocolectomy with Permanent Ileostomy (Total) 215
Splenectomy 222
Thyroidectomy 227
Transurethral Resection of the Prostate 230

Obstetric Pathways 235

Labor and Delivery 237
Newborm 241
Postpartum Vaginal Delivery 245
Postpartum Cesarean Section 249

Pediatric Pathways 257

Asthma 259
Diabetes (Type I) 263
Myringotomy and Insertion of Pressure-Equalizer Tubes 266
Pyloric Stenosis (Surgical Repair) 269
Respiratory Infection (Acute) 272
Tonsillectomy and Adenoidectomy 276

Psychiatric Pathways 279

Alcohol Withdrawal 281
Anorexia Nervosa 287
Bipolar Disorder: Manic Phase 292
Dementia 299
Depression Without Psychotic Features or Agitation 304
Panic Disorder: Outpatient Treatment 310

Index 315

Part I

Introduction

Introduction

Overview

Critical pathways are interdisciplinary client care plans that delineate assessments, interventions, treatments, and outcomes for specific health-related conditions across a designated time line. Critical pathways are also referred to as critical paths, interdisciplinary plans, anticipated recovery plans, interdisciplinary action plans, and action plans. As management tools, they can be developed for surgical procedures, medical diagnoses, and health-related interventions. They are most useful for high volume case types or situations that have relatively predictable outcomes. Extremely complex client situations with unpredictable outcomes are not usually managed with critical pathways. Critical pathways are designed through the collaboration of the health care team members involved in providing care for and managing the case type.

This type of care plan describes how clinical resources will be utilized to achieve predetermined outcomes (Giuliano & Poirier, 1991; Zander, 1991; Zander, 1992). Critical pathways establish the sequence and timing of interdisciplinary interventions, and incorporate education, discharge planning, assessments, consultations, nutrition, medications, activities, diagnostics, therapeutics, and treatments.

The goals of critical pathways include: 1) achieving realistic, expected client and family outcomes; 2) promoting professional, collaborative practice and care; 3) ensuring the continuity of care; 4) guaranteeing appropriate use of resources; 5) reducing costs and length of stay; and 6) establishing the framework for continuous quality improvement. The overall goal is to improve the quality and efficiency of client care by setting a reproducible standard of care for designated client populations.

Clinical agencies determine the process for developing critical pathways. Essential information required to develop any critical pathway includes the pertinent literature and related research, chart analyses, expert opinions, and the level of insurance reimbursement for the specific case type. A typical approach involves first identifying high-cost, high-volume, and high-risk case types for the agency. After choosing a specific case type, an interdisciplinary team, including physicians, nurses, social services, dietary and rehabilitative services, and others, develops a consensus around the management of the case type and then designs the critical pathway. Following this stage, client care units implement and pilot the pathway. The interdisciplinary team continues to refine the pathway, identifying variances and making changes as indicated, in an effort to develop a model that best meets client needs.

Historical Background

Critical pathways spring from a number of trends in health care, including case management, outcome-driven practice models, and continuous quality improvement. As a logical evolution of nursing care plans, they provide a way to integrate the traditional nursing care plan with interdisciplinary interventions.

The nursing process and nursing care plans were originally established as frameworks to address the individualized needs of clients, families, and communities. Eventually, however, the traditional nursing care plan no longer met the needs of clients or health care personnel. The traditional care plan was often based on nursing diagnoses and only included nursing interventions. Due to the variations in physicians' practice patterns, the nurse planning the care often was unaware of the planned medical interventions or length of stay. There was little interdisciplinary collaboration regarding the client or the expected outcomes. In many institutions the nursing care plan was used only by nursing staff and not even included as part of the permanent record.

Case Management

When nurses assumed case management roles, it became crucial to develop a flexible care planning and documentation system that reflected multidisciplinary efforts and addressed interventions and outcomes for a specific situation across a predetermined time line.

Nurse case managers were skilled at using the nursing process and writing intervention statements and outcomes, all components of the traditional nursing care plan. It made sense, therefore, that nurse case managers would adopt some of the components of nursing care plans when developing managed care plans. Gathering information about clients' expected length of stay and about physicians' practice patterns made it possible to place interventions and outcomes on time lines. Agencies committed to providing client-centered, interdisciplinary care empowered nurse case managers to develop managed care plans that addressed the totality of a client's needs.

Case management models and critical pathways have created new opportunities for nurses. Because they provide information crucial to the provision of nursing care, they generally free nurses from having to develop lengthy nursing care plans. Nursing time can be better spent on providing care.

Outcome-Driven Practice Models

Health care reform has furthered the development of practice models such as case management and tools such as critical pathways. Health care systems have been under increasing pressure to design cost-effective models of care. Prospective payment structures, rising numbers of elderly, quality improvement initiatives, the movement from acute care settings to home care, shrinking financial resources, and the AIDS epidemic have all contributed to changes in health care delivery. Critical pathways emerged as a cost-effective initiative that was outcome-driven, providing a framework from which to evaluate clients' responses to treatment against a time line.

Continuous Quality Improvement

Changes in quality assurance models also influenced the adoption of critical pathways. Traditional quality assurance efforts did not establish a process for quality improvement. Continuous quality improvement programs were mandated by JCAHO in 1992 (Koska, 1991), as a way to improve care through ongoing evaluation. Critical components of such programs include planning, implementing, and evaluating change.

Today, most health care agencies have adopted total quality management, quality improvement, or continuous clinical improvement programs. Critical pathways are key components of these programs. Within critical pathway models, when clients do not achieve predetermined outcomes, variances are identified. The evaluation of these variances provides the framework from which to make improvements in critical pathways, client care, and in the utilization of clinical resources.

Critical pathways and continuous improvement efforts hold health care providers responsible for both clinical and financial outcomes. Critical pathways establish a consistent methodology from which to evaluate interdisciplinary interventions, lengths of stays, readmission and complication rates, and client and staff satisfaction. Variance analyses from critical pathways assist clinicians in examining both process and outcome data for individuals and groups of clients. High-quality client outcomes are the focus of all improvement efforts.

Critical Pathways, the Nursing Process, and Nursing Diagnosis

In many acute care facilities, critical pathways have replaced traditional nursing care plans. Critical pathways or similar models are also being implemented in outpatient and long-term facilities and in the community. Despite wide acceptance of critical pathways, confusion persists in nursing education and practice about how best to represent nursing interventions and practice in pathway models.

In the 1970s and 1980s, nursing care was typically managed using nursing care plans and nursing diagnoses. Although some critical pathways reflect nursing diagnoses, they generally do not use nursing diagnoses to direct client care. In other words, the daily interdisciplinary plan of care does not necessarily reflect independent nursing interventions. Instead, categories such as tests, treatments, assessment, nutrition, activity, medications, discharge planning, teaching, psychosocial needs, and consultations serve as the framework to classify interdisciplinary interventions including dependent and interdependent nursing interventions.

As critical pathways replace nursing care plans, the struggle to clarify the independent practice of nursing continues. Within the interdisciplinary framework, nursing interventions are an essential component of the client's care. The scope of nursing includes the responsibility of identifying "human responses to actual or potential health problems" (ANA, 1980, p 9). In addition to using an established critical pathway, a nurse may identify nursing diagnoses and care specific to the client. For example, a client who is preoperative for a total hip replacement may also be blind and have family problems. In this instance, if the client's problems and needs are not addressed in the critical pathway, the nurse would identify the appropriate nursing diagnoses, such as sensory-perceptual alterations and ineffective family coping.

Variances from a critical pathway become decision points where it may be appropriate for the nurse to reassess the client, formulate a nursing diagnosis, or implement alternate interventions. For example, when a newly diagnosed diabetic does not make progress toward desired outcomes, this client variance might be related to ineffective individual coping or anger. A nursing diagnosis and a related nursing care plan could identify this client's specific needs. Client care can be improved through the use of a critical pathway and an individualized care plan, as the individualized care plan considers problems not addressed by the critical pathway.

The move toward interdisciplinary critical pathways will ensure positive client outcomes and collaborative health care. Nurses will work with all members of the health care team to develop effective approaches to managing health problems and needs. The challenge for nurses is to provide high-quality, cost-effective care that integrates human caring and concern. See Figure 1 for an example of an Interdisciplinary Client Care Plan.

Figure 1. Interdisciplinary Client Care Plan

(see Critical Pathway for Client Following Mastectomy in Part 2 on page 198)

Mrs. Deanna Fuller is an 83-year-old married female who was admitted following a right radical mastectomy. She had a positive biopsy for breast cancer two weeks prior to admission. On admission to ambulatory surgery, Mrs Fuller tells the nurse, "I have very bad cataracts. I can't even read this permit." Following surgery, Mrs Fuller repeatedly attempts to ambulate without assistance despite receiving pain medication via a PCA.

Additional Needs

Nursing Diagnosis:

- Risk for injury related to vision problems, sedation, and changes in environment

Expected Client Outcomes:

- Client will remain safe from physical injury throughout hospitalization.
- Client will identify risks that increase susceptibility to injury within 24 hours.

Nursing Interventions and Rationales:

- Assess level of orientation every shift and prn. (Changes in mental status are associated with an increased risk of falling, especially in older clients.) Reorient client to reality and immediate environment prn. (Orientation to time, place, person, and environment will reduce risk of injury associated with sensory/perceptual problems.)
- Encourage client to request assistance with activities. (Assisting the client with activities will reduce risk of injury.)
- Provide verbal instructions regarding hazards in immediate environment. (Education about potential hazards will increase compliance with injury-reduction strategies.)
- Keep rails up, bed in low position, and call bell in place when in bed. (These basic safety measures will reduce risks of falling.)
- Provide verbal instructions regarding techniques to prevent injury at home prior to discharge. (Older clients are at higher risks for falls and resultant injury. Knowledge about common hazards will decrease likelihood of falls.)

Nursing Diagnosis:

- Sensory/perceptual alterations: Visual related to cataracts and visual problems manifested by reported vision problems

Expected Client Outcomes:

- Client will remain oriented to time, place, person, and situation throughout hospital stay.
- Client will demonstrate the ability to compensate for visual problems.

Nursing Interventions and Rationales:

- Assess client for any other factors that may contribute to further sensory/perceptual alterations. (Persons with visual problems may rely on their other senses to cope with deficits. Knowledge about other problems will assist in the planning and provision of care.)
- Reorient client to reality and immediate environment with each interaction. (Illness and hospitalization may affect an individual's ability to process information.)
- Explain reasons for and location of surrounding equipment, furniture, and alarms. (Auditory information will enhance visual input.)
- Ensure access to and use of glasses. (Use of glasses will maximize remaining vision.)
- Provide all instructions verbally, and encourage client to verbalize understanding. (Clients with visual problems need to have all written instructions read aloud. Verbalizing understanding verifies level of learning.)
- Provide appropriate sensory input with social interaction, scheduled contacts, clock with large numbers, and so on. (Older adults with sensory problems may suffer from sensory deprivation. Providing appropriate sensory information will minimize risk of sensory deprivation.)

Accountability

Each organization determines the model for critical pathway implementation and the associated evaluation process. Regardless of the system, everyone involved with the case type must clearly understand the interventions, time lines, and sharing of resources. The management of the case type and the critical pathway may be evaluated by a case manager, a continuous clinical improvement team, or another designated person or group.

When critical pathways are designed and implemented, all members of the health care team share accountability. A critical pathway could be viewed as a formal agreement with a client, delineating the client's expected progress and the timing of interventions during an episode of illness or hospitalization. Members of the health care team can communicate the dimensions of the pathway with both the client and family. If goals are not achieved, variances are evaluated to determine the nature of the problem. From these variances, action plans are designed so as to improve care in the future.

Prior to the development of critical pathways, there was tremendous variability in the management of specific case types. Clients admitted with the same diagnosis could have very different length of stays and incur very different costs. Critical pathways reduce this variability and provide a user-friendly tool to help ensure financial and clinical accountability. Prospective payment schedules and fixed reimbursements necessitate controlling costs, limiting lengths of stay, and enhancing the quality of care. Critical pathways assist members of the health care team to plan and provide care, and assure that clients achieve outcomes within a prescribed time frame and established cost controls.

Case Management and Critical Pathways

Practice trends such as managed care, case management, collaborative care, and interdisciplinary managed care plans emerged concurrently. In some agencies, the term managed care is synonymous with nursing case management. Both models provide approaches to control costs and ensure quality. However, generally speaking, managed care is the system within which case management is practiced.

Professional practice models such as primary nursing evolved into nursing case management during the 1980s (Cohen & Cesta, 1993). Nursing case management models are diversified, depending on the setting, philosophy of care, and practice realities. Within hospitals, case managers may be nurses, social workers, or clinical specialists. Nursing case managers may also be employed by insurance companies or health maintenance organizations to coordinate and monitor care.

Regardless of the setting, key responsibilities for nurse case managers include 1) client assessment, 2) coordination and planning of client care, 3) collaboration with other mem-

bers of the health care team, 4) monitoring of clients' progress, 5) evaluation of outcomes, 6) communicating the client's care plan, and 7) carrying out other related responsibilities. In many settings, the role of nurse case manager continues to evolve, and one can expect marked variations in responsibilities.

The role of nurse case manager is often similar to that of an orchestra conductor. The nurse case manager works with all members of the health care team to facilitate care that reduces cost, focuses on outcomes, and enhances quality. She or he is responsible for writing a plan of care that is client- and family-centered and that synthesizes the contributions of all health care team members. While monitoring the effectiveness of the plan, the case manager ideally creates harmony among personnel in a dynamic, interactive fashion.

Strategies for Critical Pathway Development

If a national health care system is adopted, it will eventually lead to greater uniformity in health care. In terms of length of stay and costs, a person hospitalized in any area of the country would theoretically have a very similar experience to any other individual admitted with that diagnosis.

At present, however, care varies by location, practitioner, facility, and insurer. Therefore, critical pathways for specific case types are individualized to specific settings. In fact, in the same hospital one may see two different critical pathways for the same diagnosis that are labeled according to the client's physician. Although this is not ideal, we can expect future growth toward consensus and standardization.

In many instances, the health care system lacks adequate research on which to base practice decisions. Until a national research database is established, consensus among health care professionals will be used to establish critical pathways and health practices. Thus, at present, critical pathways may reflect a certain degree of variability, due to physician-specific preferences, practice settings, and rates of reimbursement.

Once individuals within a practice setting are committed to implementing critical pathways, the health care team must decide which specific diagnosis or condition will be utilized first to develop a critical pathway. Usually the team chooses high-volume cases with predictable outcomes, such as total hip replacement or anterior myocardial infarction. A case manager with expertise about the case type coordinates the development and implementation of the critical pathway. Members of the development team include all personnel who will be involved in delivering and evaluating care.

Crucial to the development of any critical pathway is physician commitment to both the concept and process. Each physician involved with the particular case type makes contributions while the critical pathway is under development. Differing physician preferences must be negotiated, reflecting individual practice differences as much as possible. The critical pathway designed by the team is for the average situation and can be individualized by the physician to meet the needs of a particular client.

Once the critical pathway is developed, most planning groups review the plan together prior to implementation. In fact, this group may be responsible for setting target dates for implementation as well as presenting the pathway to other members of the health care team. When this effort is complete, the pathway is ready for clinical testing and evaluation.

Gathering Information

Once the case type has been defined, the nurse case manager and members of the pathway team complete a thorough review of clinical cases. They collect data on the average length of stay, costs per case, interventions provided, outcomes, and demographics. When analyzed, this data provides important information about that case type in that particular setting.

Next, the pathway team completes a literature and research review. A search through both the medical and nursing information uncovers articles on critical pathway development for that case type in a variety of settings. Such articles provide samples of critical pathways that may be helpful in designing a model for the agency. The research and literature review may also stimulate ideas for development, education, and implementation. The team can offer key articles to staff as a way of introducing the concept of interdisciplinary care plans. The pathway team may use other strategies in the data collection phase, such as consulting with other institutions who have developed pathways, or adapting a commercial critical pathway system that meets its needs.

Internal and External Influences

During critical pathway development, the health care team must identify the internal and external factors that may influence development, adoption, and implementation. Internal factors include administrative support, physician backing, staff interest, and the availability of clinical resources. External factors include the clinical setting (rural vs. urban), the availability of community resources, and changes in the health care system and in reimbursement structures.

The pathway development team must address these issues, and create inventive solutions to problems. For instance, if testing equipment is available only once per week, it may not be possible for a client to have that test within 24 hours of admission. How the development team and case manager address such a problem will depend on the available resources. Indeed, what may work in one setting or with one population may be inappropriate in another situation.

Providing Information to the Client

In this era of health care reform, health care providers can expect to see clients more actively involved in their own care. Education continues to be an essential part of any health care delivery system. Critical pathways will provide information about who is responsible for specific interventions and their timing.

Ideally, the client and family should receive a simplified, written copy of the critical pathway. If this is not possible, then the plan of care should be explained verbally. Some clinicians recommend mailing preoperative clients a copy of a pathway (Mosher et al, 1992) that describes the nursing activities and client activities in lay terms. These approaches allow clients to view the totality of the care they will receive. In most critical pathway systems, clients also receive written teaching forms (See Figure 2) that address ongoing and discharge teaching needs. These standardized teaching protocols ensure high quality care and can be used to document completed teaching. Involving clients in education empowers them to participate in their own care.

Classification of Interventions

In critical pathways, the interdisciplinary interventions are classified in a way that is comfortable and applicable to the various disciplines involved in the delivery of client care. No one system is universal or appropriate to all clinical situations or settings. Categories are determined by case type, agency type, and clarity.

Nyberg and Marschke (1993) describe the use of health parameters as an organizing framework for a critical pathway classification system in a surgical setting. The categories for interdisciplinary interventions include "nutrition, elimination, structural integrity/sexual function, sensory function, neurologic-cerebral function, respiratory function, emotional response, social system, cognitive response, and health management pattern" (p 63). On a sample critical pathway provided by Nyberg and Marschke, similar headings are used with the addition of the categories of tests and consults.

Another popular classification system has been suggested by Zander (1991). This popular framework includes: "1) consults/assessments, 2) treatments, 3) nutrition, 4) medications, 5) activity/safety, 6) teaching (patient, significant others), 7) discharge planning/coordination" (p 1). Zander recommends the use of other categories such as psychosocial needs based on the needs of clients of a particular case type.

Generally speaking, the case type is the most essential determinant in terms of a classification system. For example, critical pathways for psychiatric case types are more likely to include a psychosocial category. Information about the type of agency and health care personnel may also help determine a classification system. If there is no social worker available at an

Figure 2. Sample Discharge Teaching Form

Discharge Teaching for Client Following
Mastectomy

Activity

- Gradually return to usual level of activity by increasing activity each day. Alternate activity with rest periods.
- Exercise affected arm as instructed to tolerance. Stop at the point of pain.
- Elevate affected arm several times a day, by combing hair, wall climbing, or eating with affected arm.
- Avoid heavy housework, straining, and driving for period designated by physician.

Diet

- Follow usual and customary diet.

Signs and Symptoms to Report

Notify physician if any of these symptoms occur:
- Increase in pain, redness, or swelling
- Sudden increase in wound drainage, especially if drainage has pus or a foul odor
- Chills, or fever greater than 100F or 38C

Follow-Up Care and General Health Care

- Schedule follow-up appointment with physician as directed.
- Examine remaining breast once per month.

- Refer to Reach to Recovery
- Reinforce safety precautions:
- Avoid activities that could injure arm and hand, for example: gardening, use of sharp objects
- Avoid injections or drawing blood in affected arm
- No B/P on affected arm.
- Treat burns, cuts, or scratches on affected arm immediately
- Wear gloves when working with sharp objects
- Wear loose-fitting clothing until incision heals
- Avoid sunburn
- Use a thimble when sewing
- Use an electric razor on affected underarm

Medications

- Provide written list of medications, including dose, route, frequency, and side effects.

Wound and Dressing Care

- Cleanse skin around incision daily with mild soap and water.
- If dressing present, change it daily and as often as necessary to keep dressing dry and clean.
- Remove dressing prior to showering and replace with a clean dressing afterward.
- Drainage, if present, should gradually decrease.

agency, for example, the social service category may not be appropriate. The third and perhaps most important factor is clarity: the categories should be distinct and easily understood.

Establishing Daily and Discharge Outcomes

Desired outcomes are usually established by either the case manager or the pathway development team. On the pathway, outcomes can be organized according to specific time frames such as hourly, every eight hours, or daily. Additional outcomes may be measured at the time of interagency transfers or discharge. The evaluation interval is based on the acuity of the case type and the frequency and type of interventions.

Process and outcome criteria are established by the pathway team based on clinical expertise and review of data collected during the development phase. Generally speaking, outcomes should be realistic, measurable, and understandable. They should describe desired client behavior within the specified time frames, and they should be clearly understood by all members of the health care team. The outcomes provide the basis for documenting variances and the basis for critical pathway revision and validation.

Determining the Time Line

The time frames used in a critical pathway center on the case type, the setting, and the acuity of the situation. The most common format for critical pathways is a sequential diagram where time frames are listed across the top of the page with the intervention categories listed on the left side of the diagram. Typical time categories are preadmission, admission, and each day until discharge. In some settings such as the postanesthesia care unit or emergency room, the intervals may be minutes or hours. In long-term case types, however, the time intervals may be as long as weekly. It may be appropriate in some instances to include hourly and daily time frames on the same critical pathway.

When determining the time frames, the pathway development team considers factors such as the frequency of intervention and clinical practice standards. In certain settings such as critical care units, it is appropriate to assess outcomes more frequently. The total time frame is based on the anticipated length of stay and insurance reimbursements.

Planning Interventions

The pathway team determines interventions through input from involved clinicians, chart reviews, and analysis of the literature, research, and current practice. Interventions reflect collaboration of the various disciplines involved, acknowledging the contributions of each member of the

health care team. They are focused on helping the client meet outcome goals.

Once the appropriate interventions are identified, they are classified according to the categories in use. Interventions can include assessments, diagnostics, medications, consultations, activity levels, psychosocial needs, and any other categories pertinent to the case type. Each intervention should specify the roles and responsibilities of the various disciplines and contribute to goal achievement.

Generally, intervention statements contain details such as timing and frequency and are as specific and descriptive as possible. Typical intervention statements specify what to do, when to do it, and who should do it. Any other details required to perform the intervention, including treatments and required technology, may be included.

Implementation Strategies

Once the critical pathway is completed, it is ready for implementation, clinical testing, and validation. Implementation cannot begin until staff are adequately prepared and appropriate clinical supports are in place. Key issues during the implementation phase include staff education and involvement as well as documentation systems.

Staff Education and Involvement

If critical pathways are introduced without adequate staff preparation, chaos can ensue. It is essential that all staff involved in the development and implementation of a critical pathway system learn about the process. All key members should be identified and included as clinical resources and consulted regarding development, adoption, and implementation. These individuals can assist in informing their immediate colleagues and supporting others during the implementation phase.

When a new critical pathway is introduced, "idea champions"—those who fully support the concept and process—can facilitate implementation. These individuals can support others who might be more resistant to practice changes. Those responsible for the development and implementation need to evaluate the satisfaction of staff, clients, and families. Staff need timely and positive feedback regarding their efforts and the results of this new endeavor.

Critical pathways can be instrumental in teaching new practitioners and students as well as in orienting new staff. Unlike a traditional nursing care plan, a critical pathway can assist all members of the health care team to fully understand the complexities of the client's care and the patterns of progression for specific case types. Clearly delineated outcomes and interventions will enhance each care giver's understanding of the client's holistic needs.

Communication Issues

A critical pathway provides a framework for documentation and for communication of delivered care. Whether using a computer-based documentation system or a written critical pathway, clinicians in many facilities simply initial interventions when completed. Outcomes are noted when achieved, and variances are identified when there are deviations from the critical pathway. Clinicians record variances either on the pathway or on a separate record that tracks variances for each client.

Critical pathways help facilitate intershift and interdisciplinary communication. Nurses can use the pathway when conferring with the physician and other members of the health care team regarding the client's progress. Critical pathways can also be the basis from which to discuss the interventions and the client's responses during intershift report. The variance record notes any issues that have affected the client's progress toward the predetermined outcomes.

Evaluation

Detours or Variances

Within the critical pathway system, a variance or detour is any event that affects a client's progress toward achieving predetermined outcomes. Variances are categorized as system, provider, or client variances. A system variance involves a situation in which the institution or community is unable to provide the appropriate level of care or specific intervention. A typical system variance would be the unavailability of diagnostic testing or home intravenous therapy. Provider/clinician variances occur when the health care provider's performance affects the client outcomes. Examples would be omitting a medication or respiratory treatment. A client variance relates to client factors that affect outcomes. If a client develops a complication or if an unexpected change in condition alters outcomes, a client variance is recorded. Cohen and Cesta (1993) also describe "client variance on admission" and "unmet clinical quality indicators" (p 123). Admission variances reflect client-specific assessment data, while "unmet clinical quality indicators" variances address situations in which physician-determined clinical outcomes are not achieved. See Figure 3 (beginning on page 12) for a typical variance recording sheet.

Most agencies design critical pathways so that variances can be easily recorded, although variances may not be a part of the permanent record. A typical documentation system will include a log. Once variances are recorded, they are studied concurrently and retrospectively by the nurses, case managers, and others involved in the client's care. The variances or detours provide the foundation for evaluating client care and for continuous clinical improvement.

Future Directions

Critical pathways are one approach to providing client-centered, outcome-driven interdisciplinary health care. In this era of health care reform, many other developments that facilitate the delivery of cost-effective, quality care may arise. Creative strategies that assist clients in a variety of settings will be integral to reform. Research will help determine the effectiveness of critical pathways in managing diversified health problems in diversified settings.

Clinical Applications

Although initially developed for acute hospitalizations, critical pathways are now used to manage clients in home health, outpatient, rehabilitation, and long-term agencies. A number of settings have adopted critical pathway models that reflect clients' needs in that specific setting.

Grudich (1991) implemented critical pathways as an approach to enhance the efficiency of an operating room. After careful analysis of the problems that lead to delays, scheduling, and work flow problems, the operating room department implemented a critical pathway system that guided clients' experiences through an operation. Time frames reflected certain activities around the surgical experience such as preoperative laboratory work, outpatient admission, nursing assessment, and induction. Staff found that the critical pathway system "improved efficiency" (p 714).

Nelson (1993) reports utilizing a critical pathway for chest pain in the emergency department. The sample pathway describes key assessments, treatments, medications, tests, discharge teaching, documentation, and registration. The designated time frames were minutes and hours. The interventions reflected the many different activities and disciplines involved in the care of a client in this department. This application of a critical pathway system in the emergency department has implications for all outpatient facilities.

Goodwin (1992) proposes using critical pathways and case management in home health settings. After a detailed analysis of key nursing activities, client outcomes, and the frequency of visits, a critical pathway for congestive heart failure was developed. The time frame established for the suggested pathway was based on weeks and/or number of visits. Goodwin reports that in home health settings, critical pathways might increase costs, but suggests that critical pathways may improve nursing care, ensure quality outcomes, encourage self-care, and perhaps decrease hospital admissions.

Computer Models

Computers already serve as the primary documentation system in many settings. It is hard to fully predict how computer technology and health care reform initiatives will affect health care in the future. Health information systems hold the potential to revolutionize approaches toward managing and utilizing condition- and client-specific data. In the future, vast databases will provide clinical information and assist in developing and evaluation of national standards and guidelines.

Variances from critical pathways are being analyzed using computers. With future software developments, individualized critical pathways could be developed for each client.

Validation of Time Line and Interventions

The nurse case manager is usually responsible for ensuring that the critical pathway reflects current practice and new technologies. New knowledge may indicate the need for changes in the time line or specific interventions within the pathway. As national databases of health information are compiled, trends and patterns of care will be available and can contribute toward the development of critical pathways that reflect national trends.

Health care reform will lead to the development of nationwide standards for interventions and time lines. Currently, pathways are developed using the consensus process and from available data pertinent to the case type. Physicians contributing to a pathway discuss differences in their practices and compromise to establish a pathway that can be used with the majority of their clients. Expert opinion fills the gap where there is no research base to direct clinical practice. Critical pathways should eventually reflect nationwide standards of care. Providing research-based, cost-effective, quality care is the ultimate goal of critical pathways.

References

American Nurses Association: *A social policy statement.* Kansas City, MO, 1980.

Cohen, EL, Cesta, TG: *Nursing Case Management: From Concept to Evaluation.* St. Louis: Mosby, 1993

Crummer, MB, Carter, V: Critical pathways—the pivotal tool. *Journal of Cardiovascular Nursing* 1993; 7(4):30–37.

Davis, J: Goals along the critical pathway. *Innovations* Fall 1993; (pp 2–6) St. Luke's Episcopal Hospital, Houston, TX.

Geehr, EC: The search for what works. *Healthcare Forum Journal* 1992; 35(4):28–33.

Goodwin, DR: Critical pathways in home health care. *Journal of Nursing Administration* 1992; 22(2):35–40.

Grudich, G: The critical path system: The road toward an efficient OR. *AORN Journal* 1991; 53(3):705–714.

Giulinao, KK, Poirier, CE: Nursing case management: Critical pathways to desirable outcomes. *Nursing Management* 1991; 22(3):52–55.

Koska, MT: New JCAHO standards emphasize continuous quality improvement. *Hospitals* 1991; 65(15):41–44.

Mosher, C, et al: Upgrading practice with critical pathways. *American Journal of Nursing* 1992; 92(1):41–44.

Nelson, MS: Critical pathways in the emergency department. *Journal of Emergency Nursing* 1993; 19(2):110–114.

Nyberg, D, Marschke, P: Critical pathways: Tools for continuous quality improvement. *Nursing Administration Quarterly* 1993; 17(3):62–69.

Zander, K: CareMaps: The core of cost/quality. *Definition* 1988; 6(1):1–2.

Zander, K. Managed care within acute care settings: Design and implementation via nursing case management. *Health Care Supervisor* 1988, 6(2), 27-43.

Zander, K: Quantifying, managing, and improving quality, Part I: How CareMaps link CQI to the patient. *The New Definition* 1992; 1(2):1–3.

Figure 3. Sample Variance Recording Sheet

VARIANCE REPORT

Client _____

ID Number _____

Case Type _____

Admission Date: _____ Admitting Diagnosis: _____ DRG: _____

Discharge Date: _____ Secondary Diagnosis: _____ Expected LOS: _____

Surgical Procedures: _____

A. CLIENT/FAMILY

1. Client condition
2. Client/family decision
3. Client/family availability
4. Client/family other

B. CLINICIAN

5. Physician order
6. Clinician(s) decision
7. Clinician(s) response timely
8. Clinician other

C. HOSPITAL/SYSTEM

9. Bed/appointment time availability
10. Information/data availability
11. Supplies/equipment availability
12. Department overbooked/closed
13. Hospital other

D. COMMUNITY

14. Placement/Home Care availability
15. Ambulance delay
16. Community resources
17. Equipment availability

Directions for use: Please code each entry with one of the above listed codes.

DATE	TIME	SOURCE NUMBER	DESCRIPTION	REASON	ACTION PLAN	INT.

Figure 3. Sample Variance Recording Sheet (completed)

VARIANCE REPORT

Client _____

ID Number _____

Case Type _____

Admission Date: _____   Admitting Diagnosis: _____   DRG: _____

Discharge Date: _____   Secondary Diagnosis: _____   Expected LOS: _____

Surgical Procedures: _____

A. CLIENT/FAMILY
1. Client condition
2. Client/family decision
3. Client/family availability
4. Client/family other

B. CLINICIAN
5. Physician order
6. Clinician(s) decision
7. Clinician(s) response timely
8. Clinician other

C. HOSPITAL/SYSTEM
9. Bed/appointment time availability
10. Information/data availability
11. Supplies/equipment availability
12. Department overbooked/closed
13. Hospital other

D. COMMUNITY
14. Placement/Home Care availability
15. Ambulance delay
16. Community resources
17. Equipment availability

Directions for use: Please code each entry with one of the above listed codes.

DATE	TIME	SOURCE NUMBER	DESCRIPTION	REASON	ACTION PLAN	INT.
11/19/95	1000	1.	Unable to eat ordered diet	Prolonged vomiting	MD notified — antiemetic obtained	NDB
11/20/95	2000	7	Respiratory treat- ment omitted	Clinician involved in emergency situation	Respiratory status assessed — stable — treatment rescheduled	ERB
11/21/95	1200	12	Stress test delayed 3 days	Unable to schedule during weekend	Discussed with department	MWD

Part 2

Critical Pathways

Medical Pathways

Burns, Severe Thermal   19

Cerebral Vascular Accident (CVA)   22

Congestive Heart Failure (CHF)   28

Chronic Obstructive Pulmonary Disease (COPD)   33

Deep Vein Thrombosis   38

Diabetes (Type II)   43

Diarrhea and Dehydration   48

Diverticulitis and Constipation   53

Gastrointestinal Bleeding (Upper)   58

Myocardial Infarction (Uncomplicated)   63

Osteomyelitis   68

Pneumonia   73

Sickle Cell Crisis   78

Weight Loss Program   83

Wound Management at Home   85

Critical Pathway for Client with
Severe Thermal Burns

Expected length of stay: Until stabilized for transfer to burn unit

	Date _____ Time _____ **On Admission to Emergency Department**	Date _____ Time _____ **When Stabilized and Prior to Transfer to Burn Unit**
Daily outcomes	• Client maintains a patent airway and effective breathing pattern • Interventions are initiated to stabilize vital signs • Client's condition and burns are assessed and treatment initiated • Client/family verbalizes or indicates understanding of explanations of ongoing treatment • Further trauma to skin is avoided • Client demonstrates ability to cope	• Client maintains a patent airway and effective breathing pattern, evidenced by clear lungs and ABGs within normal limits • Blood pressure, pulse, and respirations are stabilized • Client's burns receive initial treatment • Client maintains urine output of 30–50 mL/hr • Client is alert and oriented • Client/family verbalizes or indicates understanding of explanations of ongoing treatment, condition, and transfer • Client demonstrates ability to cope with ongoing stressors
Assessments, tests, and treatments	Assess and maintain patent airway Assess and monitor rhythm and rate of respirations and breath sounds Assess and monitor vital signs Administer humidified oxygen to maintain pulse oximeter >92% Monitor pulse oximeter Initiate respiratory support as indicated Keep HOB elevated unless contraindicated Assess pain level Assess level of orientation and monitor for disorientation Keep client warm Assess and monitor peripheral circulation, sensation, and motion Check peripheral pulses with Doppler Assess and monitor fluid volume status—strict intake and output Assess percentage of body surface burned Initiate venous access—administer Ringer's Lactate at 4 mL per kg of body weight per percentage of body surface area burned (2nd & 3rd degree burns) Assess location and severity (extent and depth) of burns Foley catheter Maintain body alignment Assess time and type of injury and initial treatment	Assess and maintain patent airway Assess and monitor rhythm and rate of respirations and breath sounds Assess and monitor vital signs Administer humidified oxygen to maintain pulse oximeter >92% Monitor pulse oximeter Keep HOB elevated unless contraindicated Assess pain level Assess level of orientation and monitor for disorientation Keep client warm Assess and monitor peripheral circulation, sensation, and motion Check peripheral pulses with Doppler Assess fluid volume status Strict intake and output Provide burn care: – Maintain sterile technique – Elevate burned extremities – Wash burns with warm soap and water – Dry burns and cover with topical agent (silver sulfadiazine) – Either bandage burns or leave open to the air per order – Prepare client for escharotomy if indicated – IV fluids as ordered

Severe Thermal Burns *(continued)*

	Date _____ Time _____ **On Admission to Emergency Department**	Date _____ Time _____ **When Stabilized and Prior to Transfer to Burn Unit**
Assessments, tests, and treatments (continued)	Assess client's medical history, allergies, and use of medications Laboratory Diagnostic Testing: 　CBC 　Urinalysis 　ABGs 　Type and crossmatch for specified number of units 　Serum chemistries, electrolytes 　Urine specific gravity Chest x-ray EKG Baseline physical assessment Nasogastric tube if indicated	Foley catheter Maintain body alignment Cardiac monitoring Laboratory work as ordered
Knowledge deficit	Orient to surroundings Include family in teaching Provide simple, brief instructions Review ongoing procedures Evaluate understanding of teaching	Include family in teaching Review plan of care Provide explanations for all procedures Evaluate understanding of teaching
Psychosocial	Assess anxiety Assess fears of the unknown Encourage verbalization of concerns Provide emotional support to client and family Provide information regarding injury and treatment Minimize external stimuli (eg, noise, movement)	Encourage verbalization of concerns Provide emotional support to client and family Provide information and ongoing support and encouragement
Diet	NPO Baseline nutritional assessment	NPO Mouthcare prn
Activity	Assess safety needs and implement appropriate interventions	Provide safety precautions
Medications	Assess immunization status and administer either tetanus booster or tetanus immune globulin Antibiotics as ordered IV narcotic analgesics Albumin as ordered IV fluids H_2-receptor antagonists	IV narcotic analgesics Antibiotics if ordered IV fluids
Transfer/ discharge plans	Assess adequacy of support system Initiate arrangements for transfer	Complete transfer arrangements Complete transfer summary

Severe Thermal Burns

Possible Complications

- Infection
- Respiratory distress

Health Conditions

- Pre-existing respiratory disease
- Smoker

Nursing Diagnoses

- Acute pain
- Ineffective individual or family coping

Cerebral Vascular Accident

Expected length of stay: 6–7 days

	Date _____ **Admission–Day 1**	Date _____ **Day 2**	Date _____ **Day 3**
Daily outcomes	Client will: • have stabilizing neurovital signs • have stablizing vital signs and B/P within specified range • maintain a patent airway with lungs clear to auscultation • have unlabored respirations and maintain oxygen saturation above 92% • maintain range of motion (active or passive) • indicate understanding of and demonstrate cooperation with ongoing care • maintain urine output >30 mL/hr • remain free of injury	Client will: • have stable neurovital signs • have stable vital signs and B/P within specified range • maintain a patent airway with lungs clear to auscultation • have unlabored respirations and maintain oxygen saturation above 92% • maintain range of motion • tolerate ordered diet without difficulty swallowing • indicate understanding of and demonstrate cooperation with ongoing care • participate in 25% of self-care activities • maintain urine output >30 mL/hr • demonstrate ability to cope • remain free of injury	Client will: • have stable neurovital signs • have stable vital signs and B/P within specified range • maintain a patent airway with lungs clear to auscultation • have unlabored respirations and maintain oxygen saturation above 96% on room air • maintain range of motion • tolerate ordered diet without difficulty swallowing • begin to compensate for any neurologic or sensory losses • demonstrate cooperation with ongoing care • participate in 40% of self-care activities • maintain urine output >30 mL/hr • verbalize ability to cope • remain free of injury • indicate or demonstrate beginning understanding of home care instructions
Assessments, tests, and treatments	CBC PT/PTT Chemistries Urinalysis Chest x-ray EKG CT of head ECHO & carotid Doppler Baseline physical assessment with a focus on neurologic and respiratory status Assess baseline urine and bowel elimination pattern Assess need for indwelling catheter Vital signs and O_2 saturation, neurovital signs and mental status assessment q1–2hr until stable, then q2–4hr and prn	PT/PTT if indicated Vital signs and O_2 saturation, neurovital signs and mental status assessment q4hr and prn Assess neurologic and respiratory status q4hr and prn Intake and output every shift Assess Foley catheter or voiding q4hr and prn Assess swallowing and gag reflex Oxygen as ordered to maintain O_2 saturation > 92% Protect skin per clinical practice guideline	PT/PTT if indicated Vital signs, O_2 saturation, neurovital signs, and mental status assessment q4hr and prn Assess neurovascular status and respiratory status q4hr and prn Intake and output every shift Assess Foley catheter or voiding pattern q4hr D/C oxygen if O_2 saturation > 96% on room air Protect skin per clinical practice guideline

	Date _____ **Admission–Day 1**	Date _____ **Day 2**	Date _____ **Day 3**
Assessments, tests, and treatments (continued)	Oxygen as ordered to maintain O$_2$ saturation >92% Intake and output q4–8 hr prn Maintain patent airway Assess skin and protect skin per clinical practice guidelines		
Knowledge deficit	Orient to room and surroundings Provide simple, brief instructions regarding ongoing care Evalutate understanding of teaching	Reorient to room Include family in teaching Initiate teaching regarding activity level Evaluate understanding of teaching	Reinforce earlier teaching regarding ongoing care Review teaching regarding activity level Initiate medication teaching Initiate discharge teaching Include family in teaching Evalutate understanding of teaching
Psychosocial	Assess anxiety and coping style of client and family Encourage verbalization of concerns Provide information regarding health condition Minimize external stimuli (eg, noise, movement)	Assess level of anxiety and coping style of client and family Encourage verbalization/expression of concerns Acknowledge changes in self-concept and neurologic and sensory status Provide information and ongoing support and encouragement to client and family	Encourage verbalization/expression of concerns Accept mood, affect, and behavior in a non-judgmental manner Provide ongoing support and encouragement to client and family
Diet	NPO Baseline nutritional and hydration assessment	Nutritional status assessment Begin full liquids if swallowing reflex intact	Advance diet if tolerated Encourage fluids
Activity	Assess safety needs and provide appropriate measures Bed rest with HOB elevated <30 degrees Range of motion to all extremities q2hr Turn and position q1–2hr and prn	Maintain safety precautions Up to cardiac chair BID if tolerated Range of motion to all extremities q2hr Turn and position q1–2hr and prn	Maintain safety precautions Up to cardiac chair BID if tolerated Begin ambulation with physical therapy Range of motion to all extremities q2–4hr Turn and position q1–2hr and prn
Medications	Anticoagulation therapy as indicated Routine medications as ordered Stool softeners as ordered IV therapy as ordered or IV intermittent device	Anticoagulation therapy as indicated Routine medications as ordered Stool softeners as ordered IV therapy as ordered or IV intermittent device	Anticoagulation therapy as indicated Routine medications as ordered Stool softeners as ordered IV to intermittent device or D/C Fleet enema if no BM in 3 days

Cerebral Vascular Accident (continued)

	Date _____ **Admission–Day 1**	Date _____ **Day 2**	Date _____ **Day 3**
Transfer/ discharge plans	Assess discharge plans and support system Establish discharge goals with client and family	Physical and occupational therapy referrals Speech therapy referral if indicated Review progress toward discharge goals with client and family Consult with social service regarding VNA and projected needs for home health care or transfer	Review progress toward discharge goals with client and family Establish plan for post-hospital care Make appropriate discharge referrals

	Date _____ **Day 4**	Date _____ **Day 5**	Date _____ **Day 6**
Daily outcomes	Client will: • have stable neurovital signs • have stable vital signs and B/P within specified range • maintain a patent airway with lungs clear to auscultation and unlabored respirations • tolerate diet without any difficulty swallowing • demonstrate ability to compensate for neurologic or sensory deficits • maintain range of motion • ambulate with physical therapy • demonstrate cooperation with ongoing care • participate in 60% of self-care activities • maintain urine output >30 mL/hr • verbalize/indicate ability to cope • remain free of injury • verbalize or demonstrate beginning understanding of home care instructions	Client will: • have stable neurovital signs • have stable vital signs and B/P within specified range • maintain a patent airway with lungs clear to auscultation and unlabored respirations • tolerate ordered diet without difficulty swallowing • demonstrate ability to compensate for neurologic or sensory deficits • maintain range of motion • ambulate with physical therapy • demonstrate cooperation with ongoing care • participate in 80–100% of self-care activities (or to potential) • maintain urine output >30 mL/hr • verbalize/indicate ability to cope • remain free of injury • verbalize or demonstrate understanding of home care instructions	Client has stable vital signs and neuro assessment Client's lungs are clear to auscultation Client participates in self-care to potential Client has resumed preadmission urine and bowel elimination pattern with bladder and bowel training Client maintains range of motion Client demonstrates ability to transfer and/or ambulate with assistive devices and/or assistance Client/family verbalizes or demonstrates home care instructions or need for transfer to rehab or long-term care facility Client tolerates ordered diet without difficulty swallowing Client verbalizes or demonstrates ability to cope with ongoing stressors

Cerebral Vascular Accident *(continued)*

	Date _____ **Day 4**	Date _____ **Day 5**	Date _____ **Day 6**
Assessments, tests, and treatments	PTT/PT if indicated Assess vital signs q4hr and prn Assess neurovascular status q4–8hr and prn Assess respiratory status q4–8hr and prn Intake and output every shift Remove Foley catheter and start bladder training Assess voiding pattern every shift	PT if indicated Assess vital signs q4hr and prn Assess neurovascular status q8hr and prn Assess respiratory status q4–8hr Continue bladder training	PT if indicated Assess vital signs q4–8hr Assess neurovascular status q8hr Assess respiratory status q8hr
Knowledge deficit	Include family in teaching Initiate discharge teaching regarding diet and activity Review written discharge and medication instructions with client and family Evaluate understanding of teaching	Continue discharge teaching regarding diet, signs and symptoms to report, and activity, including family Reinforce written discharge and medication instructions with client and family Evaluate understanding of teaching	Complete discharge teaching regarding diet, follow-up care, signs and symptoms to report, activity, and medications: name, purpose, dose, frequency, route, dietary interactions, and side effects Provide client with written discharge instructions Refer to appropriate agencies if knowledge deficits are present Evaluate understanding of teaching
Psychosocial	Encourage verbalization of concerns Accept mood, affect, and behavior in a non-judgmental manner Provide ongoing support and encouragement to client and family	Encourage verbalization regarding changes in neurologic and sensory status and impact on life Provide information and ongoing support and encouragement	Encourage verbalization of concerns Provide information and ongoing support and encouragement/ Refer client and family for ongoing support
Diet	Soft, regular diet as tolerated Encourage fluids	Soft, regular diet as tolerated Encourage fluids	Soft, regular diet as tolerated Encourage fluids
Activity	Maintain safety precautions Ambulate with physical therapy BID Up to cardiac chair TID and prn Range of motion to all extremities q2–4hr Turn and position q2hr and prn	Maintain safety precautions Ambulate with physical therapy TID Up to cardiac chair TID and prn Range of motion to all extremities q2–4hr Turn and position q2hr and prn	Maintain safety precautions Ambulate with physical therapy Up to cardiac chair TID and prn Range of motion to all extremities q2–4hr Turn and position q2hr and prn
Medications	Anticoagulation therapy as indicated Routine medications as ordered Stool softeners as ordered Laxative or fleet enema if no BM in 3 days	Anticoagulation therapy as indicated Routine medications as ordered Stool softeners as ordered Laxative or fleet enema if no BM in 3 days	Anticoagulation therapy as indicated Routine medications as ordered Stool softeners as ordered Laxative or fleet enema if no BM in 3 days

	Date _____ **Day 4**	Date _____ **Day 5**	Date _____ **Day 6**
Transfer/ discharge plans	Continue to review progress toward discharge goals	Finalize discharge plans Continue to review progress toward discharge goals Finalize plans for home care if needed	Complete discharge instructions

Potential Client Variances
Cerebral Vascular Accident

Possible Complications

- Seizures
- Stress ulcers
- Aspiration pneumonia
- Coma

Health Conditions

- Smoker
- Pre-existing cardiac or respiratory disease
- Diabetes

Nursing Diagnoses

- Ineffective individual or family coping
- Impaired verbal communication
- Sensory/perceptual alterations
- Ineffective management of therapeutic regimen
- Self-care deficits
- Risk for injury
- Altered thought processes

Discharge Teaching for Client Following
Cerebral Vascular Accident

Activity
- Start with the weaker side when dressing.
- Gradually return to usual level of mobility by increasing activity each day. Alternate activity with rest periods. Avoid fatigue.
- Do not drive, perform strenuous activity, or return to work until okayed by physician.
- Avoid trying to lift, carry, or hold heavy objects with the affected hand or arm.
- Use walker, cane, or crutch when walking or transferring. Cane or crutch should be used on stronger side.
- If someone is helping you in or out of a bed or chair, they should assist you on the affected side.
- Exercise your arms and legs as directed.

Diet
- Follow recommended diet. Drink plenty of fluids and eat a well-balanced diet, including fruits, meat, vegetables, bread and starches, and milk products.
- Rest after meals.
- Work towards achieving weight loss if recommended.

Signs and Symptoms to Report
Notify physician if any of these symptoms occur:
- Persistent headache
- Changes in vision
- Difficulty swallowing
- Increased weakness in the affected side or new weakness
- Increased or new difficulty with speech or slurring of speech
- Difficulty remembering

Follow-Up Care and General Health Care
- Schedule follow-up appointment with physician as directed.
- Follow bladder and bowel regimen as directed in the hospital.
- Continue therapies as directed.
- Utilize community resources for home health needs.

Medications
- Review written list of medications, including dose, frequency, food interactions, and side effects.
- Avoid over-the-counter medications unless recommended by physician.
- Ask your physician about alcohol use.

Congestive Heart Failure (CHF)

Expected length of stay: 6 days

	Date _____ **Day 1: Admission to Coronary Care Unit or Step-Down Unit**	Date _____ **Day 2**	Date _____ **Day 3: Transfer from Step-Down Unit to Floor Care**
Daily outcomes	Client will: • have stablizing vital signs and hemodynamic measures • remain alert and oriented • verbalize pain or discomfort using a 0–10 scale • verbalize understanding of ongoing treatment and need for hospitalization • demonstrate ability to adhere to activity restrictions • maintain stable respiratory rate and O_2 saturation >90% • maintain urine output >30 mL/hr • verbalize feelings regarding ongoing stressors • verbalize/demonstrate ability to cope	Client will: • have stable vital signs and hemodynamic measures • remain alert and oriented • verbalize control of chest pain • verbalize presence or absence of pain or discomfort on a 0–10 scale • verbalize understanding of ongoing treatment and need for hospitalization • demonstrate ability to adhere to activity restrictions • maintain stable respiratory rate and O_2 saturation >92% • maintain urine output >30 mL/hr • verbalize feelings regarding ongoing stressors and illness • verbalize/demonstrate ability to cope	Client will: • have stable vital signs • remain alert and oriented • verbalize presence or absence of pain or discomfort • be free of chest pain • verbalize understanding of ongoing treatment and need for hospitalization • demonstrate ability to adhere to activity restrictions • tolerate activity level without dyspnea, shortness of breath, or chest pain • have lungs clear to auscultation and maintain O_2 saturation >95% • maintain urine output >30 mL/hr • verbalize feelings regarding ongoing stressors and illness • verbalize ability to cope • verbalize understanding of transfer from CCU or step-down unit • verbalize beginning understanding of home care instructions
Assessments, tests, and treatments	CBC Electrolytes Chemistries TSH Dig level if indicated EKG PA and lateral chest x-ray ABGs Cardiac enzymes q8hr × 3 Cardiovascular and respiratory assessment q1hr and prn Assess for peripheral edema q2–4hr and prn Continuous cardiac monitoring Vital signs and O_2 saturation q1hr and prn Maintain oxygen as ordered	K^+ Vital signs and O_2 saturation, q4hr and prn Cardiovascular and respiratory assessment q4hr and prn Continuous cardiac monitoring Intake and output every shift Oxygen at 5 L to maintain O_2 saturation >92% Assist with ADLs Intake and output every shift Weight	Echocardiogram if ordered K^+ Vital signs and O_2 saturation, q4hr if stable Cardiovascular assessment q4hr and prn Continuous cardiac monitoring until transfer Intake and output every shift Oxygen to maintain O_2 saturation at 95% Assist with ADLs Transfer to floor care Weight

Congestive Heart Failure (CHF) *(continued)*

	Date _____ **Day 1: Admission to Coronary Care Unit or Step-Down Unit**	Date _____ **Day 2**	Date _____ **Day 3: Transfer from Step-Down Unit to Floor Care**
Assessments, tests, and treatments (continued)	Assist with ADLs Monitor arterial blood gases Intake and output Weight		
Knowledge deficit	Orient to room and hospital routine Review plan of care Include family in teaching Evaluate understanding of teaching	Review plan of care Brief teaching regarding CHF Include family in teaching Evaluate understanding of teaching	Reinforce earlier teaching regarding ongoing care Begin discharge teaching regarding rest, activity, and diet Begin medication teaching Include family in teaching Evaluate understanding of teaching
Psychosocial	Assess level of anxiety Encourage verbalization of concerns Provide information and ongoing support and encouragement to client and family	Assess level of anxiety Encourage verbalization of concerns Provide information and ongoing support and encouragement to client and family	Encourage verbalization of concerns Provide ongoing support and encouragement to client and family
Diet	American Heart Association diet as tolerated, providing small, frequent, nutritious feedings	American Heart Association diet as tolerated, providing small, frequent, nutritious feedings	American Heart Association diet as tolerated, providing small, frequent, nutritious feedings Provide teaching regarding diet and salt restrictions
Activity	Assess safety needs and provide appropriate precautions Bedrest with head of bed elevated Monitor responses to visitors and limit accordingly	Maintain safety precautions Bedrest with head of bed elevated Chair with legs elevated or commode privileges Provide rest periods Monitor responses to visitors and limit accordingly	Maintain safety precautions Chair with legs elevated Ambulate in room Provide rest periods
Medications	IV KVO IV nitro as ordered IV diuretics as ordered Digoxin if ordered Pre-load/after-load reducers as indicated Stool softener	IV KVO IV nitro as ordered Diuretics as ordered Digoxin if ordered Pre-load/after-load reducers as indicated K^+ replacements as indicated Stool softener	Intermittent IV device D/C nitro Diuretics as ordered Digoxin if ordered Pre-load/after-load reducers as indicated K^+ replacements as indicated Stool softener Laxative if no BM in 3 days
Transfer/ discharge plans	Establish discharge goals with client and family Consult with social service regarding VNA projected needs for home health care (if any)	Review progress towards discharge goals with client and family Referral to cardiac rehab if indicated	Review progress toward discharge goals with client and family Cardiac rehab evaluation completed

➤

	Date _____ **Day 4**	Date _____ **Day 5**	Date _____ **Day 6**
Daily outcomes	Client will: • be afebrile and have stable vital signs and hemodynamic measures • verbalize understanding and demonstrate cooperation with ongoing treatment and care • demonstrate ability to adhere to activity restrictions • tolerate activity level without dyspnea, shortness of breath, or chest pain • have lungs clear to auscultation • maintain urine output >30 mL/hr • verbalize feelings regarding ongoing stressors • verbalize/demonstrate ability to cope • verbalize beginning understanding of illness • verbalize beginning understanding of home care instructions	Client will: • be afebrile and have stable vital signs • verbalize understanding and demonstrate cooperation with ongoing treatment and care • demonstrate ability to adhere to activity restrictions • tolerate activity level without dyspnea, shortness of breath, or chest pain • have lungs clear to auscultation • maintain urine output >30 mL/hr • verbalize feelings regarding ongoing stressors • verbalize/demonstrate ability to cope • verbalize understanding of home care instructions	Client is afebrile and has stable vital signs Client has lungs that are clear to auscultation Client is independent in self-care Client is fully ambulatory Client tolerates activity level without dyspnea, shortness of breath, or chest pain Client has resumed preadmission urine and bowel elimination pattern Client verbalizes/demonstrates home care instructions Client tolerates ordered diet Client verbalizes/demonstrates ability to cope with ongoing stressors Client verbalizes understanding of illness and discharge care Client and family verbalize strategies to reduce risk factors for heart disease, including diet, medication, activity restrictions, signs and symptoms to report
Assessments, tests, and treatments	K^+ Vital signs and O_2 saturation, q4hr and prn Cardiac and respiratory assessment q4hr and prn D/C intake and output Weight D/C oxygen if O_2 saturation >96% on room air	K^+ BUN Creatinine Chest x-ray Vital signs and O_2 saturation, q4hr and prn Cardiac and respiratory assessment q4hr Weight	K^+ Vital signs and O_2 saturation, q4hr and prn Cardiac and respiratory assessment q4hr
Knowledge deficit	Reinforce earlier teaching regarding ongoing care Review written discharge instructions regarding diet, exercise and medication Include family in teaching Evaluate understanding of teaching	Reinforce earlier teaching regarding ongoing care Reinforce written discharge instructions with client and family Include family in teaching Evaluate understanding of teaching	Reinforce earlier teaching regarding ongoing care Complete discharge teaching to include diet, follow-up care, signs and symptoms to report, follow-up MD visit, activity, and medications: name, purpose, dose, frequency, route, dietary interactions, and side effects Provide client with written discharge instructions Include family in teaching Evaluate understanding of teaching Refer client if knowledge deficits continue

Congestive Heart Failure (CHF) *(continued)*

	Date _____ **Day 4**	Date _____ **Day 5**	Date _____ **Day 6**
Psychosocial	Encourage verbalization of concerns Provide ongoing support and encouragement to client and family	Encourage verbalization of concerns Provide ongoing support and encouragement to client and family	Encourage verbalization of concerns Provide ongoing support and encouragement to client and family
Diet	American Heart Association diet as tolerated, providing small, frequent, nutritious feedings	American Heart Association diet as tolerated, providing small, frequent, nutritious feedings	American Heart Association diet as tolerated, providing small, frequent, nutritious feedings
Activity	Ambulate in room 3–4 times/day Ambulate in hallway 1–2 times/day Maintain safety precautions	Ambulate in room 3–4 times/day Ambulate in hallway 2–3 times/day Start stair walking Maintain safety precautions	Ambulate in room 3–4 times/day Ambulate in hallway Maintain safety precautions
Medications	D/C intermittent IV device Diuretics as ordered Cardiac medications as ordered K^+ as ordered Stool softener	Diuretics as ordered Cardiac medications as ordered K^+ as ordered Stool softener	Diuretics as ordered Cardiac medications as ordered K^+ as ordered Stool softener
Transfer/ discharge plans	Continue to review progress toward discharge goals Finalize discharge plans Finalize referral to cardiac rehab Continue discharge teaching	Finalize plans for home care if needed Make any other appropriate referrals Continue discharge teaching	Complete any appropriate referrals Complete discharge teaching

Potential Client Variances
Congestive Heart Failure (CHF)

Possible complications

- Cardiogenic shock
- Renal failure
- Respiratory failure
- Cardiac dysrhythmias

Health Conditions

- Smoker
- Pre-existing cardiac or respiratory disease
- Chronic renal failure

Nursing Diagnoses

- Activity intolerance
- Anxiety
- Ineffective management of therapeutic regimen
- Self-care deficits
- Sleep pattern disturbances
- Altered thought processes

Discharge Teaching for Client With
Congestive Heart Failure (CHF)

Activity

- Gradually return to usual level of activity by increasing activity each day. Alternate activity with rest periods. Avoid fatigue. Plan rest periods each day.
- Gradually increase your walking and other activities. Monitor your response to activity and stop activity if shortness of breath, palpitations, or severe fatigue occur.
- No strenuous activity or return to work until okayed by physician.
- Check with your physician about heavy housework or straining.

Diet

- Follow American Heart Association diet. Restrict sodium as instructed. Drink plenty of fluids and eat a well-balanced diet, including fruits, meat, vegetables, bread and starches, and milk products.
- Plan rest periods after meals.

Signs and Symptoms to Report

Notify physician if any of these symptoms occur:

- Shortness of breath, chest pain, difficulty breathing, increasing fatigue, weakness, increased coughing, voiding more frequently at night, breathing more rapidly, increased pulse rate.
- Weight gain over 2 pounds per day.
- Swollen ankles, feet, or fingers.
- Needing extra pillows at night to assist breathing when sleeping.

Follow-Up Care and General Health Care

- Schedule follow-up appointment with physician as directed.
- Attend cardiac rehab as directed.
- Notify physician if activity intolerance occurs.

Medications

- Review written list of medications, including dose, frequency, food interactions, and side effects.
- Carry a list of medication and doses.
- Avoid over-the-counter medications unless recommended by physician.
- Discuss alcohol use with physician.

Critical Pathway for Client with

Chronic Obstructive Pulmonary Disease (COPD)

Expected length of stay: 6 days

	Date _____ **Day 1**	Date _____ **Day 2**	Date _____ **Day 3**
Daily outcomes	Client will: • have stable vital signs • maintain a patent airway and effective breathing pattern at rest • verbalize understanding and demonstrates cooperation with respiratory therapy • have a productive cough • have an intake of 2000 mL/day (IV/PO) • demonstrate ability to cope	Client will: • have stable vital signs • maintain a patent airway and effective breathing pattern at rest • ABGs within client's usual range • verbalize understanding and demonstrates cooperation with respiratory therapy • have a productive cough • have an intake of 2000 mL/day (IV/PO) • verbalize understanding of disease process and its chronic nature • demonstrate effective breathing techniques • demonstrate ability to cope	Client will: • be afebrile, have stable vital signs • maintain a patent airway and effective breathing pattern with activity • verbalize understanding and demonstrate cooperation with respiratory therapy • have a productive cough • have an intake of 2000 mL/day (PO) • demonstrate ability to cope • verbalize understanding of energy-conserving measures and reconditioning exercises • verbalize beginning understanding of home care instructions
Assessments, tests, and treatments	CBC with differential PA and lateral chest x-ray EKG ABGs Blood culture × 2, if temp over 101F Sputum for gram stain and C & S Vital signs and O_2 saturation, q4hr and prn Assess respiratory status q4hr and prn Assess mental status q4hr and prn Nebulizer therapy q4hr Intake and output every shift Position client in semi-Fowler's or high Fowler's position Assist with nebulizer treatments Administer oxygen per nasal cannula to maintain: saturation at 93–96% if PCO_2 <45 saturation at 88–90% if PCO_2 >45 Assist with ADLs	ABGs if ordered Vital signs and O_2 saturation, q4hr and prn Assess respiratory status q4hr and prn Assess mental status q4hr and prn Intake and output every shift Nebulizer therapy q4hr Chest physical therapy Position client in semi-Fowler's or high Fowler's position Assist with nebulizer treatments Assist with ADLs Administer oxygen per nasal cannula to maintain: saturation at 93-96% if PCO_2 <45 saturation at 88-90% if PCO_2 >45	Vital signs and O_2 saturation, q4hr and prn Assess respiratory status q4hr and prn Assess mental status q4hr and prn Intake and output every shift Nebulizer therapy q4hr Chest physical therapy Position client in semi-Fowler's or high Fowler's position Assist with nebulizer treatments Administer oxygen per nasal cannula to maintain: saturation at 93–96% if PCO_2 <45 saturation at 88–90% if PCO_2 >45 Assist with ADLs Check culture and sensitivities

Chronic Obstructive Pulmonary Disease (COPD) *(continued)*

	Date _____ **Day 1**	Date _____ **Day 2**	Date _____ **Day 3**
Knowledge deficit	Orient to room and hospital routine Review plan of care Assess use of inhalers and instruct as needed regarding proper technique Include family in teaching Evaluate understanding of teaching	Review plan of care Assess knowledge regarding COPD Assess smoking history Respiratory consult to review breathing techniques Include family in teaching Evaluate understanding of teaching	Reinforce earlier teaching regarding ongoing care Begin discharge teaching regarding rest, activity, and diet Discuss strategies to conserve energy and reconditioning exercises Include family in teaching Evaluate understanding of teaching
Psychosocial	Assess level of anxiety Encourage verbalization of concerns Provide information and ongoing support and encouragement to client and family	Assess level of anxiety Encourage verbalization of concerns Provide information and ongoing support and encouragement to client and family	Encourage verbalization of concerns Provide ongoing support and encouragement to client and family
Diet	Diet as tolerated, providing small, frequent, nutritious feedings Encourage fluid intake of 2000 mL/day	Diet as tolerated, providing small, frequent, nutritious feedings Consult with dietitian Encourage fluid intake of 2000 mL/day	Diet as tolerated, providing small, frequent, nutritious feedings Encourage fluid intake of 2000 mL/day
Activity	Assess safety needs and provide appropriate precautions Bathroom privileges with assistance Provide rest periods	Maintain safety precautions Bathroom privileges with assistance Up to chair BID Provide rest periods	Maintain safety precautions Ambulate 4 times with assistance Provide rest periods
Medications	IV fluids IV aminophylline IV steroid IV antibiotics Inhalers as ordered Expectorants as ordered Tylenol 650 mg q4hr po for temp over 101F	IV fluids IV aminophylline IV steroid (begin taper) IV antibiotics Inhalers as ordered Expectorants as ordered Tylenol 650 mg q4hr po for temp over 101F	Convert IV to IV intermittent device D/C IV aminophylline Start oral theophylline as ordered IV steroid or begin po steroid IV antibiotics Inhalers as ordered Expectorants as ordered Tylenol 650 mg q4hr po for temp over 101F
Transfer/ discharge plans	Establish discharge goals with client and family Consult with social service regarding VNA projected needs for home health care (if any)	Review progress toward discharge goals with client and family Identify potential referrals If smoking, refer for smoking cessation	Review progress toward discharge goals with client and family Refer to pulmonary rehab Assess need for home oxygen therapy

Chronic Obstructive Pulmonary Disease (COPD) *(continued)*

	Date _____ **Day 4**	Date _____ **Day 5**	Date _____ **Day 6**
Daily outcomes	Client will: • be afebrile, and have stable vital signs • maintain a patent airway and tolerate activity • verbalize understanding and demonstrate cooperation with respiratory therapy • have an oral intake of 2000 mL/day • demonstrate energy conserving measures and reconditioning exercises • verbalize feelings regarding chronic nature of illness • demonstrate ability to cope • verbalize understanding of home care instructions	Client will: • be afebrile, and have stable vital signs • maintain a patent airway and tolerate activity • verbalize understanding and demonstrate cooperation with respiratory therapy • have an oral intake of 2000 mL/day • demonstrate energy conserving measures and reconditioning exercises • demonstrate ability to cope • verbalize understanding of home care instructions	Client is afebrile and has stable vital signs Client has a patent airway and unlabored respirations with activity Client is independent in self-care Client is fully ambulatory Client tolerates ordered activity without dyspnea, shortness of breath, or chest pain Client has resumed preadmission urine and bowel elimination pattern Client verbalizes/demonstrates home care instructions, including strategies to reduce exposure to infectious illnesses Client tolerates usual diet and has an oral intake of 2000 mL/day Client verbalizes ability to cope with lifestyle changes and effects of chronic illness Client demonstrates/verbalizes ability to cope with ongoing stressors

Assessments, tests, and treatments	Theophylline level
	Vital signs and O_2 saturation, q4hr and prn
	Assess respiratory status q4hr and prn
	Assess mental status q4hr and prn
	Intake and output every shift
	Nebulizer therapy q4hr
	Position client in semi-Fowler's or high Fowler's position
	Administer oxygen per nasal cannula to maintain:
	  saturation at 93–96% if PCO_2 <45
	  saturation at 88–90% if PCO_2 >45
	D/C oxygen per order
		CBC
		Vital signs and O_2 saturation, q4hr and prn
		Assess respiratory status q4hr and prn
		Assess mental status q4hr and prn
		Intake and output every shift
		Nebulizer therapy q4hr prn
		Position client in semi-Fowler's or high Fowler's position
		Administer oxygen per nasal cannula to maintain:
		  saturation at 93–96% if PCO_2 <45
		  saturation at 88–90% if PCO_2 >45
		D/C oxygen per order
			Vital signs and O_2 saturation, q4hr and prn
			Assess respiratory status q4hr and prn
			Assess mental status q4hr and prn

Chronic Obstructive Pulmonary Disease (COPD) *(continued)*

	Date _____ **Day 4**	Date _____ **Day 5**	Date _____ **Day 6**
Knowledge deficit	Reinforce earlier teaching regarding ongoing care Review written discharge instructions with client and family Include family in teaching Evaluate understanding of teaching	Reinforce earlier teaching regarding ongoing care Review written discharge instructions with client and family Include family in teaching Evaluate understanding of teaching	Reinforce earlier teaching regarding ongoing care Complete discharge teaching to include diet, follow-up care, signs and symptoms to report, follow-up MD visit, activity, and medications: name, purpose, dose, frequency, route, dietary interactions, and side effects Provide client with written discharge instructions Include family in teaching Evaluate understanding of teaching
Psychosocial	Encourage verbalization of concerns Provide ongoing support and encouragement to client and family	Encourage verbalization of concerns Provide ongoing support and encouragement to client and family	Encourage verbalization of concerns Provide ongoing support and encouragement to client and family
Diet	Diet as tolerated, providing small, frequent, nutritious feedings Encourage fluid intake of 2000 mL/day	Diet as tolerated, providing small, frequent, nutritious feedings Encourage fluid intake of 2000 mL/day	Diet as tolerated, providing small, frequent, nutritious feedings Encourage fluid intake of 3000 mL/day
Activity	Ambulate independently at least 4 times Maintain safety precautions	Ambulate as tolerated Maintain safety precautions	Fully ambulatory
Medications	D/C IV device Antibiotics as ordered Theophylline as ordered Inhalers as ordered Steroids as ordered Expectorants as ordered Tylenol 650 mg q4hr po for temp over 101F	Antibiotics as ordered Theophylline as ordered Steroids (taper) as ordered Inhalers as ordered Expectorants as ordered Tylenol 650 mg q4hr po for temp over 101F	Antibiotics as ordered Theophylline as ordered Steroids (taper) as ordered Inhalers as ordered Expectorants as ordered Tylenol 650 mg q4hr po for temp over 101F
Transfer/ discharge plans	Continue to review progress toward discharge goals Review discharge plans Refer to Better Breathers Club	Continue to review progress toward discharge goals Finalize discharge plans Make appropriate referrals	Finalize plans for home care if needed Make any appropriate referrals Complete discharge teaching

Chronic Obstructive Pulmonary Disease (COPD)

Possible Complications

- Spontaneous pneumothorax
- Pneumonia
- Systemic infection
- Cor pulmonale
- Respiratory failure

Health Conditions

- Smoker
- Malnutrition
- Genetic deficiency of alpha$_1$-antitrypsin

Nursing Diagnoses

- Activity intolerance
- Anxiety
- Ineffective management of therapeutic regimen
- Ineffective individual coping
- Self-care deficits

Discharge Teaching for Client With
Chronic Obstructive Pulmonary Disease (COPD)

Activity

- Gradually return to usual level of activity by increasing activity each day. Alternate activity with rest periods. Avoid fatigue.
- No strenuous activity or return to work until okayed by physician.
- Check with your physician about heavy housework or straining.
- Do your breathing exercises as instructed.

Diet

- Follow usual and customary diet. Drink plenty of fluids and eat a well-balanced diet, including fruits, meat, vegetables, bread and starches, and milk products.
- Plan rest period after meals.

Signs and Symptoms to Report

Notify physician if any of these symptoms occur:
- Shortness of breath, difficulty breathing
- Chills, or fever greater than 100F or 38C
- Cough, sore throat, runny nose, ear ache

Follow-Up Care and General Health Care

- Schedule follow-up appointment with physician as directed.
- Avoid individuals with respiratory infections.
- Dispose of your tissues in a paper or plastic trash bag.
- Avoid cigarettes, cigarette smoke, dust, fumes, perfumes, and sprays.

Medications

- Review written list of medications, including dose, frequency, food interactions, and side effects.
- Avoid over-the-counter medications unless recommended by physician.
- Ask your physician about flu and pneumonia vaccines.

Critical Pathway for Client with

Deep Vein Thrombosis

Expected length of stay: 7 days

	Date _____ **Day 1**	Date _____ **Days 2–3**	Date _____ **Day 4**
Daily outcomes	Client will: • have stable vital signs • be alert and oriented • verbalize understanding and demonstrate cooperation with ongoing care • verbalize control of pain • experience diminished pain, swelling and tenderness of affected extremity • have lungs clear to auscultation • remain free of respiratory distress • remain free of bleeding • have an intake of 2000–3000 mL/day (IV/PO) • maintain urine output >30mL/hr • verbalize ability to cope	Client will: • have stable vital signs • be alert and oriented • verbalize understanding and demonstrate cooperation with ongoing care • verbalize control of pain • experience diminished pain, swelling, and tenderness of affected extremity • have lungs clear to auscultation • remain free of respiratory distress • remain free of bleeding • have an intake of 2000–3000 mL/day (IV/PO) • maintain urine output >30 mL/hr • verbalize ability to cope	Client will: • be afebrile and have stable vital signs • be alert and oriented • verbalize understanding and demonstrate cooperation with ongoing care • verbalize control of pain • experience diminished pain, swelling and tenderness of affected extremity • have lungs clear to auscultation • remain free of respiratory distress • remain free of bleeding • have an intake of 2000–3000 mL/day (IV/PO) • maintain urine output >30 mL/hr • verbalize ability to cope • verbalize beginning understanding of home care instructions

Assessments, tests, and treatments	Laboratory/diagnostic tests:
	  CBC
	  PA and lateral chest x-ray
	  ABGs
	  PT/PTT
	  Venogram
	  Doppler ultrasound
	  Diagnostic imaging as ordered
	Vital signs and O_2 saturation, q4hr and prn
	Intake and output every shift
	Assess CSMs q2–4hr and prn
	Assess level of pain, circumference, swelling, tenderness, and warmth of affected extremity
	Monitor for signs and symptoms of pulmonary embolus
	Assess respiratory status and respiratory movements q4hr and prn
		PT, PTT
		Vital signs and O_2 saturation, q4hr and prn
		Monitor for signs and symptoms of pulmonary embolus
		Assess respiratory status q4hr and prn
		Intake and output every shift
		Assess CSMs q4hr and prn
		Assess level of pain, circumference, swelling, tenderness, and warmth of affected extremity
		Encourage deep breathing q2hr and prn
		Oxygen to maintain O_2 saturation at 92%
		Assist with ADLs
		Continuous warm compresses to affected extremity
			PT, PTT
			Vital signs and O_2 saturation, q4hr and prn
			Assess respiratory status q4hr and prn
			Monitor for signs and symptoms of pulmonary embolus
			Intake and output every shift
			Assess CSMs q4hr and prn
			Assess level of pain, circumference, swelling, tenderness, and warmth of affected extremity
			Encourage deep breathing q2hr and prn
			Oxygen to maintain O_2 saturation at 92%
			Assist with ADLs
			Continuous warm compresses to affected extremity

	Date _____ **Day 1**	Date _____ **Days 2–3**	Date _____ **Day 4**
Assessments, tests, and treatments (continued)	Encourage deep breathing q1–2hr Oxygen so as to maintain O_2 saturation at 92% Assist with ADLs Monitor arterial blood gases as ordered Continuous warm compresses to affected extremity		
Knowledge deficit	Orient to room and hospital routine Review plan of care Include family in teaching Evaluate understanding of teaching	Review plan of care and continued importance of increased fluids, activity, turning, coughing, deep breathing, and incentive spirometer Include family in teaching Evaluate understanding of teaching	Reinforce earlier teaching regarding ongoing care Begin discharge teaching regarding rest, activity, and diet Begin coumadin teaching Include family in teaching Evaluate understanding of teaching
Psychosocial	Assess level of anxiety Encourage verbalization of concerns Provide information and ongoing support and encouragement to client and family	Assess level of anxiety Encourage verbalization of concerns Provide information and ongoing support and encouragement to client and family	Encourage verbalization of concerns Provide ongoing support and encouragement to client and family
Diet	Diet as tolerated, providing small, frequent, nutritious feedings Encourage fluid intake of 2000–3000 mL/day	Diet as tolerated, providing small, frequent, nutritious feedings Encourage fluid intake of 2000–3000 mL/day	Diet as tolerated, providing small, frequent, nutritious feedings Encourage fluid intake of 2000–3000 mL/day
Activity	Assess safety needs and provide appropriate precautions Bed rest with legs elevated Instruct not to cross legs and not to gatch knees Provide rest periods	Maintain safety precautions Bed rest with legs elevated Provide rest periods	Maintain safety precautions Bed rest with legs elevated Provide rest periods
Medications	IV heparin as ordered Colace 100 mg BID Consider thrombolytic therapy Tylenol 650 mg q4hr po prn for discomfort	IV heparin as ordered Coumadin as ordered Colace 100 mg BID Tylenol 650 mg q4hr po prn for discomfort	IV heparin as ordered Coumadin as ordered Colace 100 mg BID Tylenol 650 mg q4hr po prn for discomfort
Transfer/ discharge plans	Establish discharge goals with client and family Consult with social service regarding VNA projected needs for home health care	Review progress toward discharge goals with client and family Identify potential referrals	Review progress toward discharge goals with client and family

	Date _____ **Day 5**	Date _____ **Day 6**	Date _____ **Day 7**
Daily outcomes	Client will: • be afebrile with stable vital signs • be alert and oriented • verbalize understanding and demonstrate cooperation with ongoing care • verbalize control of pain • experience diminished pain, swelling, and tenderness of affected extremity • have lungs clear to auscultation • remain free of respiratory distress • remain free of bleeding • have an intake of 2000–3000 mL/day (IV/po) • maintain urine output >30 mL /hr • verbalize ability to cope • verbalize beginning understanding of home care instructions	Client will: • be afebrile with stable vital signs • be alert and oriented • verbalize understanding and demonstrate cooperation with ongoing care • verbalize control of pain • experience diminished pain, swelling, and tenderness of affected extremity • have lungs clear to auscultation • remain free of respiratory distress • remain free of bleeding • have an intake of 2000–3000 mL/day (IV/po) • maintain urine output >30mL/hr • verbalize ability to cope • verbalize beginning understanding of home care instructions	Client is afebrile and has stable vital signs Client has unlabored respirations and lungs are clear to auscultation Client has adequate CSMs to affected extremity Client is independent in self-care Client is fully ambulatory Client has resumed preadmission urine and bowel elimination pattern Client verbalizes/demonstrates home care instructions Client verbalizes understanding of precautions related to taking anticoagulants Client verbalizes strategies to promote venous return and prevent future thrombus formation Client tolerates usual diet and has an intake of 2000-3000 mL/day Client verbalizes ability to cope with ongoing stressors
Assessments, tests, and treatments	PT/PTT Vital signs and O_2 saturation, q4hr and prn Assess respiratory status q4hr and prn Monitor for signs and symptoms of pulmonary embolus Assess CSMs q4 hr and prn Assess level of pain, circumference, swelling, tenderness, and warmth of affected extremity Encourage deep breathing q2hr and prn D/C oxygen if O_2 saturation at 92% Assist with ADLs Continuous warm compresses to affected extremity	PT/PTT Vital signs and O_2 saturation, q4hr and prn Assess respiratory status q4hr and prn Monitor for signs and symptoms of pulmonary embolus Assess CSMs q4hr and prn Assess level of pain, circumference, swelling, tenderness, and warmth of affected extremity Encourage deep breathing q2–4hr and prn Assist with ADLs Continuous warm compresses to affected extremity	PT Vital signs and O_2 saturation, q4hr and prn Assess respiratory status q4hr and prn Monitor for signs and symptoms of pulmonary embolus Assess CSMs q4hr and prn Assess level of pain, circumference, swelling, tenderness, and warmth of affected extremity

	Date _____ **Day 5**	Date _____ **Day 6**	Date _____ **Day 7**
Knowledge deficit	Reinforce earlier teaching regarding ongoing care and discharge care Begin discharge teaching regarding prevention strategies: TED stockings, avoiding prolonged sitting or standing, the importance of regular exercise, and avoiding smoking and oral contraceptives Review coumadin teaching Include family in teaching Evaluate understanding of teaching	Reinforce earlier teaching regarding ongoing care and discharge care Begin discharge teaching regarding follow-up care, medications, and signs and symptoms to report Reinforce and complete coumadin teaching Include family in teaching Evaluate understanding of teaching	Reinforce earlier teaching regarding ongoing care and discharge care Complete discharge teaching to include diet, follow-up care, signs and symptoms to report, follow-up MD visit, activity, and medications: name, purpose, dose, frequency, route, dietary interactions, and side effects Provide client with written discharge instructions Include family in teaching Evaluate understanding of teaching
Psychosocial	Encourage verbalization of concerns Provide ongoing support and encouragement to client and family	Encourage verbalization of concerns Provide ongoing support and encouragement to client and family	Encourage verbalization of concerns Provide ongoing support and encouragement to client and family
Diet	Diet as tolerated, providing small, frequent, nutritious feedings Encourage fluid intake of 2000–3000 mL/day	Diet as tolerated, providing small, frequent, nutritious feedings Encourage fluid intake of 2000–3000 mL/day	Diet as tolerated, providing small, frequent, nutritious feedings Encourage fluid intake of 2000–3000 mL/day
Activity	Maintain safety precautions Bed rest with legs elevated and begin ambulation in room to tolerance for short periods Provide rest periods	Maintain safety precautions Bed rest with legs elevated Begin ambulation in room and hallway to tolerance for short periods Provide rest periods	Fully ambulatory
Medications	IV heparin as ordered Coumadin as ordered Colace 100 mg BID Laxative if no BM in 3 days Tylenol 650 mg q4hr po prn for discomfort	IV heparin: D/C per order Coumadin as ordered Colace 100 mg BID Tylenol 650 mg q4hr po prn for discomfort	Coumadin as ordered Colace 100 mg BID Tylenol 650 mg q4hr po prn for discomfort
Transfer/ discharge plans	Review progress toward discharge goals with client and family Consult with social service regarding projected needs for home health care	Review progress toward discharge goals with client and family Make appropriate referrals	Finalize plans for home care if needed Complete appropriate referrals Complete discharge teaching

Deep Vein Thrombosis

Possible Complications
- Pulmonary embolism
- Bleeding related to anticoagulant therapy

Health Conditions
- Immobility
- Orthopedic surgery
- Urological surgery
- Fracture of lower extremity
- Oral contraceptives
- Pregnancy
- Malignancy

Nursing Diagnoses
- Acute pain
- Anxiety
- Impaired physical mobility
- Self-care deficits
- Ineffective management of therapeutic regimen

Discharge Teaching for Client Following
Deep Vein Thrombosis

Activity
- Gradually return to usual level of activity by increasing activity each day. Alternate activity with rest periods. Avoid fatigue.
- No strenuous activity or return to work until okayed by physician.
- Check with your health care provider regarding driving.
- Avoid heavy housework or straining for the period designated by your physician.
- Avoid prolonged sitting or standing.
- Avoid crossing legs or placing a pillow under knees.
- Check with health care provider regarding a regular exercise program.

Diet
- Follow usual and customary diet. Drink plenty of fluids and eat a well-balanced diet including fruits, meat, vegetables, bread and starches, and milk products.
- Try to achieve and/or maintain ideal body weight.

Signs and Symptoms to Report
Notify physician if any of these symptoms occur:
- Shortness of breath or difficulty breathing
- Worsening pain, tenderness, or swelling in affected area
- Unexpected or prolonged bleeding (if taking anticoagulants)

Follow-Up Care and General Health Care
- Schedule follow-up appointment with physician as directed.
- Schedule follow-up laboratory appointments for coagulation studies.
- Wear non-constrictive clothing.
- Wear support stockings or compression hose as directed.
- Avoid smoking and second-hand smoke.
- Avoid use of oral contraceptives.
- Notify physician if pregnancy is suspected or planned.
- Wear a medical alert tag identifying the use of anticoagulants.

Medications
- Review written list of medications, including dose, frequency, food interactions, and side effects.
- Avoid over-the-counter medications, especially aspirin or those containing aspirin or other salicylates, unless recommended by physician.
- Review teaching regarding anticoagulant therapy.
- Ask your physician about alcohol use.

New Onset Diabetes (Type II)

Expected length of stay: 5 days

	Date _____ **Day 1**	Date _____ **Day 2**	Date _____ **Day 3**
Daily outcomes	Client will: • have stable vital signs • verbalize beginning understanding and importance of diet compliance and regular blood sugar testing • have episodes of hypo- or hyperglycemia detected early • verbalize beginning ability to cope with diagnosis	Client will: • have stable vital signs • verbalize understanding and importance of diet compliance and regular blood sugar testing • if overweight, have weight loss of 1/2 pound • have episodes of hypo- or hyperglycemia detected early • demonstrate ability to cope • verbalize beginning understanding of home care instructions	Client will: • have stable vital signs • verbalize understanding and importance of diet compliance and regular blood sugar testing • if overweight, have weight loss of 1/2 pound • have episodes of hypo- or hyperglycemia detected early • demonstrate ability to cope • verbalize willingness to participate in a regular exercise program • identify eating behaviors that lead to weight gain • demonstrate ability to self-administer insulin and perform self monitoring of blood glucose safely and correctly with minimal supervision • verbalize beginning understanding of home care instructions
Assessments, tests, and treatments	CBC Fasting blood sugar Glycosylated hemoglobin Baseline laboratory work Vital signs q4hr and prn Daily weight Fingerstick blood sugar ac, hs, and prn; if blood glucose over 240 mg, then obtain serum glucose Monitor for signs and symptoms of hypo- and hyperglycemia and implement appropriate protocol if signs or symptoms are present Intake and output every shift	Fasting blood sugar Vital signs q4hr and prn Daily weight Fingerstick blood sugar ac, hs, and prn Monitor for signs and symptoms of hypo- and hyperglycemia and follow appropriate protocol if symptoms occur Intake and output every shift	Fasting blood sugar Vital signs q4hr and prn Daily weight Fingerstick blood sugar ac, hs, and prn Monitor for signs and symptoms of hypo- and hyperglycemia and follow appropriate protocol if symptoms occur Intake and output every shift

➤

	Date _____ **Day 1**	Date _____ **Day 2**	Date _____ **Day 3**
Knowledge deficit	Orient to room and hospital routine Review plan of care Assess readines for teaching Include family in teaching program Review steps of insulin administration and provide written instruction sheets Review steps of self monitoring of blood glucose (SMBG) Consult with diabetic nurse educator Consult with registered dietitian for instruction in diet and exchange lists Evaluate understanding of teaching	Reorient to room and hospital routine Review plan of care Include family in teaching Review steps of insulin administration and SMBG Encourage client to practice with related equipment Show client and significant other videotapes related to Type II diabetes and self-care practices Evaluate understanding of teaching	Reorient to room and hospital routine Review plan of care Include family in teaching Supervise client in self-administration of insulin and performing SMBG Client attends classes on general health care practices and foot care and watches video related to identifying and managing hypo- and hyperglycemia and sick day management Evaluate understanding of teaching
Psychosocial	Assess level of anxiety Encourage verbalization of concerns Provide ongoing support and encouragement to client and family	Assess level of anxiety Encourage verbalization of concerns Provide ongoing support and encouragement to client and family	Encourage verbalization of concerns Provide ongoing support and encouragement to client and family
Diet	Dietary consult ADA diet as ordered Encourage fluid intake of 2000 mL/day Assess for causes of excessive weight gain (if overweight) Encourage client to identify activities and foods that contribute to excessive intake	ADA diet as ordered Encourage fluid intake of 2000 mL/day Encourage client to identify activities and foods that contribute to excessive intake Identify behavior modification strategies to assist in weight loss	ADA diet as ordered Encourage fluid intake of 2000 mL/day Encourage client to identify activities and foods that contribute to excessive intake Encourage client to utilize behavior modification strategies Explain the relationships between regular physical exercise, weight loss, and weight control Encourage client to establish regular exercise program
Activity	Assess safety needs and provide appropriate precautions Bathroom privileges OOB ad lib in room Provide rest periods	Maintain safety precautions OOB ad lib Encourage rest periods	Maintain safety precautions Ambulate ad lib Encourage rest periods
Medications	Regular insulin to scale ac and hs Oral agents as ordered	Regular insulin to scale ac and hs Oral agents as ordered, or NPH insulin per order	Regular insulin to scale ac and hs Oral agents if ordered, or NPH insulin per order

New Onset Diabetes (Type II) *(continued)*

	Date _____ **Day 1**	Date _____ **Day 2**	Date _____ **Day 3**
Transfer/ discharge plans	Establish discharge goals with client and family Consult with social service regarding VNA and projected needs for home health care (if any)	Review progress toward discharge goals with client and family Assess need for referrals	Review progress toward discharge goals with client and family Refer to diabetic support group Refer to diabetic nurse educator for continued teaching after discharge Make any appropriate referrals

	Date _____ **Day 4**	Date _____ **Day 5**
Daily outcomes	Client will: • have stable vital signs • verbalize understanding and importance of diet compliance and regular blood sugar testing • if overweight have weight loss of 1/2 pound • verbalize responsibility for weight loss • have episodes of hypo- or hyperglycemia detected early • demonstrate ability to cope • verbalize understanding of home care instructions	Client is afebrile and has stable vital signs Client has a normal blood sugar Client is independent in self-care Client is fully ambulatory Client verbalizes responsibility for weight loss Client verbalizes plan to exercise 15–20 min 3–4 times/week Client has resumed preadmission urine and bowel elimination pattern Client verbalizes/demonstrates home care instructions, including aspects of diabetic care: 1) diet control, 2) SMBG, 3) insulin care and administration, 4) foot care, 5) general health care rules, and 6) S & S of hypo- and hyperglycemia, and management of those problems Client verbalizes importance of ongoing nursing and medical care Client tolerates ordered diet and has an intake of 2000 mL/day Client demonstrates/verbalizes ability to cope with ongoing stressors

➤

	Date _____ **Day 4**	Date _____ **Day 5**
Assessments, tests, and treatments	Fasting blood sugar Vital signs q4hr and prn Weight Fingerstick blood sugar ac, hs, and prn Monitor for signs and symptoms of hypo- and hyperglycemia and follow appropriate protocol if symptoms occur D/C intake and output if stable	Fasting blood sugar Vital signs q4hr and prn Weight Fingerstick blood sugar ac, hs, and prn Monitor for signs and symptoms of hypo- and hyperglycemia and follow appropriate protocol if symptoms occur
Knowledge deficit	Include family in teaching Reinforce earlier teaching regarding ongoing care Review written discharge instructions with client and family Attend diabetic classes per diabetic nurse educator Evaluate understanding of teaching	Include family in teaching Reinforce earlier teaching regarding ongoing care Complete discharge teaching to include diet, follow-up care, signs and symptoms to report, follow-up appointment, activity, and medications: dose, frequency, route, name, purpose, and side effects Provide client with written discharge instructions specific to care and management of diabetes Evaluate understanding of teaching Refer any knowledge deficits to diabetic nurse educator
Psychosocial	Encourage verbalization of concerns Provide ongoing support and encouragement to client and family	Encourage verbalization of concerns Provide ongoing support and encouragement to client and family
Diet	ADA diet as ordered Encourage fluid intake of 2000 mL/day Encourage client to utilize behavior modification strategies Encourage client to establish regular exercise program following discharge	ADA diet as ordered Encourage fluid intake of 2000 mL/day Encourage client to utilize behavior modification strategies Encourage client to establish regular exercise program after discharge
Activity	Fully ambulatory	Fully ambulatory
Medications	Regular insulin to scale ac and hs Oral agents if ordered, or NPH insulin per order	Regular insulin to scale ac and hs Oral agents if ordered, or NPH insulin per order

	Date _____ **Day 4**	Date _____ **Day 5**
Transfer/ *discharge plans*	Continue to review progress to- ward discharge goals Finalize discharge plans	Finalize plans for home care if needed Complete discharge teaching

Potential Client Variances
New Onset Diabetes (Type II)

Possible Complications

- Hyperosmolar nonketotic coma
- Hypoglycemia
- Hyperglycemia
- Infection
- Altered tissue perfusion

Health Conditions

- Vision problems
- Neurologic deficits

Nursing Diagnoses

- Risk for infection
- Ineffective management of therapeutic regimen
- Impaired skin integrity
- Altered nutrition: more than body requirements

Discharge Teaching for Client with
New Onset Diabetes (Type II)

Activity

- Continue exercise program as recommended by your physician.

Diet

- Follow prescribed diabetic diet as instructed. (Diet plan and exchange lists provided)

Signs and Symptoms to Report

Notify physician if any of these symptoms occur:
- Episodes of hypoglycemia or hyperglycemia
- Blood sugars over 240 mg
- Any evidence of infections or skin problems

Follow-Up Care and General Health Care

- Schedule follow-up appointment with physician as directed.
- Continue blood sugar testing as recommended and maintain record.
- Perform foot care as instructed.
- Wear a MedicAlert tag or bracelet.

Medications

- Review written list of medications, including dose, route, frequency, food interactions, and side effects.

Critical Pathway for Client Following

Diarrhea and Dehydration

Expected length of stay: 5 days

	Date _____ **Day 1**	Date _____ **Day 2**	Date _____ **Day 3**
Daily outcomes	Client will: • have stable vital signs • have an intake of 2000 mL/day (IV) • remain free of nausea and vomiting • verbalize understanding of ongoing care • have a soft, non-distended abdomen • demonstrate ability to cope	Client will: • have stable vital signs • have an intake of 2000 mL/day (IV) • remain free of nausea and vomiting • verbalize understanding of ongoing care • have moist mucous membranes and skin • have a urine output of at least 30 mL/hr • have a soft, non-distended abdomen • demonstrate ability to cope	Client will: • have stable vital signs • have an intake of 2000 mL/day (IV/PO) • verbalize understanding of ongoing care • have a soft, non-distended abdomen and active bowel sounds • tolerate clear liquids without nausea and vomiting • have balanced fluid and electrolyte status • have urine output of at least 30 mL/hr • demonstrate ability to cope • verbalize/demonstrate beginning understanding of home care instructions
Assessments, tests, and treatments	CBC with differential Electrolytes Abdominal x-rays Stools for OB × 3 Blood culture × 2, if temp over 101F Vital signs q4hr and prn Assess gastrointestinal status q4hr and prn Intake and output every shift Daily weight Monitor serum electrolytes Assess mental status every shift Assist with/provide perianal care after each loose stool Monitor stools for color and consistency, and measure volume Stool cultures as ordered Assess usual bowel elimination pattern Report worsening abdominal pain, nausea, vomiting, diarrhea, or increasing abdominal distention	Electrolytes Blood culture × 2, if temp over 101F Vital signs q4hr and prn Assess gastrointestinal status q4hr and prn Intake and output every shift Monitor stools for color and consistency, and measure volume Daily weight Monitor serum electrolytes Assess mental status every shift Assist with/provide perianal care after each loose stool Report worsening abdominal pain, nausea, vomiting, diarrhea, or increasing abdominal distention	Electrolytes Blood culture × 2, if temp over 101F Vital signs q4hr and prn Assess gastrointestinal status q4hr and prn Intake and output every shift Monitor stools for color and consistency, and measure volume Daily weight Monitor serum electrolytes Assess mental status every shift Assist with/provide perianal care after each loose stool Report worsening abdominal pain, nausea, vomiting, diarrhea or increasing abdominal distention

	Date _____ **Day 1**	Date _____ **Day 2**	Date _____ **Day 3**
Knowledge deficit	Orient to room and hospital routine Review plan of care and importance of bowel rest, bed rest, and emotional rest Include family in teaching Evaluate understanding of teaching	Review plan of care and continued importance of bowel rest, bed rest, and emotional rest Include family in teaching Evaluate understanding of teaching	Reinforce earlier teaching regarding ongoing care Begin discharge teaching regarding rest, activity, and diet Include family in teaching Evaluate understanding of teaching
Psychosocial	Assess level of anxiety Encourage verbalization of concerns Provide information regarding illness Provide ongoing support and encouragement	Assess level of anxiety Encourage verbalization of concerns Provide information regarding treatment Provide ongoing support and encouragement	Encourage verbalization of concerns Provide ongoing support and encouragement
Diet	NPO Mouth care q2hr and prn NG to low suction with persistent vomiting	NPO Mouth care q2hr and prn D/C NG if no vomiting and active bowel sounds	Begin clear liquids to tolerance Mouth care prn
Activity	Assess safety needs and provide appropriate precautions Bedrest with commode privileges Provide rest periods Assist with ADLs	Maintain safety precautions Bathroom privileges with assistance Provide rest periods Assist with ADLs	Maintain safety precautions Up to chair ad lib Provide rest periods Assist with ADLs
Medications	IV fluids with electrolyte replacement as ordered Antidiarrheal drugs as ordered Tylenol 650 mg q4hr PR for temp over 101F	IV fluids with electrolyte replacement as ordered Antidiarrheal drugs as ordered Tylenol 650 mg q4hr PR for temp over 101F If indicated, initiate treatment based on stool cultures	IV fluids with electrolyte replacement as ordered Antidiarrheal drugs as ordered Tylenol 650 mg q4hr po for temp over 101F
Transfer/ discharge plans	Establish discharge goals with client and family Consult with social service regarding VNA and projected needs for home health care (if any)	Review progress toward discharge goals with client and family	Review progress toward discharge goals with client and family Make appropriate referrals

➤

Diarrhea and Dehydration *(continued)*

	Date _____ **Day 4**	Date _____ **Day 5**
Daily outcomes	Client will: • have stable vital signs • have an oral intake of 2000 mL/day • remain free of nausea and vomiting • verbalize understanding of ongoing care • have a soft, non-distended abdomen, and active bowel sounds • pass soft, brown stools • tolerate ordered diet without nausea and vomiting • demonstrate ability to cope • verbalize/demonstrate beginning understanding of home care instructions	Client is afebrile and has stable vital signs Client has a soft, non-distended abdomen and passes soft, brown stools each day Client is independent in self-care Client is fully ambulatory Client has resumed preadmission urine elimination pattern Client verbalizes/demonstrates home care instructions Client tolerates ordered diet and has an oral intake of 2000 mL/day Client demonstrates ability to cope with ongoing stressors
Assessments, tests, and treatments	Blood culture × 2, if temp over 101F Vital signs q4hr and prn Electrolytes Daily weight Assess gastrointestinal status q4hr and prn Intake and output every shift Assess gastrointestinal status q4hr and prn Report worsening abdominal pain, nausea, vomiting, diarrhea, or increasing abdominal distention	Blood culture × 2, if temp over 101F Daily weight Vital signs q4hr and prn Assess gastrointestinal status q4hr and prn Intake and output every shift
Knowledge deficit	Reinforce earlier teaching regarding ongoing care Review written discharge instructions with client and family Discuss need to eat 3 to 4 regularly scheduled meals Teach client signs and symptoms requiring follow-up: worsening abdominal pain, nausea, vomiting, change in bowel habits, and/or fever Include family in teaching Evaluate understanding of teaching	Reinforce earlier teaching regarding ongoing care Complete discharge teaching to include diet, follow-up care, signs and symptoms to report, activity, and medications: name, purpose, dose, frequency, route, food interactions, and side effects Include family in teaching Provide client with written discharge instructions Evaluate understanding of teaching

Diarrhea and Dehydration *(continued)*

	Date _____ **Day 4**	Date _____ **Day 5**
Psychosocial	Encourage verbalization of concerns Provide ongoing support and encouragement	Encourage verbalization of concerns Provide ongoing support and encouragement
Diet	Full liquids to soft diet as tolerated, providing small, frequent, nutritious feedings Encourage fluid intake of 2000 mL/day	Soft diet as tolerated, providing small, frequent, nutritious feedings Encourage fluid intake of 2000 mL/day
Activity	Self-care Ambulate independently at least 4 times	Self-care Fully ambulatory
Medications	D/C IV if oral intake >2000 mL/day Tylenol 650 mg q4hr po for temp over 101F	Tylenol 650 mg q4hr po for temp over 101F
Transfer/ discharge plans	Continue to review progress toward discharge goals Finalize discharge plans	Finalize plans for home care if needed Complete discharge teaching

Potential Client Variances
Diarrhea and Dehydration

Possible Complications

- Fluid and electrolyte disturbances

Health Conditions

- Pre-existing mobility problems

Nursing Diagnoses

- Risk for altered skin integrity
- Risk for injury

Discharge Teaching for Client Following
Diarrhea and Dehydration

Activity

- Gradually return to usual level of activity by increasing activity each day. Alternate activity with rest periods. Avoid fatigue.
- Avoid overexertion until your strength returns.
- Return to work following your physician's approval.

Diet

- Eat a well-balanced diet, including all food groups. Continue soft diet for 3 to 5 days and begin to gradually introduce fresh fruits and vegetables. Avoid foods that cause GI distress such as fatty or spicy foods
- Report nausea, vomiting, or change in bowel habits
- Drink 6–8 glasses of fluid each day

Signs and Symptoms to Report

Notify physician if any of these symptoms occur:
- Abdominal pain or recurrent diarrhea
- Blood in stools or dark-colored stools
- Chills, or fever greater than 100F or 38C

Follow-Up Care and General Health Care

- Schedule follow-up appointment with physician as directed.
- Wash and dry perianal area after each bowel movement.

Medications

- Review written list of medications, including dose, route, frequency, food interactions, and side effects.
- Avoid alcohol if taking medication.

Diverticulitis and Constipation

Expected length of stay: 5–6 days

	Date _____ **Day 1**	Date _____ **Day 2**	Date _____ **Day 3**
Daily outcomes	Client will: • have stable vital signs • have an intake of 2000 mL/day (IV) • remain free of nausea and vomiting • state control of pain • verbalize understanding of ongoing care • have a soft, non-distended abdomen • demonstrate ability to cope	Client will: • have stable vital signs • have an intake of 2000 mL/day (IV) • remain free of nausea and vomiting • state control of pain • verbalize understanding of ongoing care • have a soft, non-distended abdomen • demonstrate ability to cope	Client will: • have stable vital signs • have an intake of 2000 mL/day (IV/PO) • state control of pain • verbalize understanding of ongoing care • have a soft, non-distended abdomen, and active bowel sounds • tolerate clear liquids without nausea or vomiting • demonstrate ability to cope • verbalize/demonstrate beginning understanding of home care instructions
Assessments, tests, and treatments	CBC with differential Electrolytes Abdominal x-rays as ordered Colonoscopy if ordered Blood culture × 2, if temp over 101F Vital signs q4hr and prn Assess gastrointestinal status q4hr and prn Intake and output every shift	Blood culture × 2, if temp over 101F Vital signs q4hr and prn Assess gastrointestinal status q4hr and prn Intake and output every shift Enemas if ordered	Blood culture × 2, if temp over 101F Vital signs q4hr and prn Assess gastrointestinal status q4hr and prn Intake and output every shift
Knowledge deficit	Orient to room and hospital routine Review plan of care and importance of bowel rest, bed rest, and emotional rest Include family in teaching Evaluate understanding of teaching	Review plan of care and continued importance of bowel rest, bed rest, and emotional rest Include family in teaching Evaluate understanding of teaching	Reinforce earlier teaching regarding ongoing care Begin discharge teaching regarding rest, activity, and diet Include family in teaching Evaluate understanding of teaching
Psychosocial	Assess level of anxiety Encourage verbalization of concerns Provide information Provide ongoing support and encouragement	Assess level of anxiety Encourage verbalization of concerns Provide information Provide ongoing support and encouragement	Encourage verbalization of concerns Provide ongoing support and encouragement
Diet	NPO Mouth care q2hr and prn	NPO Mouth care q2hr and prn	Begin warm, clear liquids to tolerance

Diverticulitis and Constipation *(continued)*

	Date _____ **Day 1**	Date _____ **Day 2**	Date _____ **Day 3**
Activity	Assess safety needs and provide appropriate precautions Bedrest with commode privileges Provide rest periods Assist with ADLs	Maintain safety precautions Bathroom privileges with assistance Provide rest periods Assist with ADLs	Maintain safety precautions Up to chair ad lib Provide rest periods Assist with ADLs
Medications	IV fluids IV antibiotics IM/IV analgesics Laxatives if ordered Tylenol 650 mg q4hr PR for temp over 101F	IV fluids IV antibiotics IM/IV analgesics Laxatives if ordered Tylenol 650 mg q4hr PR for temp over 101F	IV fluids IV antibiotics IM analgesics Tylenol 650 mg q4hr po for temp over 101F
Bowel management	Assess usual bowel elimination pattern Assess gastrointestinal status q4hr and prn Observe stools for color, consistency, frequency, and amount Report worsening abdominal pain, nausea, vomiting, or increasing abdominal distention	Assess gastrointestinal status q4hr and prn Observe stools for color, consistency, frequency, and amount Report worsening abdominal pain, nausea, vomiting or increasing abdominal distention	Assess gastrointestinal status q4hr and prn Observe stools for color, consistency, frequency, and amount Report worsening abdominal pain, nausea, vomiting or increasing abdominal distention
Transfer/ discharge plans	Establish discharge goals with client and family Consult with social service regarding VNA and projected needs for home health care (if any)	Review progress toward discharge goals with client and family	Review progress toward discharge goals with client and family Make appropriate referrals

Diverticulitis and Constipation *(continued)*

	Date _____ **Day 4**	Date _____ **Days 5–6**
Daily outcomes	Client will: • have stable vital signs • have an oral intake of 2000 mL/day • remain free of nausea and vomiting • state control of pain • verbalize understanding of ongoing care • have a soft, non-distended abdomen, and active bowel sounds • pass soft, brown stools • tolerate ordered diet without nausea and vomiting • demonstrate ability to cope • verbalize/demonstrate understanding of home care instructions	Client is afebrile and has stable vital signs Client has a soft, non-distended abdomen and passes soft, brown stools each day Client is independent in self-care Client is fully ambulatory Client has resumed preadmission urine elimination pattern Client verbalizes/demonstrates home care instructions Client tolerates ordered diet and has an intake of 2000 mL/day Client demonstrates ability to cope with ongoing stressors
Assessments, tests, and treatments	Blood culture × 2, if temp over 101F Vital signs q4hr and prn Assess gastrointestinal status q4hr and prn Intake and output every shift	Blood culture × 2, if temp over 101F Vital signs q4hr and prn Assess gastrointestinal status q4hr and prn Intake and output every shift
Knowledge deficit	Reinforce earlier teaching regarding ongoing care Review written discharge instructions with client and family Include family in teaching Evaluate understanding of teaching	Reinforce earlier teaching regarding ongoing care Complete discharge teaching to include diet, follow-up care, signs and symptoms to report, activity, and medications: name, purpose, dose, frequency, route, food interactions, and side effects Provide client with written discharge instructions Include family in teaching Evaluate understanding of teaching
Psychosocial	Encourage verbalization of concerns Provide ongoing support and encouragement	Encourage verbalization of concerns Provide ongoing support and encouragement

➤

Diverticulitis and Constipation *(continued)*

	Date _____ **Day 4**	Date _____ **Days 5–6**
Diet	Full liquids to soft diet as tolerated, providing small, frequent, nutritious feedings Encourage fluid intake of 2000 mL/day	Soft diet as tolerated, providing small, frequent, nutritious feedings Encourage fluid intake of 2000 mL/day
Activity	Maintain safety precautions Self-care Ambulate independently at least 4 times	Maintain safety precautions Self-care Fully ambulatory
Medications	D/C IV if oral intake >2000 mL/day Oral antibiotics Oral analgesics Tylenol 650 mg q4hr po for temp over 101F	Oral antibiotics Tylenol 650 mg q4hr po for temp over 101F
Bowel management	Assess gastrointestinal status q4hr and prn Report worsening abdominal pain, nausea, vomiting or increasing abdominal distention Offer warm liquids early each morning Discuss need to eat 3–4 regularly scheduled meals Encourage increased physical activity Teach client signs and symptoms requiring follow-up: worsening abdominal pain, nausea, vomiting, change in bowel habits, and/or fever Encourage client to eat a well-balanced diet, including all food groups, after this acute episode Instruct regarding the importance of increasing fiber from whole grains, fruits, and vegetables while avoiding nuts, seeds, and berries Encourage client to avoid straining for a BM and to avoid constipation using a hydrophyllic colloid laxative Instruct client to avoid strong laxatives and enemas, constipation, restrictive clothing, and any activities that increase intra-abdominal pressure (lifting, bending, and coughing)	Assess gastrointestinal status q4hr and prn Report worsening abdominal pain, nausea, vomiting or increasing abdominal distention Offer warm liquids early each morning Reinforce the following instructions: – need to eat 3–4 regularly scheduled meals per day – the importance of increased physical activity Review signs and symptoms requiring follow-up: worsening abdominal pain, nausea, vomiting, change in bowel habits, and/or fever Reinforce importance of eating a well-balanced diet and the importance of increasing fiber from whole grains, fruits, and vegetables while avoiding nuts, seeds and berries

	Date _____ **Day 4**	Date _____ **Days 5–6**
Transfer/ discharge plans	Continue to review progress toward discharge goals Finalize discharge plans	Finalize plans for home care if needed Complete discharge teaching

Potential Client Variances
Diverticulitis and Constipation

Possible Complications
- Bowel obstruction
- Bowel perforation
- Peritonitis
- Sepsis

Health Conditions
- Undernutrition
- Steroid dependency

Nursing Diagnoses
- Acute pain
- Constipation

Discharge Teaching for Client With
Diverticulitis and Constipation

Activity
- Gradually return to usual level of activity by increasing activity each day. Alternate activity with rest periods. Avoid fatigue.
- Avoid overexertion for the period of time designated by your physician.

Diet
- Eat a well-balanced diet, including all food groups.
- Continue to gradually add fiber to diet in the form of fruits, vegetables, and whole grain cereals, and bran. Avoid foods with seeds, nuts, and berries.
- Drink 6–8 glasses of fluid each day.

Signs and Symptoms to Report
Notify physician if any of these symptoms occur:
- Abdominal pain
- Nausea or vomiting
- Change in bowel habits
- Chills, or fever greater than 100F or 38C
- Blood in stools or dark-colored stools.

Follow-Up Care and General Health Care
- Schedule follow-up appointment with physician as directed.
- Wash and dry perineal area after each bowel movement.

Medications
- Review written list of medications including dose, route, frequency, food interactions, and side effects.
- Avoid alcohol if taking medication.

Critical Pathway for Client with

Upper Gastrointestinal Bleeding

Expected length of stay: 6 days

	Date _____ Admission–Day 1	Date _____ Day 2	Date _____ Day 3
Daily outcomes	Client will: • have stabilizing vital signs and remain hemodynamically stable • remain alert and oriented • verbalize understanding and demonstrate cooperation with ongoing care • verbalize control of pain • demonstrate ability to cope • have a patent NG tube and treatment initiated to control bleeding • maintain urine output >30 mL/hr • have lungs clear to auscultation	Client will: • have stable vital signs • remain alert and oriented • verbalize understanding and demonstrate cooperation with ongoing care • verbalize control of pain • have active bowel sounds • remain free of uncontrolled bleeding • demonstrate ability to cope • have a patent NG tube • maintain urine output >30 mL/hr • have lungs clear to auscultation	Client will: • have stable vital signs • remain alert and oriented • demonstrate cooperation with ongoing care • demonstrate ability to cope • verbalize control of pain • remain free of uncontrolled bleeding • tolerate ordered diet without nausea or vomiting • have active bowel sounds • verbalize beginning understanding of home care instructions • have a patent NG tube • maintain urine output >30 mL/hr • have lungs clear to auscultation
Assessments, tests, and treatments	CBC Serum chemistries Urinalysis Chest x-ray PT/PTT Type and screen Vital signs q15min until stable—include orthostatic signs; O_2 saturation q1–2hr and prn until stable Baseline physical assessment with a focus on respiratory status, mental status, and gastrointestinal function Oxygen to maintain O_2 saturation >95% Intake and output q2hr and prn Assess patency of NG tube q1hr, noting volume and character of drainage q2hr Assess respiratory status and gastrointestinal function q2–4hr and prn Gastric lavage if ordered Assess voiding pattern q4hr and prn	CBC PT/PTT Endoscopy Vital signs and O_2 saturation q4hr and prn Assess respiratory status and gastrointestinal function q4hr and prn Oxygen to maintain O_2 saturation >95% Intake and output every shift Assess patency of NG tube q2hr, noting volume and character of drainage q2hr Report any nausea or vomiting Assess voiding pattern every shift Assess and record the description, location, duration, and characteristics of client's pain q 2–4 hr and prn Encourage verbalization of pain and discomfort	CBC Other diagnostic tests as ordered Vital sign assessment q4hr and prn Assess respiratory status and gastrointestinal function q4hr and prn Oxygen to maintain O_2 saturation >95% Intake and output every shift Assess patency and output of NG tube q4hr noting volume and character of drainage q2hr Discontinue NG tube when ordered Assess voiding pattern every shift Assess and record the description, location, duration, and characteristics of client's pain q4hr and prn Encourage verbalization of pain and discomfort

Upper Gastrointestinal Bleeding (continued)

	Date _____ **Admission**	Date _____ **Day 2**	Date _____ **Day 3**
Assessments, tests, and treatments (continued)	Assess and record the description, location, duration, and characteristics of client's pain q2–4hr and prn Instruct in relaxation and distraction techniques as an adjunct to pain medications	Reduce or eliminate pain-producing factors and employ distraction or relaxation techniques Provide back rubs	Reduce or eliminate pain-producing factors, employ distraction or relaxation techniques, and offer back rubs
Knowledge deficit	Orient to room and surroundings Provide simple, brief instructions including hospital and ongoing care Discuss tubes: nasogastric (NG) and intravenous (IV), pain management Include family in teaching Evaluate understanding of teaching	Review plan of care and importance of early mobilization Review importance of NG and IV, pain management Include family in teaching Evaluate understanding of teaching Review pain management strategies	Reinforce earlier teaching regarding ongoing care Begin discharge teaching regarding diet and signs and symptoms of bleeding Initiate medication teaching Include family in teaching Evaluate understanding of teaching
Psychosocial	Assess anxiety related to diagnosis Encourage verbalization of concerns Offer emotional support Provide information regarding diagnosis and treatment Provide support to family Establish and provide quiet, calm restful environment Minimize external stimuli (eg, noise, movement)	Assess level of anxiety Encourage verbalization of concerns Provide information, ongoing support and encouragement to client and family Maintain restful environment	Encourage verbalization of concerns Provide information, ongoing support and encouragement to client and family Maintain restful environment Explore ongoing stressors and initiate teaching regarding stress-reducing strategies
Diet	NPO Baseline nutritional assessment	NPO NG tube	NPO until NG tube removed Start small amounts of fluids if ordered Avoid gastric irritants such as coffee or caffeinated colas
Activity	Assess safety needs and provide safety precautions Bedrest with HOB up 30 degrees	Maintain safety precautions Bathroom privileges with assistance if no active bleeding	Maintain safety precautions Begin activity to tolerance if no active bleeding
Medications	Administer prescribed IM or IV analgesics and record response IV fluids Blood products if ordered Vitamin K if ordered IV H_2-receptor antagonists Antacids as ordered	Administer prescribed IM or IV analgesics and record response IV fluids Blood products if ordered IV H_2-receptor antagonists Antacids as ordered	Administer oral analgesics and record response IV fluids IV or po H_2-receptor antagonists Antacids as ordered

➤

	Date _____ **Admission**	Date _____ **Day 2**	Date _____ **Day 3**
Transfer/ discharge plans	Assess potential discharge needs and support system Establish discharge goals with client and family	Review progress toward discharge goals with client and family Consult with social service re- garding projected needs for home health care (if any)	Review progress toward discharge goals with client and family

	Date _____ **Day 4**	Date _____ **Day 5**	Date _____ **Day 6**

Daily outcomes	Client will:
	• have stable vital signs
	• remain alert and oriented
	• tolerate ordered diet without
	  nausea or vomiting
	• have active bowel sounds
	• remain free of uncontrolled
	  bleeding
	• maintain urine output
	  >30 mL/hr
	• have lungs clear to auscultation
	• participate in self-care activities
	  and ambulation without signs
	  of activity intolerance
	• verbalize control of pain
	• demonstrate ability to cope
	• verbalize beginning under-
	  standing of home care
	  instructions
		Client will:
		• have stable vital signs
		• remain alert and oriented
		• tolerate ordered diet without
		  nausea or vomiting
		• have active bowel sounds
		• remain free of uncontrolled
		  bleeding
		• maintain urine output
		  >30 mL/hr
		• have lungs clear to auscultation
		• participate in self-care activities
		  and ambulation without signs
		  of activity intolerance
		• verbalize control of pain
		• demonstrate ability to cope
		• verbalize understanding of
		  home care instructions
			Client has stable vital signs
			Client manages any pain with
			  non-pharmacologic measures
			Client is independent in self-care
			Client is fully ambulatory without
			  evidence of activity intolerance
			Client has resumed preadmission
			  urine and bowel elimination
			  pattern
			Client has no signs of active
			  bleeding
			Client verbalizes home care
			  instructions
			Client tolerates ordered diet
			Client demonstrates ability to
			  cope with ongoing stressors

*Assessments, tests,
and treatments*
	Assess vital signs q4hr and prn
	Intake and output every shift
	Assess voiding pattern every shift
	Assess respiratory status, mental
	  status, and gastrointestinal
	  function q4–8hr and prn
	D/C oxygen if O$_2$ saturation >98%
	  on room air
	Assess and record description,
	  location, duration, and charac-
	  teristics of client's pain q4hr
	  and prn
	Encourage client to employ
	  distraction or relaxation
	  techniques
		Assess vital signs q4hr and prn
		Assess respiratory status, mental
		  status, and gastrointestinal
		  function q8hr and prn
		Assess and record description,
		  location, duration, and charac-
		  teristics of client's pain q4hr
		  and prn
		Encourage client to employ
		  distraction or relaxation
		  techniques
			Assess vital signs q4hr and prn
			Assess respiratory status, mental
			  status, and gastrointestinal
			  function
			Assess and record description,
			  location, duration, and charac-
			  teristics of client's pain q4hr
			  and prn
			Encourage client to employ
			  distraction or relaxation
			  techniques

	Date _____ **Day 4**	Date _____ **Day 5**	Date _____ **Day 6**
Knowledge deficit	Review discharge teaching regarding diet and signs and symptoms of bleeding Review medication teaching Review stress-reducing strategies Reinforce written discharge instructions with client and family Evaluate understanding of teaching	Reinforce discharge teaching regarding diet and signs and symptoms of bleeding Reinforce medication teaching Reinforce stress reducing strategies Discuss interventions to minimize recurrence of bleeding Review written discharge instructions with client and family Evaluate understanding of teaching	Complete discharge teaching to include diet, follow-up care, signs and symptoms to report, activity, and medications: dose, frequency, route, food interactions, and side effects Review stress-reducing strategies Provide client with written discharge instructions Evaluate understanding of teaching
Psychosocial	Encourage verbalization of concerns Provide ongoing support and encouragement Maintain restful environment	Encourage verbalization of concerns Provide ongoing support and encouragement Maintain restful environment	Encourage verbalization of concerns Provide ongoing support and encouragement Maintain restful environment
Diet	Ordered or bland, soft diet in small amounts as tolerated	Ordered or bland, soft diet Visit with dietitian for meal planning at home	Ordered or bland, soft diet
Activity	Activity to tolerance	Activity to tolerance	Activity to tolerance
Medications	Provide ordered analgesics Intermittent IV device Oral H_2-receptor antagonists Antacids as ordered	D/C intermittent IV device Oral H_2-receptor antagonists Antacids as ordered	Oral H_2-receptor antagonists Antacids as ordered
Transfer/ discharge plans	Continue to review progress toward discharge goals	Finalize discharge plans Continue to review progress toward discharge goals Finalize plans for home care if needed	Complete discharge instructions Complete appropriate referrals

Upper Gastrointestinal Bleeding

Possible Complications
- Hypovolemic shock
- Aspiration
- Perforated ulcer

Health Conditions
- Undernutrition
- Ulcer disease
- Impaired physical mobility
- Anemia
- Alcoholism

Nursing Diagnoses
- Altered nutrition: less than body requirements
- Ineffective individual coping
- Anxiety
- Noncompliance

Discharge Teaching for Client Following
Upper Gastrointestinal Bleeding

Activity
- Gradually return to usual level of activity by increasing activity each day. Alternate activity with rest periods. Avoid fatigue.
- Avoid heavy housework, straining, heavy lifting, and driving for the period designated by your physician.
- Return to work following physician approval.

Diet
- Follow diet instructions given by dietitian. Avoid foods that you find spicy or gas-producing.
- If you experience discomfort during meals, decrease the amount of food consumed.
- Eat frequent, small meals.
- Avoid stress during and after meals.
- Rest after meals.

Signs and Symptoms to Report
Notify physician if any of these symptoms occur:
- Pain, abdominal distention, nausea, vomiting or diarrhea
- Blood in stools or dark-colored stools

Follow-Up Care and General Health Care
- Schedule follow-up appointment with physician as directed.
- Avoid smoking.
- Utilize strategies to reduce stress.

Medications
- Review written list of medications, including dose, route, frequency, food interactions, and side effects.
- Check with your physician regarding alcohol use.
- Avoid aspirin or aspirin-containing medications.
- Avoid over-the-counter drugs and nonsteroidal anti-inflammatory medications unless ordered by your physician.

Critical Pathway for Client Following

Myocardial Infarction (Uncomplicated)

Expected length of stay: 6 days

	Date _____ **Day 1: Admission to Coronary Care Unit**	Date _____ **Day 2**	Date _____ **Day 3: Transfer to Stepdown Unit**
Daily outcomes	Client will: • have stabilizing vital signs and hemodynamic measures • remain alert and oriented • verbalize pain or discomfort using a 0–10 scale • verbalize control of chest pain • verbalize understanding of ongoing treatment and need for hospitalization • demonstrate ability to adhere to activity restrictions • have lungs clear to auscultation • maintain urine output >30 mL/hr • verbalize feelings regarding ongoing stressors • verbalize/demonstrate ability to cope	Client will: • have stable vital signs and hemodynamic measures • remain alert and oriented • verbalize control of chest pain • verbalize presence or absence of pain or discomfort on a 0–10 scale • verbalize understanding of ongoing treatment and need for hospitalization • demonstrate ability to adhere to activity restrictions • have lungs clear to auscultation • maintain urine output >30 mL/hr • verbalize feelings regarding ongoing stressors and illness • verbalize/demonstrate ability to cope	Client will: • be afebrile, with stable vital signs • remain alert and oriented • verbalize presence or absence of pain or discomfort • be free of chest pain • verbalize understanding of ongoing treatment and need for hospitalization • demonstrate ability to adhere to activity restrictions • tolerate activity level without dyspnea, shortness of breath, or chest pain • have lungs clear to auscultation • maintain urine output >30 mL/hr • verbalize feelings regarding ongoing stressors and illness • verbalize ability to cope • verbalize understanding of transfer to stepdown unit • verbalize beginning understanding of home care instructions
Assessments, tests, and treatments	CBC EKG PA and lateral chest x-ray ABGs PT/PTT Cardiac enzymes q8hr x 3 Cardiovascular assessment q4hr and prn Continuous cardiac monitoring Vital signs and O_2 saturation, q4hr and prn Incentive spirometer q2hr Oxygen to maintain O_2 saturation > 95% Assist with ADLs Monitor arterial blood gases Weight	Vital signs and O_2 saturation, q4hr and prn Cardiovascular assessment q4hr and prn Continuous cardiac monitoring Intake and output every shift Oxygen to maintain O_2 saturation > 95% Weight	Vital signs and O_2 saturation, q4hr and prn Cardiovascular assessment q4hr and prn Continuous cardiac monitoring Intake and output every shift Oxygen to maintain O_2 saturation > 96% Assist with ADLs Transfer to stepdown unit as ordered Weight

	Date _____ **Day 1: Admission to Coronary Care Unit**	Date _____ **Day 2**	Date _____ **Day 3: Transfer to Stepdown Unit**
Knowledge deficit	Orient to room and hospital routine Review plan of care Include family in teaching Evaluate understanding of teaching	Review plan of care Brief MI teaching Include family in teaching Evaluate understanding of teaching	Reinforce earlier teaching regarding ongoing care Begin discharge teaching using MI teaching packet regarding rest, activity, and diet Include family in teaching Evaluate understanding of teaching
Psychosocial	Assess level of anxiety Encourage verbalization of concerns Provide information and ongoing support and encouragement to client and family	Assess level of anxiety Encourage verbalization of concerns Provide information and ongoing support and encouragement to client and family	Encourage verbalization of concerns Provide ongoing support and encouragement to client and family
Diet	American Heart Association diet as tolerated, providing small, frequent, nutritious feedings Avoid extremes in temperatures	American Heart Association diet as tolerated, providing small, frequent, nutritious feedings Avoid extremes in temperatures	American Heart Association diet as tolerated, providing small, frequent, nutritious feedings Avoid extremes in temperatures
Activity	Assess safety needs and provide appropriate precautions Bed rest Assist with ADLs Provide rest periods Monitor responses to visitors and limit accordingly	Maintain safety precautions Bed rest with commode privileges Assist with ADLs Transfer to chair, as tolerated Provide rest periods Monitor responses to visitors and limit accordingly	Maintain safety precautions Chair, ambulate in room Assist with ADLs Provide rest periods Monitor responses to activity
Medications	IV KVO Consider thrombolytics IV heparin as ordered Aspirin as ordered IV nitro as ordered IV beta blockers as ordered Sleeping medication if ordered	IV KVO IV heparin as ordered Aspirin as ordered IV nitro as ordered and then begin weaning per order IV beta blockers as ordered Sleeping medication if ordered Stool softener	Intermittent IV device IV heparin as ordered Aspirin as ordered Cardiac meds as ordered Sleeping medication if ordered Stool softener Laxative if no BM in 3 days
Transfer/ discharge plans	Establish discharge goals with client and family Consult with social service regarding VNA projected needs for home health care (if any)	Review progress toward discharge goals with client and family Referral to cardiac rehab	Review progress toward discharge goals with client and family Cardiac rehab evaluation completed

Myocardial Infarction (Uncomplicated) *(continued)*

	Date _____ **Day 4**	Date _____ **Day 5**	Date _____ **Day 6**
Daily outcomes	Client will: • be afebrile and have stable vital signs • verbalize understanding and demonstrate cooperation with ongoing care • verbalize presence/absence of chest pain • verbalize understanding of ongoing treatment and care • demonstrate ability to adhere to activity restrictions • tolerate activity level without dyspnea, shortness of breath, or chest pain • have lungs clear to auscultation • maintain urine output >30 mL/hr • verbalize feelings regarding ongoing stressors • verbalize/demonstrate ability to cope • verbalize beginning understanding of illness and benefits of cardiac rehab • verbalize beginning understanding of home care instructions	Client will: • be afebrile and have stable vital signs • verbalize understanding and demonstrate cooperation with ongoing care • verbalize presence/absence of chest pain • verbalize understanding of ongoing treatment and care • demonstrate ability to adhere to activity restrictions • tolerate activity level without dyspnea, shortness of breath, or chest pain • have lungs clear to auscultation • maintain urine output >30 mL/hr • verbalize feelings regarding ongoing stressors • verbalize/demonstrate ability to cope • verbalize understanding of illness and benefits of cardiac rehab • verbalize understanding of home care instructions	Client is afebrile and has stable vital signs Client has lungs that are clear to auscultation Client is independent in self-care Client is fully ambulatory Client tolerates activity level without dyspnea, shortness of breath, or chest pain Client has resumed preadmission urine and bowel elimination pattern Client verbalizes/demonstrates home care instructions Client tolerates ordered diet Client verbalizes/demonstrates ability to cope with ongoing stressors Client verbalizes understanding of illness and discharge care Client and family verbalize strategies to reduce risk factors for heart disease, including diet, medication, activity restrictions, signs and symptoms to report
Assessments, tests, and treatments	Vital signs and O_2 saturation, q4hr and prn Cardiac assessment q4hr and prn Intake and output every shift Continuous cardiac monitoring D/C oxygen if O_2 saturation 98% on room air	Vital signs and O_2 saturation, q4hr and prn Cardiac assessment q4hr and prn Intake and output every shift Discontinue continuous cardiac monitoring Schedule stress test	Vital signs and O_2 saturation, q4hr and prn Cardiac assessment q4hr and prn
Knowledge deficit	Reinforce earlier teaching regarding ongoing care Review written discharge instructions from MI teaching packet with client and family Include family in teaching Evaluate understanding of teaching	Reinforce earlier teaching regarding ongoing care Review written discharge instructions with client and family Include family in teaching Evaluate understanding of teaching	Reinforce earlier teaching regarding ongoing care Complete discharge teaching to include diet, follow-up care, signs and symptoms to report, follow-up MD visit, activity, and medications: name, purpose, dose, frequency, route, dietary interactions, and side effects Provide client with written discharge instructions Include family in teaching Evaluate understanding of teaching

	Date _____ **Day 4**	Date _____ **Day 5**	Date _____ **Day 6**
Psychosocial	Encourage verbalization of concerns Provide ongoing support and encouragement to client and family	Encourage verbalization of concerns Provide ongoing support and encouragement to client and family	Encourage verbalization of concerns Provide ongoing support and encouragement to client and family
Diet	American Heart Association diet as tolerated, providing small, frequent, nutritious feedings	American Heart Association diet as tolerated, providing small, frequent, nutritious feedings	American Heart Association diet as tolerated, providing small, frequent, nutritious feedings
Activity	Ambulate in room 3–4 times/day Ambulate in hallway Maintain safety precautions Monitor responses to activity	Ambulate in room 3–4 times/day Ambulate in hallway Start stair walking Maintain safety precautions Monitor responses to activity	Ambulate in room 3–4 times/day Ambulate in hallway Maintain safety precautions Monitor responses to activity
Medications	Intermittent IV device D/C heparin Aspirin as ordered Sleeping medication if ordered Stool softener Cardiac meds as ordered	D/C intermittent IV device Aspirin as ordered Sleeping medication if ordered Stool softener Cardiac meds as ordered	Aspirin as ordered Sleeping medication if ordered Stool softener Cardiac meds as ordered
Transfer/ discharge plans	Continue to review progress toward discharge goals Finalize discharge plans Finalize referral to cardiac rehab Continue discharge teaching	Finalize plans for home care if needed Make any other appropriate referrals Continue discharge teaching	Finalize plans for home care if needed Make any appropriate referrals Complete discharge teaching

Potential Client Variances
Myocardial Infarction (Uncomplicated)

Possible Complications

- Dysrhythmias
- Congestive heart failure
- Pericarditis
- Extension of MI

Health Conditions

- Diabetes
- Hypertension
- Kidney failure
- Pre-existing coronary or respiratory disease

Nursing Diagnoses

- Acute pain
- Anxiety
- Fear
- Ineffective individual coping
- Decreased cardiac output
- Activity intolerance
- Ineffective management of therapeutic regimen

Discharge Teaching for Client Following
Myocardial Infarction (Uncomplicated)

Activity

- Gradually return to usual level of activity by increasing activity each day. Alternate activity with rest periods. Avoid fatigue.
- Continue exercise program as instructed by physical therapist or cardiac rehabilitation nurse.
- Avoid sitting or standing for long periods.
- Do not cross your legs.
- No strenuous activity until okayed by physician.
- Avoid heavy housework, straining, and driving for the period designated by your physician.
- Check with physician as to when to resume sexual activity.
- Check with your physician about driving or other traveling.

Diet

- Eat a well-balanced diet, including all food groups. Continue any recommended dietary restrictions (usually low fat, low cholesterol, and low sodium).
- Avoid large meals and alcohol.
- Rest after meals.
- Lose weight if your physician recommends this to you.

Signs and Symptoms to Report

Notify physician if any of these symptoms occur:
- Chest pain, dyspnea, shortness of breath, weight gain, or decrease in exercise tolerance.
- Side effects from medications.
- Chest pain unrelieved by medications.
- Pain that radiates to jaw or arm(s).

Follow-Up Care and General Health Care

- Schedule follow-up appointment with physician as directed.
- Do not smoke and avoid second-hand smoke.
- Discuss alcohol use with your physician.
- Begin cardiac rehabilitation program as directed.
- If you experience chest pain, stop what you are doing and rest and take medication if ordered.
- Notify your physician or go to the nearest emergency room if you have chest pain unrelieved by rest and/or medication or you experience sweating, nausea, vomiting, shortness of breath with the pain, or pain that radiates.

Medications

- Review written list of medications, including dose, frequency, food interactions, and side effects.
- Review medication teaching sheets.
- Make a list of medications and doses and carry it with you.

Critical Pathway for Client with

Osteomyelitis

Expected length of stay: 5 days

	Date _____ Day 1	Date _____ Day 2	Date _____ Day 3
Daily outcomes	Client will: • have stable vital signs • verbalize understanding of diagnosis and planned treatment • have an intake of 3000 mL/day (IV/po) unless contraindicated • demonstrate ability to cope	Client will: • have stable vital signs • have an intake of 3000 mL/day (IV/po) unless contraindicated • demonstrate ability to cope	Client will: • be afebrile, have stable vital signs • demonstrate ability to cope • verbalize beginning understanding of home care instructions • demonstrate beginning competence in self-IV therapy • have an intake of 3000 mL/day (IV/po) unless contraindicated
Assessments, tests, and treatments	CBC with differential Erythrocyte sedimentation rate Prepare for x-rays, bone scanning, CT or MRI as ordered Blood culture × 2, if temp over 101F Wound smear for gram stain and C & S Vital signs and q4hr and prn Assess respiratory status q4hr and prn Intake and output every shift Immobilize affected area Assess distal pulses q2-4hr and prn Assess affected area for redness, swelling, drainage, and pain Maintain sterile technique for any dressing changes Assess pain level q2hr and prn	Vital signs q4hr and prn Assess respiratory status q4hr and prn Immobilize affected area Assess distal pulses q2–4hr and prn Assess affected area for redness, swelling, drainage, and pain Maintain sterile technique for any dressing changes Assess pain level q2hr and prn Intake and output every shift	Vital signs q4hr and prn Assist with ADLs Check culture and sensitivities Immobilize affected area Assess distal pulses q2–4hr and prn Assess affected area for redness, swelling, drainage, and pain Maintain sterile technique for any dressing changes Assess pain level q2hr and prn Intake and output every shift
Knowledge deficit	Orient to room and hospital routine Review plan of care and the importance of long-term antibiotic therapy Include family in teaching Evaluate understanding of teaching	Review plan of care Initiate teaching regarding home IV therapy Encourage client to observe IV–related care Include family in teaching Evaluate understanding of teaching	Reinforce earlier teaching regarding ongoing care Begin discharge teaching regarding activity, diet, and the need for long-term antibiotic therapy at home Review teaching regarding home IV therapy Include family in teaching Evaluate understanding of teaching

Osteomyelitis *(continued)*

	Date _____ **Day 1**	Date _____ **Day 2**	Date _____ **Day 3**
Psychosocial	Assess level of anxiety Encourage verbalization of concerns Provide information and ongoing support and encouragement to client and family	Assess level of anxiety Encourage verbalization of concerns Provide information and ongoing support and encouragement to client and family	Encourage verbalization of concerns Provide ongoing support and encouragement to client and family
Diet	Diet as tolerated providing small, frequent, nutritious feedings Encourage fluid intake of 2000 mL/day unless contraindicated	Diet as tolerated providing small, frequent, nutritious feedings Encourage fluid intake of 2000–3000 mL/day unless contraindicated	Diet as tolerated providing small, frequent, nutritious feedings Encourage fluid intake of 2000–3000 mL/day unless contraindicated
Activity	Assess safety needs and provide appropriate precautions Bathroom privileges with assistance Provide rest periods	Maintain safety precautions Bathroom privileges with assistance Provide rest periods	Maintain safety precautions Ambulate as ordered Provide rest periods
Medications	IV fluids IV antibiotics as ordered Tylenol 650 mg q4hr po for temp over 101F	IV fluids/intermittent IV device IV antibiotics as ordered Tylenol 650 mg q4hr po for temp over 101F	Intermittent IV device IV antibiotics as ordered Tylenol 650 mg q4hr po for temp over 101F
Transfer/ discharge plans	Establish discharge goals with client and family Consult with social service regarding VNA projected needs for home health care (if any)	Review progress toward discharge goals with client and family Identify potential referrals	Review progress toward discharge goals with client and family

	Date _____ **Day 4**	Date _____ **Day 5**
Daily outcomes	Client will: • be afebrile and have stable vital signs • have an oral intake of 3000 mL/day unless contraindicated • demonstrate ability to cope • verbalize understanding of home care instructions • verbalize understanding of home IV therapy • demonstrate competence in IV therapy	Client is afebrile and has stable vital signs Client has a WBC <11,000 and negative wound cultures Client is independent in self-care Client is fully ambulatory Client has resumed preadmission urine and bowel elimination pattern Client verbalizes/demonstrates home care instructions Client demonstrates care of IV catheter and administration of antibiotics safely and correctly Client tolerates usual diet and has an oral intake of 3000 mL/day Client demonstrates ability to cope with ongoing stressors
Assessments, tests, and treatments	Vital signs q4hr if stable Assess respiratory status q4hr and prn Immobilize affected area Assess distal pulses q2–4hr and prn Assess affected area for redness, swelling, drainage, and pain Maintain sterile technique for any dressing changes Assess pain level q2hr and prn	Vital signs q4hr if stable Assess respiratory status q4hr and prn Immobilize affected area Assess distal pulses q2–4hr and prn Assess affected area for redness, swelling, drainage, and pain Maintain sterile technique for any dressing changes Assess pain level q2hr and prn
Knowledge deficit	Reinforce earlier teaching regarding ongoing care Reinforce instructions regarding care of the IV and antibiotic administration Provide client with opportunities to demonstrate self-administration of IV antibiotics Review written discharge instructions with client and family Include family in teaching Evaluate understanding of teaching	Reinforce earlier teaching regarding ongoing care Complete discharge teaching to include diet, follow-up care, signs and symptoms to report, follow-up MD visit, activity, and medications: name, purpose, dose, frequency, route, dietary interactions, and side effects Provide client with written discharge instructions Include family in teaching Evaluate understanding of teaching
Psychosocial	Encourage verbalization of concerns Provide ongoing support and encouragement to client and family	Encourage verbalization of concerns Provide ongoing support and encouragement to client and family

	Date _____ **Day 4**	Date _____ **Day 5**
Diet	Diet as tolerated, providing small, frequent, nutritious feedings Encourage fluid intake of 3000 mL/day unless contraindicated	Diet as tolerated, providing small, frequent, nutritious feedings Encourage fluid intake of 3000 mL/day unless contraindicated
Activity	Activity as ordered Maintain safety precautions	Activity as ordered
Medications	IV antibiotics as ordered Tylenol 650 mg q4hr po for temp over 101F	IV antibiotics as ordered Tylenol 650 mg q4hr po for temp over 101F
Transfer/ discharge plans	Continue to review progress toward discharge goals Finalize discharge plans	Finalize plans for home care if needed Make any appropriate referrals Complete discharge teaching

Potential Client Variances
Osteomyelitis

Possible complications
- Systemic infection/sepsis
- Vascular insufficiency
- Amputation
- Pathological fractures

Health Conditions
- Immunosuppression
- Peripheral vascular disease
- Pre-existing renal disease
- Diabetes

Nursing Diagnoses
- Pain
- Ineffective management of therapeutic regimen
- Self-care deficits
- Risk for injury
- Impaired physical mobility

Discharge Teaching for Client Following
Osteomyelitis

Activity

- Avoid activities that would result in unnecessary stretching, pulling, or injury to the area of infection and/or wound, or soiling of the dressing or wound.
- Return to work only as advised by your physician.

Diet

- Eat a well-balanced diet, including all food groups.
- Drink 6–8 glasses of fluid each day.

Signs and Symptoms to Report

Notify physician if any of these symptoms occur:
- Chills, or fever greater than 100F or 38C
- Decreased motion in the affected area.
- Worsening pain or discomfort in the affected area.
- Increase in drainage, swelling, or tenderness, or foul-smelling drainage.

Follow-Up Care and General Health Care

- Schedule follow-up appointment with physician as directed.
- Maintain schedule for follow-up laboratory work and/or audiograms.
- Check with your physician if you have any problems or questions.

Medications

- Review written list of medications, including dose, route, frequency, food interactions, and side effects.
- Review the importance of long-term antibiotic therapy to prevent recurrence or extension of the infection.
- Review instructions for IV administration of medications at home if ordered.

Wound and Dressing Care

- Perform wound care as directed.
- Keep dressing dry and clean.
- If there is a marked increase in drainage, swelling, tenderness, fever, or if drainage is foul-smelling, notify physician.

Critical Pathway for Client with

Pneumonia

Expected length of stay: 5 days

	Date _____ **Day 1**	Date _____ **Day 2**	Date _____ **Day 3**
Daily outcomes	Client will: • have stabilizing vital signs • verbalize understanding and demonstrate cooperation with turning and splinting • cough and deep breathe purposefully q1–2hr during day • have a productive cough • have an intake of 3000 mL/day (IV/po) unless contraindicated • verbalize ability to cope	Client will: • have stable vital signs and un-labored respirations at rest • verbalize understanding and demonstrate cooperation with turning and splinting • cough and deep breathe purposefully q1–2hr during day • have a productive cough • have an intake of 3000 mL/day (IV/po) unless contraindicated • verbalize ability to cope	Client will: • be afebrile, have stable vital signs and unlabored respirations with activity • verbalize understanding and demonstrate cooperation with turning and splinting • cough and deep breathe purposefully q1–2hr during day • have a productive cough • have an oral intake of 3000 mL/day unless contraindicated • verbalize ability to cope • verbalize beginning understanding of home care instructions
Assessments, tests, and treatments	CBC with differential PA and lateral chest x-ray ABGs Blood culture × 2, if temp over 101F Sputum for gram stain and C & S Vital signs and O_2 saturation, q4hr and prn Assess respiratory status q4hr and prn Incentive spirometer q2hr Nebulizer therapy q4hr Chest physical therapy Intake and output every shift Assess respirations and respiratory movements q4hr and prn Encourage coughing and deep breathing q1–2hr Demonstrate effective coughing while splinting client's chest Position client in semi-Fowler's or high Fowler's position Assist with postural drainage 3 times daily Assist with nebulizer treatments Oxygen as ordered to maintain O_2 saturation >95% Assist with ADLs Monitor arterial blood gases/pulse oximeter	Vital signs and O_2 saturation, q4hr and prn Assess respiratory status q4hr and prn Incentive spirometer q2hr Intake and output every shift Assess respirations and respiratory movements q4hr and prn Nebulizer therapy q4hr Chest physical therapy Encourage coughing and deep breathing q1–2hr Demonstrate effective coughing while splinting client's chest Position client in semi-Fowler's or high Fowler's position Assist with postural drainage 3 times daily Assist with nebulizer treatments Oxygen as ordered to maintain O_2 saturation >95% Assist with ADLs	Vital signs and O_2 saturation, q4hr and prn Assess respiratory status q4hr and prn Incentive spirometer q2hr Intake and output every shift Assess respirations and respiratory movements q4hr and prn Nebulizer therapy q4hr Chest physical therapy Encourage coughing and deep breathing q1–2hr Position client in semi-Fowler's or high Fowler's position Assist with postural drainage 3 times daily Assist with nebulizer treatments Oxygen to maintain pulse oximeter > 95% Assist with ADLs Check culture and sensitivities

Pneumonia *(continued)*

	Date _____ **Day 1**	Date _____ **Day 2**	Date _____ **Day 3**
Knowledge deficit	Orient to room and hospital routine Review plan of care and importance of increased fluids, activity, turning, coughing, deep breathing, and incentive spirometer Include family in teaching Evaluate understanding of teaching	Review plan of care and continued importance of increased fluids, activity, turning, coughing, deep breathing, and incentive spirometer Include family in teaching Evaluate understanding of teaching	Reinforce earlier teaching regarding ongoing care Begin discharge teaching regarding rest, activity, and diet Include family in teaching Evaluate understanding of teaching
Psychosocial	Assess level of anxiety Encourage verbalization of concerns Provide information and ongoing support and encouragement to client and family	Assess level of anxiety Encourage verbalization of concerns Provide information and ongoing support and encouragement to client and family	Encourage verbalization of concerns Provide ongoing support and encouragement to client and family
Diet	Diet as tolerated providing small, frequent, nutritious feedings Encourage fluid intake of 2000 mL/day unless contraindicated	Diet as tolerated providing small, frequent, nutritious feedings Encourage fluid intake of 2000–3000 mL/day unless contraindicated	Diet as tolerated providing small, frequent, nutritious feedings Encourage fluid intake of 2000–3000 mL/day unless contraindicated
Activity	Assess safety needs and provide appropriate precautions Bathroom privileges with assistance Assist with ADLs Provide rest periods	Maintain safety precautions Bathroom privileges with assistance Assist with ADLs Ambulate in room with assistance Provide rest periods	Maintain safety precautions Ambulate 4 times with assistance Assist with ADLs Provide rest periods
Medications	IV fluids IV antibiotics as ordered Bronchodilators as ordered Tylenol 650 mg q4hr po for temp over 101F	IV fluids/intermittent IV device IV antibiotics as ordered Bronchodilators as ordered Tylenol 650 mg q4hr po for temp over 101F	Intermittent IV device: D/C if IV antibiotics D/C Antibiotics as ordered Bronchodilators as ordered Tylenol 650 mg q4hr po for temp over 101F
Transfer/ discharge plans	Establish discharge goals with client and family Consult with social service regarding VNA projected needs for home health care (if any)	Review progress toward discharge goals with client and family Identify potential referrals	Review progress toward discharge goals with client and family

Pneumonia *(continued)*

	Date _____ **Day 4**	Date _____ **Day 5**
Daily outcomes	Client will: • be afebrile, with stable vital signs and unlabored respirations with activity • verbalize understanding and demonstrate cooperation with turning and splinting • cough and deep breathe purposefully q1–2hr during day • have an oral intake of 3000 mL/day unless contraindicated • verbalize ability to cope • verbalize understanding of home care instructions	Client is afebrile and has stable vital signs Client has unlabored respirations and lungs clear to auscultation Client is independent in self-care Client is fully ambulatory Client has resumed preadmission urine and bowel elimination pattern Client verbalizes/demonstrates home care instructions Client tolerates usual diet and has an oral intake of 3000 mL/day unless contraindicated Client verbalizes ability to cope with ongoing stressors
Assessments, tests, and treatments	Vital signs and O_2 saturation, q4hr and prn Assess respiratory status q4hr and prn Incentive spirometer q2hr Intake and output every shift Assess respirations and respiratory movements q4hr and prn Nebulizer therapy q4hr Chest physical therapy Encourage coughing and deep breathing q1–2hr while awake Assist with postural drainage 3 times daily Assist with nebulizer treatments D/C oxygen if O_2 saturation 98% on room air	Vital signs and O_2 saturation, q4hr and prn Assess respiratory status q4hr and prn Incentive spirometer q2hr Intake and output every shift Assess respirations and respiratory movements q4hr and prn Nebulizer therapy q4hr Chest physical therapy Encourage coughing and deep breathing q1–2hr while awake
Knowledge deficit	Reinforce earlier teaching regarding ongoing care Review written discharge instructions with client and family Include family in teaching Evaluate understanding of teaching	Reinforce earlier teaching regarding ongoing care Complete discharge teaching to include diet, follow-up care, signs and symptoms to report, follow-up MD visit, activity, and medications: name, purpose, dose, frequency, route, dietary interactions, and side effects Provide client with written discharge instructions Include family in teaching Evaluate understanding of teaching

➤

Pneumonia *(continued)*

	Date _____ **Day 4**	Date _____ **Day 5**
Psychosocial	Encourage verbalization of concerns Provide ongoing support and encouragement to client and family	Encourage verbalization of concerns Provide ongoing support and encouragement to client and family
Diet	Diet as tolerated, providing small, frequent, nutritious feedings Encourage fluid intake of 3000 mL/day unless contraindicated	Diet as tolerated, providing small, frequent, nutritious feedings Encourage fluid intake of 3000 mL/day unless contraindicated
Activity	Ambulate independently at least 4 times Maintain safety precautions	Fully ambulatory
Medications	Antibiotics as ordered Bronchodilators as ordered Tylenol 650 mg q4hr po for temp over 101F	Antibiotics as ordered Bronchodilators as ordered Tylenol 650 mg q4hr po for temp over 101F
Transfer/ discharge plans	Continue to review progress toward discharge goals Finalize discharge plans	Finalize plans for home care if needed Make any appropriate referrals Complete discharge teaching

Potential Client Variances
Pneumonia

Possible complications

- Pleural effusion
- Systemic infection

Health Conditions

- Pre-existing respiratory conditions
- Chronic obstructive pulmonary disease (COPD)
- Smoker

Nursing Diagnoses

- Activity intolerance
- Ineffective breathing pattern
- Sleep pattern disturbance
- Ineffective management of therapeutic regimen

Discharge Teaching for Client Following
Pneumonia

Activity
- Gradually return to usual level of activity by increasing activity each day. Alternate activity with rest periods. Avoid fatigue.
- No strenuous activity or return to work until okayed by physician.
- Avoid heavy housework or straining for the period designated by your physician.

Diet
- Follow usual and customary diet. Drink plenty of fluids and eat a well-balanced diet including fruits, meat, vegetables, bread and starches, and milk products.

Signs and Symptoms to Report
Notify physician if any of these symptoms occur:
- Shortness of breath, difficulty breathing
- Chills, or fever greater than 100F or 38C

Follow-Up Care and General Health Care
- Schedule follow-up appointment with physician as directed.
- Avoid individuals with respiratory infections.
- Cover your mouth and turn your head away from others when you cough.
- Dispose of your tissues in a paper or plastic trash bag.
- Avoid cigarette smoke, dust, fumes, and sprays.

Medications
- Review written list of medications including dose, frequency, food interactions, and side effects.
- Avoid over-the-counter medications unless recommended by physician.
- Ask your physician about flu and pneumonia vaccines.

Sickle Cell Crisis

Expected length of stay: 6–8 days

	Date _____ **Day 1**	Date _____ **Day 2**	Date _____ **Days 3–4**
Daily outcomes	Client will: • have stable vital signs • have an intake of 3000 mL/day unless contraindicated • remain free of nausea and vomiting • verbalize understanding of ongoing care • verbalize control of pain and understanding of pain relief measures • demonstrate ability to cope with current hospitalization • have intact skin • maintain urine output >30 mL/hr	Client will: • have stable vital signs • have an intake of 3000 mL/day unless contraindicated • remain free of nausea and vomiting • verbalize understanding of ongoing care • verbalize control of pain and understanding of pain relief measures • demonstrate ability to cope with current hospitalization • have intact skin • maintain urine output >30 mL/hr	Client will: • have stable vital signs • have an intake of 3000 mL/day unless contraindicated • verbalize understanding of ongoing care • verbalize control of pain and understanding of pain relief measures • demonstrate ability to cope with current hospitalization • verbalize ability to cope with chronic illness • verbalize/demonstrate beginning understanding of home care instructions • have intact skin • maintain urine output >30 mL/hr
Assessments, tests, and treatments	CBC with differential Chemistry profile Urinalysis Folic acid Reticulocyte count Chest x-ray Vital signs q4hr if stable Intake and output every shift Assess pallor, fatigue, and dyspnea on exertion Assess pain—location, type, and severity Oxygen to maintain O_2 saturation > 95% Transfuse as ordered Pulse oximeter q4hr and prn Provide quiet, restful environment with dimmed lights Protect from exposure to infection Pain management techniques, including massage, heat, relaxation, and guided imagery	Vital signs q4hr and prn Intake and output every shift Oxygen to maintain O_2 saturation > 95% Pulse oximeter q4hr and prn Assess pallor, fatigue, and dyspnea Assess pain—location, type, and severity Provide quiet, restful environment with dimmed lights Protect from exposure to infection Pain management techniques, including massage, heat, relaxation, and guided imagery	CBC Routine vital signs Intake and output every shift Oxygen to maintain O_2 saturation > 95% Pulse oximeter q4hr and prn Assess pallor, fatigue, and dyspnea Assess pain—location, type, and severity Transfuse as ordered Provide quiet, restful environment with dimmed lights Protect from exposure to infection Pain management techniques, including massage, heat, relaxation, and guided imagery

Sickle Cell Crisis *(continued)*

	Date _____ **Day 1**	Date _____ **Day 2**	Date _____ **Days 3–4**
Knowledge deficit	Orient to room and hospital routine Review plan of care Include family in teaching Evaluate understanding of teaching	Review plan of care Include family in teaching Evaluate understanding of teaching	Reinforce earlier teaching regarding ongoing care Begin discharge teaching regarding rest, activity, and diet Include family in teaching Evaluate understanding of teaching
Psychosocial	Assess level of anxiety Encourage verbalization of concerns Provide ongoing support and encouragement	Assess level of anxiety Encourage verbalization of concerns Provide ongoing support and encouragement	Encourage verbalization of concerns Provide ongoing support and encouragement
Diet	Regular diet—encourage foods high in folic acid, iron, protein, minerals, and vitamins Offer oral fluids q1hr	Regular diet—encourage foods high in folic acid, iron, protein, minerals, and vitamins Offer oral fluids q1hr	Regular diet—encourage foods high in folic acid, iron, protein, minerals, and vitamins Offer oral fluids q1hr
Activity	Assess safety needs and provide appropriate precautions Activity to tolerance, encouraging change of position Provide rest periods Encourage ROM to unaffected joints	Maintain safety precautions Activity to tolerance, encouraging change of position Provide rest periods Encourage ROM to unaffected joints	Maintain safety precautions Up ad lib to tolerance Encourage rest periods Encourage ROM to unaffected joints
Medications	IV fluids as ordered IV antibiotics as ordered Folic acid 1 mg po QD Colace 100 mg BID Motrin or Toradol as ordered Narcotic analgesic via PCA q15 minute bolus × 24 hr Antipyretics as ordered	IV fluids as ordered IV antibiotics as ordered Folic acid 1 mg po QD Colace 100 mg BID Motrin or Toradol as ordered Narcotic analgesic via PCA q20 minute bolus × 24 hr Antipyretics as ordered	IV fluids as ordered IV antibiotics as ordered Folic acid 1 mg po QD Colace 100 mg BID Motrin or Toradol as ordered Narcotic analgesic via PCA q30–60 minute bolus × 24 hr Antipyretics as ordered
Transfer/ discharge plans	Establish discharge goals with client and family Consult with social service regarding VNA and projected needs for home health care (if any)	Review progress toward discharge goals with client and family	Review progress toward discharge goals with client and family Make appropriate referrals

Sickle Cell Crisis *(continued)*

	Date _____ **Day 5**	Date _____ **Day 6**	Date _____ **Days 7–8**
Daily outcomes	Client will: • have stable vital signs • have an intake of 3000 mL/day unless contraindicated • verbalize understanding of ongoing care • demonstrate ability to cope with current hospitalization and chronic nature of illness • verbalize/demonstrate beginning understanding of home care instructions • have intact skin • maintain urine output >30 mL/hr	Client will: • have stable vital signs • have an intake of 3000 mL/day unless contraindicated • verbalize understanding of ongoing care • demonstrate ability to cope with current hospitalization and chronic nature of illness • verbalize/demonstrate beginning understanding of home care instructions • have intact skin • maintain urine output >30 mL/hr • verbalize willingness to follow treatment plan • verbalize understanding of precipitating factors	Client is afebrile and has stable vital signs Client is independent in self-care Client is fully ambulatory Client has resumed preadmission urine and bowel elimination pattern Client verbalizes/demonstrates home care instructions Client tolerates ordered diet and has an intake of 3000 mL/day Client demonstrates ability to cope with ongoing stressors Client has intact skin Client maintains urine output >30 mL/hr Client identifies support system Client verbalizes understanding of precipitating factors and plans to follow recommendations to prevent future episodes of sickle cell crisis
Assessments, tests, and treatments	CBC Routine vital signs Intake and output Assess pallor, fatigue, and dyspnea Assess pain—location, type, and severity Oxygen therapy until O_2 saturation >95% on room air Provide quiet, restful environment with dimmed lights Protect from exposure to infection Pain management techniques including massage, heat, relaxation, and guided imagery	Routine vital signs Intake and output Assess pallor, fatigue, and dyspnea Assess pain—location, type and severity Oxygen therapy until O_2 saturation >95% on room air Provide quiet, restful environment with dimmed lights Protect from exposure to infection Pain management techniques including massage, heat, relaxation, and guided imagery	CBC Routine vital signs Protect from exposure to infection Pain management techniques including massage, heat, relaxation, and guided imagery

	Date _____ **Day 5**	Date _____ **Day 6**	Date _____ **Days 7–8**
Knowledge deficit	Reinforce earlier teaching regarding ongoing care Review written discharge instructions with client and significant other including signs and symptoms requiring follow-up Review the importance of avoiding infections, strenuous activity, stress, smoking, inadequate hydration, and cold exposure Discuss need to eat 3 to 4 regularly scheduled meals Include family in teaching Evaluate understanding of teaching	Reinforce earlier teaching regarding ongoing care Include family in teaching Provide client with written discharge instructions Evaluate understanding of teaching	Reinforce earlier teaching regarding ongoing care Complete discharge teaching to include diet, follow-up care, signs and symptoms to report, activity, and medications: name, purpose, dose, frequency, route, food interactions, and side effects Include family in teaching Provide client with written discharge instructions Evaluate understanding of teaching
Psychosocial	Encourage verbalization of concerns Provide ongoing support and encouragement	Encourage verbalization of concerns Provide ongoing support and encouragement	Encourage verbalization of concerns Provide ongoing support and encouragement
Diet	Regular diet—encourage foods high in folic acid, iron, protein, minerals, and vitamins Encourage fluid intake of 3000 mL/day unless contraindicated	Regular diet—encourage foods high in folic acid, iron, protein, minerals, and vitamins Encourage fluid intake of 3000 mL/day unless contraindicated	Regular diet—encourage foods high in folic acid, iron, protein, minerals, and vitamins Encourage fluid intake of 3000 mL/day unless contraindicated
Activity	Self-care Fully ambulatory	Self-care Fully ambulatory	Self-care Fully ambulatory
Medications	D/C IV if oral intake >2000 mL/day Folic acid 1 mg po QD Colace 100 mg BID Motrin or Toradol as ordered Oral antibiotic as ordered Narcotic analgesic via PCA—no bolus Begin oral analgesic	Folic acid 1 mg po QD Colace 100 mg BID Motrin or Toradol as ordered Oral antibiotic as ordered Taper narcotic analgesic via PCA—no bolus Continue oral analgesic	Folic acid 1 mg po QD Colace 100 mg BID Motrin or Toradol as ordered Oral antibiotic as ordered D/C PCA Oral analgesics
Transfer/ discharge plans	Continue to review progress toward discharge goals Finalize discharge plans	Finalize plans for home care if needed Complete discharge teaching Discuss referral to support group	Finalize plans for home care if needed Complete discharge teaching

Potential Client Variances
Sickle Cell Crisis

Possible Complications

- Uncontrolled pain
- Neurovascular compromise
- Osteomyelitis
- Hemiplegia
- Dysrhythmias
- Heart failure

Health Conditions

- Undernutrition
- Dehydration
- Infectious disease(s)
- Hypothermia
- Smoker
- Physical/psychologic stressors

Nursing Diagnoses

- Acute pain
- Ineffective individual coping
- Impaired physical mobility
- Impaired skin integrity

Discharge Teaching for Client Following
Sickle Cell Crisis

Activity

- Gradually return to usual level of activity by increasing activity each day. Alternate activity with rest periods. Avoid fatigue.
- Avoid strenous activity.

Diet

- Eat a well-balanced diet that includes all food groups. Be sure to include foods high in folic acid, iron, protein, minerals, and vitamins.
- Drink at least 10–12 glasses of fluid each day.

Signs and Symptoms to Report

Notify physician if any of these symptoms occur:
- Increase in pain
- Difficulty breathing or shortness of breath
- Chills, or fever greater than 100F or 38C

Follow-Up Care and General Health Care

- Schedule follow-up appointment with physician as directed.
- Avoid individuals with infections.
- Manage stress.
- No smoking.
- Avoid second-hand smoke.
- Consider support group.
- Avoid cold exposure.

Medications

- Review written list of medications, including dose, route, frequency, food interactions, and side effects.
- Avoid alcohol if taking medication.

Weight Loss Program

Expected length of treatment: 1 week for each 1/2 to 1 pound weight loss, then maintenance for life

	Initial visit and initiation of weight loss program	Ongoing weekly visits	Maintenance program when weight goal achieved
Outcomes	Client verbalizes commitment to regular exercise program Client verbalizes understanding of dietary plan and behavior modification strategies to change eating habits Client verbalizes feelings regarding weight	Client maintains exercise diary and exercises aerobically at least 30 minutes every other day Client maintains diet diary and discusses strategies to reshape eating habits Client loses up to 1 pound each week Blood pressure remains in normal range	Client continues aerobic exercise at least 30 minutes every other day Client maintains a low-calorie, low-fat diet Client's weight remains stable, within a 5-pound range
Assessments, tests, and treatments	Height and weight Blood pressure Bioelectrical impedance and skin fold Thyroid profile Serum glucose, lipid profile Electrocardiogram	Weight Blood pressure Review laboratory results and any required therapies and goals of weight loss	Monthly weights and blood pressures by office nurse Follow-up laboratory testing based on any previously detected abnormalities
Psychosocial	Encourage to verbalize feelings regarding weight Set small, achievable goals Discuss cues to eating Explore the possibility of psychologic counseling	Continue encouraging client to discuss feelings regarding weight Continue to identify strategies to eliminate or reduce eating cues Discuss feelings regarding weight loss and changes in self-concept Discuss availability of support systems in weight loss efforts	Client continues use of identified strategies for behavior modification Client receives continued assistance from support persons
Diet	Calculate calorie needs Instruct in low-calorie, low-fat diet Stress the importance of a well-balanced diet Instruct to maintain diet diary	Assess ability to adhere to low-calorie, low-fat diet and any problems incurred since modifying diet Assess diet diary for compliance and discuss related problems Continue strategizing meals and food selection	Client continues low-calorie, low-fat diet Client manages social situations by making low-calorie, low-fat choices Client fully integrates behavior modification strategies into daily life

	Initial visit and initiation of weight loss program	Ongoing weekly visits	Maintenance program when weight goal achieved
Activity/Exercise	Discuss current and past exercise patterns Explore aerobic exercise interests Establish contract with client that delineates a regular exercise program, such as walking 30 minutes every other day	Review the importance of regular aerobic exercise and its relationship to weight loss and control Encourage client to maintain exercise diary considering intensity and duration Explore ways to increase overall level of activity (such as stair-walking, parking further away from the store, etc)	Client continues aerobic exercise 30 minutes every other day Client increases duration and intensity of exercise when calorie or fat intake is higher than usual Client fully integrates increased activity into daily life

Potential Client Variances
Weight Loss Program

Possible Complications

- Anorexia
- Electrolyte disturbances
- Bulimia

Health Conditions

- Gall bladder disease
- Activity intolerance

Nursing Diagnoses

- Self-concept disturbance
- Ineffective management of therapeutic regimen
- Altered nutrition: Less than body requirements

Discharge Teaching for Client in
Weight Loss Program

Activity

- Include 30 minutes of aerobic exercise at least 5 days a week.

Diet

- Follow low-fat, low-calorie diet as instructed.
- Maintain diet diary, recording time of eating, foods eaten, mood, and feelings.
- Drink 8–10 glasses of fluid each day.

Follow-up Care and General Health Care

- Schedule follow-up appointment with physician as directed.

Medications

- Review written list of medications, including dose, route, frequency, food interactions, and side effects.

Wound Management at Home

Expected length of treatment: 7–10 days

	Date _____ **Outpatient Setting**	Date _____ **Daily for 10 Days** **(Client activities)**
Daily outcomes	Client verbalizes understanding of teaching, including wound care, signs and symptoms to report, and follow-up care	At time of suture removal: Client is afebrile Client has a dry, clean wound with edges well-approximated, healing by first intention
Knowledge deficit	Provide simple, brief instructions regarding injury and treatment Encourage client to ask questions and seek assistance Assess the client's knowledge about wound care Review written instruction sheet for wound care with client and provide copy Evaluate understanding of teaching	Follow written discharge teaching regarding wound care/dressing change Call physician with questions/problems Return to office in 10 days for suture removal
Diet	Instruct client about foods high in protein and vitamin C and encourage adequate intake	Diet high in protein and vitamin C Cultural remedies that will not interfere with healing
Wound care	Irrigate and cleanse wound with normal saline and peroxide Surgical consultation for wound closure Following wound closure, apply dry sterile dressing	Change dressing daily and prn to keep dressing dry and clean Inspect wound daily and report any signs and symptoms of infection (redness, pain, warmth, drainage or fever)
Medications	Tetanus toxoid if indicated	Only if ordered

Potential Client Variances
Wound Management at Home

Possible Complications

- Infection local/systemic

Health Conditions

- Diabetes
- Steroid dependency

Nursing Diagnoses

- Risk for infection
- Risk for injury

Wound Management at Home

Activity

- Return to usual level of activity. Avoid activities that would result in unnecessary stretching or pulling in the area of the wound or soiling of the dressing or wound.
- Return to work as designated by your physician.

Diet

- Eat a well-balanced diet, including all food groups.
- Drink 6–8 glasses of fluid each day.

Signs and Symptoms to Report

Notify physician if any of these symptoms occur:
- Chills, or fever greater than 100F or 38C
- Increase in pain, redness, or swelling
- Increase in wound drainage, especially if drainage has pus or a foul odor

Follow-Up Care and General Health Care

- Schedule follow-up appointment with your physician as directed.
- Check with your physician if you have any problems or questions.

Medications

- Review written list of medications including dose, route, frequency, food interactions, and side effects.

Wound and Dressing Care

- Cleanse skin around wound daily with mild soap and water.
- Change dressing daily and as often as necessary to keep dressing dry and clean.
- Remove dressing prior to showering and replace with a clean dressing afterward.
- Drainage, if present, should gradually decrease.
- If there is a marked increase in drainage, swelling, tenderness, fever, or if drainage is foul-smelling, notify physician.

Surgical Pathways

Abdominal Aortic Aneurysm Repair   89

Appendectomy   95

Arm Fracture (Upper) with Open Reduction   99

Carotid Endarectomy   103

Cataract Surgery   108

Cholecystectomy (Laparoscopic)   111

Colon Resection   114

Coronary Angioplasty, Percutaneous Transluminal   120

Coronary Artery Bypass Surgery   123

Craniotomy for Brain Tumor   131

Cystectomy with Ileal Conduit   135

Femoral Popliteal Bypass Graft   141

Gastrectomy, Partial   146

Hernia Repair (Laparoscopic)   152

Hip Pinning (Fractured Hip with
Prosthesis or Internal Fixation)   155

Hip Replacement (Total)   163

Hysterectomy (Abdominal)   168

Hysterectomy (Vaginal)   172

Knee Replacement (Total)   176

Laminectomy (Lumbar)   182

Laryngectomy   186

Lower Leg Fracture (Open Reduction and Internal Fixation)   194

Mastectomy 198

Microdiskectomy 202

Nephrectomy 205

Permanent Pacemaker Insertion 211

Proctocolectomy with Permanent Ileostomy (Total) 215

Splenectomy 222

Thyroidectomy 227

Transurethral Resection of the Prostate 230

Abdominal Aortic Aneurysm Repair

Expected length of stay: 6–7 days

	Date _____ **Preoperative**	Date _____ **1st 24 Hours Postoperative**	Date _____ **2nd–3rd Days Postoperative**
Daily outcomes	Client verbalizes understanding of preoperative teaching, including: turning, coughing, deep breathing, incentive spirometer, mobilization, possible tubes (nasogastric tube, IV, Foley catheter, penrose or other drains), and pain management Client demonstrates ability to cope Client verbalizes understanding of procedure Obtain informed consent	Client will: • have stable vital signs • have adequate CSMs • have a clean, dry wound with edges well-approximated, healing by first intention • recover from anesthesia as evidenced by VS return to baseline, and being awake, alert, and oriented • verbalize understanding and demonstrate cooperation with turning, coughing, deep breathing and splinting • lungs clear to auscultation • maintain urine output >30 mL/hr • demonstrate ability to use PCA if in use • verbalize control of incisional pain with epidural, PCA, or ordered medications • transfer out of bed with assistance 2–3 times • demonstrate ability to cope	Client will: • be afebrile and have stable vital signs • have adequate CSMs • remain alert and oriented • have a clean, dry wound with edges well-approximated, healing by first intention • have active bowel sounds • tolerate ordered diet without vomiting • demonstrate cooperation with turning, coughing, deep breathing, and splinting • have lungs clear to auscultation • maintain urine output >30 mL/hr • ambulate 4 times • verbalize control of incisional pain • verbalize ability to cope • verbalize beginning understanding of home care instructions
Assessments, tests, and treatments	CBC Urinalysis Chest x-ray Flat plate of the abdomen Abdominal ultrasound CT of abdomen Baseline physical assessment with a focus on respiratory status and gastrointestinal function Assess and record the description, location, duration, and characteristics of client's pain Reduce or eliminate pain-producing factors such as fear and anxiety	CBC Electrolytes Vital signs and O_2 saturation, neurovascular assessment, CSMs, dressing and wound drainage assessment q15min × 4; q30min × 4; q1hr × 4 and then q4hr and prn Assess respiratory status and gastrointestinal function q4hr and prn Incentive spirometer q1–2hr Intake and output every shift Assess patency of NG tube q2hr, noting volume q4–8hr	Vital signs and dressing and wound drainage assessment q4hr and prn Assess neurovascular status and CSMs q2–4hr and prn Assess respiratory status and gastrointestinal function q4hr Incentive spirometer q2hr until fully ambulatory O_2 as indicated Intake and output every shift If still in place, assess patency and output of NG tube q4–8hr Assess voiding pattern every shift Using sterile asepsis change dressing, assess wound healing and wound drainage

➤

Abdominal Aortic Aneurysm Repair *(continued)*

	Date _____ **Preoperative**	Date _____ **1st 24 Hours Postoperative**	Date _____ **2nd–3rd Days Postoperative**
Assessments, tests, and treatments (continued)		Assess Foley catheter or voiding—if unable to void, try suggestive voiding techniques or catheterize q8hr or prn Assess and record the description, location, duration, and characteristics of client's pain q2–4hr and prn Encourage verbalization of pain and discomfort Reduce or eliminate pain-producing factors and employ distraction or relaxation techniques Provide back rubs Encourage client to request analgesic or use PCA before pain becomes severe	Assess and record the description, location, duration, and characteristics of client's pain q4hr and prn Reduce or eliminate pain-producing factors, employ distraction or relaxation techniques, and offer back rubs
Knowledge deficit	Orient to room and surroundings Provide simple, brief instructions Review preoperative preparation including hospital and surgical routines, and possibility of ICU post-operatively Include family in teaching Discuss surgery and specific postoperative care: turning, coughing, deep breathing, splinting incision, incentive spirometer, mobilization, possible tubes (nasogastric [NG] and intravenous [IV]), and pain management (PCA, epidural, or prn medications) Instruct regarding distraction techniques, such as slow rhythmic breathing and guided imagery, to produce pain relief Instruct in relaxation techniques, such as tensing and relaxing muscle groups and rhythmic breathing Evaluate understanding of teaching	Reorient to room and postoperative routine Include family in teaching Review plan of care and importance of early mobilization Review importance of turning, coughing, deep breathing, splinting incision, incentive spirometer, mobilization, drainage tubes (Foley catheter and intravenous), and pain management (PCA, epidural, or prn medications) Evaluate understanding of teaching	Reinforce earlier teaching regarding ongoing care Include family in teaching Begin discharge teaching regarding wound care/dressing change and activity Evaluate understanding of teaching

	Date ___ **Preoperative**	Date ___ **1st 24 Hours Postoperative**	Date ___ **2nd–3rd Days Postoperative**
Psychosocial	Assess anxiety related to diagnosis and pending surgery Assess fears of the unknown related to surgery Encourage verbalization of concerns Minimize external stimuli (eg, noise, movement)	Assess level of anxiety Encourage verbalization of concerns Provide information and ongoing support and encouragement to client and family	Assess level of anxiety Encourage verbalization of concerns Provide ongoing support and encouragement
Diet	NPO Baseline nutritional and hydration assessment	NPO NG tube until return of bowel sounds	When NG tube removed, begin clear liquids to tolerance
Activity	Assess safety needs and provide appropriate measures Activity as ordered	Maintain safety precautions Assist to chair 2–3 times	Maintain safety precautions Ambulate 4 times with assistance
Medications	Preoperative medications as ordered	IV fluids Antihypertensives as ordered Analgesics as ordered	IV fluids Antihypertensives as ordered Analgesics as ordered With return of bowel sounds, start Colace 100 mg BID prn
Transfer/ discharge plans	Assess discharge plans and support system Establish discharge goals with client and family	Review progress toward discharge goals with client and family Consult with social service regarding VNA and projected needs for home health care (if any)	Review progress toward discharge goals with client and family Make appropriate discharge referrals

	Date ___ **4th Day Postoperative**	Date ___ **5th Day Postoperative**	Date ___ **6th–7th Days Postoperative**
Daily outcomes	Client will: • be afebrile and have stable vital signs • have adequate CSMs • have a clean, dry wound with edges well-approximated, healing by first intention • tolerate ordered diet without nausea or vomiting • ambulate 4–6 times • verbalize control of incisional pain	Client will: • be afebrile and have stable vital signs • have adequate CSMs • have a clean, dry wound with edges well-approximated, healing by first intention • tolerate ordered diet without nausea or vomiting • ambulate 4–6 times • verbalize control of incisional pain	Client is afebrile and has stable vital signs Client has adequate CSMs Client has a dry, clean wound with edges well-approximated, healing by first intention Client manages pain with non-pharmacologic measures and any ordered oral medications Client is independent in self-care

	Date _____ **4th Day Postoperative**	Date _____ **5th Day Postoperative**	Date _____ **6th–7th Days Postoperative**
Daily outcomes (continued)	• have lungs clear to auscultation • have active bowel sounds • maintain urine output >30 mL/hr • verbalize ability to cope • verbalize beginning understanding of home care instructions	• have lungs clear to auscultation • have active bowel sounds and have a soft, formed bowel movement • maintain urine output >30 mL/hr • verbalize ability to cope • verbalize beginning understanding of home care instructions	Client is fully ambulatory Client has resumed preadmission urine and bowel elimination pattern Client verbalizes home care instructions Client tolerates usual diet Client verbalizes ability to cope with ongoing stressors
Assessments, tests, and treatments	Vital signs and dressing and wound drainage assessment q4hr and prn Assess neurovascular status and CSMs q4–8hr and prn Incentive spirometer q2hr until fully ambulatory O_2 if indicated Intake and output every shift Assess voiding pattern every shift Assess respiratory status and gastrointestinal function q4–8hr Using sterile asepsis, change dressing, assess wound healing and wound drainage Assess and record description, location, duration, and characteristics of client's pain q4hr and prn Encourage client to employ distraction or relaxation techniques	Vital signs and dressing and wound drainage assessment q4hr and prn Assess neurovascular status and CSMs q8hr and prn Assess respiratory status and gastrointestinal function q4–8hr Remove dressing and assess wound healing and drainage Assess and record description, location, duration, and characteristics of client's pain q4hr and prn Encourage client to employ distraction or relaxation techniques	Vital signs and dressing and wound drainage assessment q4–8hr Assess neurovascular status and CSMs q8hr Assess respiratory status and gastrointestinal function Assess wound healing Assess and record description, location, duration, and characteristics of client's pain q4hr and prn Encourage client to employ distraction or relaxation techniques
Knowledge deficit	Include family in teaching Initiate discharge teaching regarding wound care, diet, and activity Review written discharge instructions with client and family Evaluate understanding of teaching	Continue discharge teaching to client and family regarding wound care, diet, signs and symptoms to report, medications, and activity Review written discharge instructions with client and family Evaluate understanding of teaching	Complete discharge teaching to include wound care, diet, follow-up care, signs and symptoms to report, activity, and medications: name, purpose, dose, frequency, route, dietary interactions, and side effects Provide client with written discharge instructions Evaluate understanding of teaching
Psychosocial	Encourage verbalization of concerns Provide ongoing support and encouragement	Encourage verbalization of concerns Provide ongoing support and encouragement	Encourage verbalization of concerns Provide ongoing support and encouragement
Diet	If tolerating clear liquids, advance to full liquids as tolerated	Advance diet to soft, regular diet as tolerated	Regular diet as tolerated

	Date _____ **4th Day Postoperative**	Date _____ **5th Day Postoperative**	Date _____ **6th–7th Days Postoperative**
Activity	Ambulate independently at least 4 times Maintain safety precautions	Fully ambulatory Maintain safety precautions	Fully ambulatory
Medications	Analgesics as ordered Intermittent IV device for any IV medications—D/C when so ordered Colace 100 mg BID prn	Oral analgesics Colace 100 mg BID prn Laxative if no BM in 3 days	Oral analgesics
Transfer/ discharge plans	Continue to review progress toward discharge goals	Finalize discharge plans Continue to review progress toward discharge goals Finalize plans for home care if needed	Complete discharge instructions

Potential Client Variances
Abdominal Aortic Aneurysm Repair

Possible Complications
- Graft occlusion
- Arterial embolization — lower extremities
- Hemorrhage
- Bowel ischemia
- Renal ischemia

Health Conditions
- Diabetes
- Smoker
- Advanced peripheral vascular disease
- Clotting disorders
- Pre-existing respiratory or cardiac disorders
- Renal disorders

Nursing Diagnoses
- Acute pain
- Risk for impaired skin integrity
- Risk for injury
- Altered tissue perfusion

Discharge Teaching for Client Following
Abdominal Aortic Aneurysm Repair

Activity

- Gradually return to usual level of activity by increasing activity each day. Alternate activity with rest periods. Avoid fatigue.
- No sitting or standing for long periods.
- Do not cross your legs.
- No strenuous activity until okayed by physician.
- Avoid heavy housework, straining, lifting, sexual intercourse, strenuous activity, and driving for the period designated by your physician.

Diet

- Eat a well-balanced diet, including all food groups. Maintain any recommended dietary prescription.
- Drink 6–8 glasses of fluid each day.
- Eat food high in fiber such as fresh fruits and vegetables.

Signs and Symptoms to Report

Notify physician if any of these symptoms occur:
- Increase in pain, redness, or swelling
- Increase in wound drainage, especially if drainage has pus or a foul odor
- Chills, or fever greater than 100F or 38C
- Pain in your legs with or without numbness or tingling, calf pain when walking, cool feet or legs, pale or dusky-colored feet
- Worsening pain in abdomen, back, or groin
- Persistent diarrhea
- Impotence

Follow-Up Care and General Health Care

- Schedule follow-up appointment with physician as directed.
- Do not smoke and avoid second-hand smoke.
- Discuss alcohol use with your physician.
- Do not wear restrictive or tight clothing.

Medications

- Review written list of medications, including dose, frequency, food interactions, and side effects.

Wound and Dressing Care

- Cleanse skin around incision daily with mild soap and water.
- If you still need a dressing, change it daily and as often as necessary to keep dressing dry and clean.
- Remove dressing prior to showering and replace with a clean dressing afterward.
- Drainage, if present, should gradually decrease.
- If there is a marked increase in drainage, swelling, tenderness, fever, or if drainage is foul-smelling, notify physician.

Critical Pathway for Client Following
Appendectomy

Expected length of stay following surgery: 3 days

	Date _____ **Preoperative**	Date _____ **1st Day Postoperative**
Daily outcomes	Client verbalizes understanding of preoperative teaching including: turning, coughing, deep breathing, incentive spirometer, mobilization, possible tubes (nasogastric [NG] and intravenous [IV]), and pain management (PCA or prn medications) Client verbalizes ability to cope Client verbalizes understanding of procedure Obtain informed consent	Client will: • have stable vital signs • have clean, dry wound with edges well-approximated, healing by first intention • recover from anesthesia as evidenced by VS return to baseline, and being awake, alert, and oriented • verbalize understanding and demonstrate cooperation with turning, coughing, deep breathing, and splinting • tolerate ordered diet without nausea and vomiting • verbalize control of incisional pain • demonstrate ability to cope
Assessments, tests, and treatments	CBC Urinalysis Emergency surgery Baseline physical assessment with a focus on respiratory status and gastrointestinal function Assess hydration level Monitor intake and output	CBC Electrolytes if on NG suction Vital signs and O_2 saturation, neurovascular assessment, and dressing and wound drainage assessment q15min × 4; q30min × 4; q1hr × 4 and then q4hr and prn Assess respiratory status and gastrointestinal function q4hr and prn Incentive spirometer q2hr Intake and output every shift Assess voiding—if unable to void, try suggestive voiding techniques or catheterize q8hr or prn Change dressing daily and prn—monitor and record any drainage
Knowledge deficit	Orient to room and surroundings Provide simple, brief instructions Review preoperative preparation including hospital and surgical routines Include family in teaching Discuss surgery and specific postoperative care: turning, coughing, deep breathing, incentive spirometer, mobilization, possible tubes (nasogastric [NG] and intravenous [IV]), and pain management (PCA or prn medications) Evaluate understanding of teaching	Reorient to room and postoperative routine Include family in teaching Review plan of care and importance of early mobilization Begin discharge teaching regarding wound care and dressing care Evaluate understanding of teaching

Appendectomy *(continued)*

	Date _____ **Preoperative**	Date _____ **1st Day Postoperative**
Psychosocial	Assess anxiety related to diagnosis and pending surgery Assess fears of the unknown related to surgery Encourage verbalization of concerns Provide emotional support to client and family Minimize external stimuli (eg, noise, movement)	Assess level of anxiety Encourage verbalization of concerns Provide ongoing support and encouragement to client and family
Diet	NPO Baseline nutritional and fluid balance assessment	Advance to clear liquids if NG not ordered or discontinued
Activity	Assess safety needs and provide appropriate precautions Bed rest or bathroom privileges with assistance	Maintain safety precautions Bathroom privileges with assistance Ambulate 4 times with assistance
Medications	After diagnosis made: IM or IV analgesics Pre-op medications IV fluids IV antibiotics	Analgesics as ordered IV antibiotics IV fluid or intermittent IV device Antipyretics as ordered
Transfer/ discharge plans	Assess potential discharge needs and support system at home	Assess need for referral to appropriate home care agencies Begin home care teaching with client and/or family

	Date _____ **2nd Day Postoperative**	Date _____ **3rd Day Postoperative**
Daily outcomes	Client will: • have stable vital signs • have clean, dry wound with edges well-approximated, healing by first intention • demonstrate cooperation with turning, coughing, deep breathing, and splinting • tolerate ordered diet without nausea and vomiting • ambulate 4 times per day • verbalize control of incisional pain • demonstrate ability to cope • verbalize beginning understanding of home care instructions	Client is afebrile Client has a dry, clean wound with edges well-approximated, healing by first intention Client manages pain with non-pharmacologic measures and prn medication Client has resumed preadmission urine and bowel elimination patterns Client verbalizes home care instructions Client tolerates usual diet Client demonstrates ability to cope with ongoing stressors
Assessments, tests, and treatments	Vital signs and dressing and wound drainage assessment q4hr and prn Assess respiratory status and gastrointestinal function q4hr Incentive spirometer q2hr until fully ambulatory Intake and output every shift Assess voiding pattern every shift Change dressing daily and prn	WBC if ordered Vital signs and dressing and wound drainage assessment q4hr Assess respiratory status and gastrointestinal function

	Date _____ **2nd Day Postoperative**	Date _____ **3rd Day Postoperative**
Knowledge deficit	Continue discharge teaching regarding wound care, diet, and activity Review written discharge instructions Include family in teaching Evaluate understanding of teaching	Complete discharge teaching to include wound care, diet, follow-up care, signs and symptoms to report, activity, and medications: name, purpose, dose, frequency, route, food interactions, and side effects Provide client with written discharge instructions Include family in discharge teaching Evaluate client understanding of teaching
Psychosocial	Assess level of anxiety Encourage verbalization of concerns Provide ongoing support and encouragement to client and family	Encourage verbalization of concerns Provide ongoing support and encouragement
Diet	If tolerating clear liquids or NG removed, advance to full liquids/regular diet as tolerated	Regular diet as tolerated
Activity	Maintain safety precautions Ambulate independently at least 4 times	Fully ambulatory
Medications	Analgesics as ordered IV antibiotics Intermittent IV device Antipyretics as ordered	Oral analgesics Oral antibiotics if ordered D/C intermittent IV device
Transfer/ discharge plans	Complete discharge plans Continue home care instructions Make appropriate referrals	Complete discharge instructions Contact appropriate agency for follow-up care if indicated

Potential Client Variances
Appendectomy

Possible Complications
- Peritonitis
- Ileus

Health Conditions
- Respiratory problems
- Undernutrition

Nursing Diagnoses
- Risk for infection
- Acute pain

Discharge Teaching for Client Following
Appendectomy

Activity
- Gradually return to usual level of activity by increasing activity each day. Alternate activity with rest periods. Avoid fatigue.
- You may go up and down stairs.
- Avoid heavy housework, straining, heavy lifting, and driving for the period designated by your physician.

Diet
- Eat a well balanced diet, including all food groups.
- Report nausea, vomiting, or change in bowel habits.
- Drink 6–8 glasses of fluid each day.

Signs and Symptoms to Report
Notify physician if any of these symptoms occur:
- Increase in pain or any redness or swelling in wound
- Sudden increase in wound drainage, especially if drainage has pus or a foul odor
- Chills, or fever greater than 100F or 38C

Follow-Up Care and General Health Care
- Schedule follow-up appointment with physician as directed.

Medications
- Review written list of medications, including dose, route, frequency, food interactions, and side effects.
- Avoid alcohol if taking medication.

Wound and Dressing Care
- Cleanse skin around incision daily with mild soap and water.
- If you still need a dressing, change it daily and as often as necessary to keep dressing dry and clean.
- Remove dressing prior to showering and replace with a clean dressing afterward.
- Drainage, if present, should gradually decrease.
- If there is a marked increase in drainage, swelling, tenderness, fever, or if drainage is foul-smelling, notify physician.

Upper Arm Fracture with Open Reduction

Expected length of stay: 3–4 days following surgery

	Date _____ **1st 24 Hours Postoperative**	Date _____ **2nd Day Postoperative**
Daily outcomes	Client will: • have stable vital signs • recover from anesthesia as evidenced by VS return to baseline, and being awake, alert, and oriented, with clear lungs • verbalize understanding and demonstrate cooperation with turning, coughing, deep breathing, and prescribed activity level • state pain controlled with ordered medication • tolerate ordered diet without nausea and vomiting • verbalize ability to cope	Client will: • have stable vital signs, with clear lungs, and be alert and oriented • verbalize understanding and demonstrate cooperation with turning, coughing, deep breathing, and prescribed activity level • state pain controlled with ordered medication • tolerate ordered diet without nausea and vomiting • verbalize ability to cope
Assessments, tests, and treatments	Hct/Hgb Vital signs and O_2 saturation, neurovascular assessment and cast/dressing assessment q15min × 4; q30min × 4; q1hr × 4 and then q4hr and prn Head to toe assessment q4–8hr Incentive spirometer q2hr Intake and output every shift	Vital signs and O_2 saturation, neurovascular assessment and cast/dressing assessment q4hr and prn Head to toe assessment every shift and prn Incentive spirometer q2hr Intake and output every shift
Knowledge deficit	Orient to room and surroundings Provide simple, brief instructions Review plan of care and importance of specific postoperative care: turning, coughing, deep breathing, incentive spirometer, mobilization, possible tubes and intravenous, and pain management Include family in teaching Evaluate understanding of teaching	Review plan of care and importance of early mobilization Begin discharge teaching regarding cast/dressing care and mobility Include family in teaching Evaluate understanding of teaching
Psychosocial	Assess anxiety related to diagnosis and surgery Assess fears of the unknown related to surgery Encourage verbalization of concerns Minimize external stimuli (eg, noise, movement)	Assess level of anxiety Encourage verbalization of concerns Provide ongoing support and encouragement
Diet	Advance from clear liquids to full liquids as tolerated Baseline nutritional assessment	Advance from full liquids to regular diet as tolerated Offer supplemental feedings high in protein and vitamins Encourage fluids

➤

Upper Arm Fracture with Open Reduction *(continued)*

	Date _____ **1st 24 Hours Postoperative**	Date _____ **2nd Day Postoperative**
Activity	Assess safety needs and provide appropriate precautions Reposition q2hr and prn Assist client with full range of motion to all unaffected extremities 3 or 4 times daily Instruct client regarding isometric exercises for upper arm Encourage client to participate in activities of daily living as much as possible Keep extremity elevated	Maintain safety precautions Encourage client to participate in activities of daily living as much as possible Ambulate in room qid Sling for casted extremity when ambulatory, otherwise elevate extremity
Medications	Analgesics as ordered IV antibiotics IV fluids Antipyretics as ordered Tetanus toxoid if indicated	Analgesics as ordered IV antibiotics IV fluids or intermittent IV device Antipyretics as ordered
Transfer/ discharge plans	Assess potential discharge needs and support system	Determine needs for referrals at time of discharge Begin home care teaching

	Date _____ **3rd Day Postoperative**	Date _____ **4th–5th Days Postoperative**
Daily outcomes	Client will: • have stable vital signs and clear lungs • demonstrate cooperation with turning, coughing, deep breathing, and prescribed activity level • state pain controlled with ordered medication • tolerate ordered diet without nausea and vomiting • verbalize ability to cope • verbalize beginning understanding of home care instructions	Client is afebrile, with stable vital signs and clear lungs Client has intact neurovascular status to affected extremity Client manages pain with oral medications Client is independent in self-care Client is fully ambulatory Client has resumed preadmission urine and bowel elimination patterns Client verbalizes/demonstrates understanding of home care instructions Client tolerates usual diet Client verbalizes ability to cope with ongoing stressors
Assessments, tests, and treatments	Vital signs q4hr and prn Head to toe assessment every shift and prn Incentive spirometer q2hr until fully ambulatory Intake and output every shift Neurovascular and cast assessment q4hr and prn	Vital signs assessment q4hr Neurovascular and cast/dressing assessment q4hr and prn Head to toe assessment every shift Incentive spirometer q2hr until fully ambulatory D/C intake and output if taking adequate fluids and balanced with output

	Date _____ **3rd Day Postoperative**	Date _____ **4th–5th Days Postoperative**
Knowledge deficit	Initiate discharge teaching regarding diet, signs and symptoms to report, cast/dressing care, and activity level Review written discharge instructions Include family in teaching Evaluate understanding of teaching	Provide client with written discharge instructions that discuss: 1) signs and symptoms of infection related to internal fixation device, 2) importance of regular follow-up care, 3) care of cast/dressing, and 4) monitoring neurovascular status Complete discharge teaching to include diet, follow-up care, signs and symptoms to report, activity, and medications: name, purpose, dose, frequency, route, food interactions, and side effects Include family in teaching Evaluate understanding of teaching
Psychosocial	Encourage verbalization of concerns Provide ongoing support and encouragement	Encourage verbalization of concerns Provide ongoing support and encouragement to client and family
Diet	Regular diet as tolerated Encourage fluid intake of 2000 mL per day Offer supplemental feedings high in protein and vitamins	Regular diet as tolerated Encourage fluids to 2000 mL/24 hr Offer supplemental feedings high in protein and vitamins
Activity	Maintain safety precautions Encourage client to participate in activities of daily living as much as possible Ambulate ad lib Sling for casted extremity when ambulatory, otherwise elevate extremity	Provide safety precautions Encourage ambulation ad lib Extremity elevated or in sling Encourage client to participate in activities of daily living as much as possible
Medications	Analgesics as ordered IV antibiotics Intermittent IV device	Oral analgesics as ordered D/C intermittent IV device
Transfer/ discharge plans	Complete discharge plans Make appropriate referrals Continue home care instructions	Complete discharge instructions

Potential Client Variances
Upper Arm Fracture with Open Reduction

Possible Complications
- Infection
- Compartment syndrome

Health Conditions
- Pre-existing mobility problems
- Sensory perceptual alterations

Nursing Diagnoses
- Risk for injury
- Self-care deficits

Discharge Teaching for Client Following
Upper Arm Fracture with Open Reduction

Activity
- Gradually return to usual level of activity by increasing activity each day. Alternate activity with rest periods. Avoid fatigue.
- To prevent swelling keep arm elevated at all times. When in bed or on couch, elevate arm on pillow. Use a sling when walking or sitting, keeping fingers elevated toward ceiling.
- No strenuous activity until okayed by physician.
- Avoid driving for the period designated by your physician.
- Continue exercises as recommended by your physician.

Diet
- Eat a well-balanced diet, including all food groups.
- Drink 6–8 glasses of fluid each day.

Signs and Symptoms to Report
Notify physician if any of these symptoms occur:
- Increase in pain, redness, or swelling
- Sudden increase in wound drainage, especially if drainage has pus or a foul odor
- Chills or fever greater than 100F or 38C

Follow-Up Care and General Health Care
- Schedule follow-up appointment with physician as directed.
- Have someone remove scatter rugs from floors at home.
- Have someone remove any potential safety hazards from home.
- Wear an apron or shoulder bag to carry small objects from room to room.

Medications
- Review written list of medications including dose, frequency, food interactions, and side effects.

Wound and Dressing Care
If dressing is present:
- Cleanse skin around incision daily with mild soap and water.
- Change dressing daily and as often as necessary to keep dressing dry and clean.
- Drainage, if present, should gradually decrease.
- If there is a marked increase in drainage, swelling, tenderness, fever, or if drainage is foul-smelling, notify physician.
If cast is present:
- Keep cast dry.
- Do not put any objects or material under cast.
- When cast is removed, minimize exposure to sun.

Carotid Endarterectomy

Expected length of stay: 3–4 days

	Date _____ **Preoperative**	Date _____ **1st 24 Hours Postoperative**
Daily outcomes	Client verbalizes understanding of preoperative teaching, including: turning, coughing, and deep breathing, IV therapy, JP drain, mobilization, telemetry, O_2 therapy and pain management Client demonstrates ability to cope Client verbalizes understanding of procedure Obtain informed consent	Client will: • maintain adequate cerebral blood flow as evidenced by stable vital signs, being alert and oriented, and maintaining usual sensory and motor function • maintain cranial nerve function • have stable vital signs and B/P within specified range • have lungs clear to auscultation • have unlabored respirations and maintain oxygen saturation >95% • have clean, dry dressing • recover from anesthesia • verbalize understanding and demonstrate cooperation with turning, deep breathing, coughing, and splinting • tolerate ordered diet without nausea or vomiting • verbalize control of incisional pain with ordered medications • demonstrate ability to cope
Assessments, tests, and treatments	CBC Urinalysis CXR EKG Arteriogram Carotid ultrasound Baseline physical assessment with focus on respiratory, cardiovascular, and neuro function	Vital signs and O_2 saturation, neurovascular assessment, and dressing and wound drainage assessment q15min × 4; q30min × 4; q1hr × 24 and prn Maintain patency of drain Assess cranial nerve function q2–4hr and prn Monitor for bleeding and/or cerebral ischemia Assess respiratory status q4hr and prn Oxygen as ordered to maintain O_2 saturation >92% Incentive spirometer q2hr Intake and output every shift Assess voiding—if unable to void, try suggestive voiding techniques or if still unable, catheterize q8hr or prn
Knowledge deficit	Orient to surroundings and room Provide simple, brief instructions Preoperative teaching as ordered	Orient to room and surroundings Provide simple, brief instructions Include family in teaching Review specific postoperative care: turning, coughing, deep breathing, incentive spirometer, mobilization, intravenous, and pain management (prn medications or PCA) Instruct client regarding the importance of supporting head and neck during position changes Evaluate understanding of teaching

Carotid Endarterectomy *(continued)*

	Date _____ **Preoperative**	Date _____ **1st 24 Hours Postoperative**
Psychosocial	Assess anxiety regarding impending surgery Assess fears of unknown related to surgery Offer emotional support Encourage verbalization of concerns Provide information regarding surgical experience Minimize external stimuli (noise, movement)	Assess level of anxiety Assess coping status of client and family Encourage verbalization of concerns Provide information and ongoing support and encouragement to client and family
Diet	NPO Baseline nutritional and hydration assessment	Prior to offering food or fluids, assess return of gag and ability to chew and swallow HOB up for all meals unless contraindicated Clear liquids to diet as tolerated

Activity	Assess potential safety needs and provide appropriate
	   safety measures
		Assess safety needs and provide adequate precautions
		HOB up 30 degrees, support head and neck when
		   changing positions
		Dangle/chair evening of surgery if stable

Medications	Preoperative medications per anesthesia	Analgesics as ordered IV fluids Antihypertensives as ordered
Transfer/ discharge plans	Assess potential discharge needs and support system Establish discharge goals with client and family	Establish discharge objectives with client and family Determine discharge needs and support system with client and family Begin home care instructions

	Date _____ **2nd Day Postoperative**	Date _____ **3–4 Days Postoperative**
Daily outcomes	Client will: • maintain adequate cerebral blood flow as evidenced by stable vital signs, being alert and oriented, and maintaining usual sensory and motor function • maintain cranial nerve function • have stable vital signs and B/P within specified range • have lungs clear to auscultation • have unlabored respirations and maintain oxygen saturation >95% • have clean, dry wound with edges well-approximated, healing by first intention • demonstrate cooperation with turning, deep breathing, coughing, and splinting • tolerate ordered diet without nausea and vomiting • ambulate 4 times per day in hallway • verbalize control of incisional pain • demonstrate ability to cope • verbalize/demonstrate beginning understanding of home care instructions	Client is afebrile Client maintains adequate cerebral blood flow as evidenced by stable vital signs, being alert and oriented, and maintaining usual sensory and motor function Client maintains cranial nerve function Client has stable vital signs and B/P within specified range Client has lungs clear to auscultation and unlabored respiration with an oxygen saturation >95% Client has clean, dry wound with edges well-approximated, healing by first intention Client manages pain with oral medications and/or non-pharmacologic measures Client is independent in self-care Client is fully ambulatory Client has resumed preadmission urine and bowel elimination pattern Client verbalizes/demonstrates home care instructions Client tolerates low-salt, low-saturated fat, and low-cholesterol diet or diet as ordered Client demonstrates ability to cope with ongoing stressors
Assessments, tests, and treatments	Vital signs, neurovascular and cranial nerve assessment, O_2 saturation and dressing and wound drainage assessment q2–4 hr and prn Monitor for bleeding and/or cerebral ischemia Assess respiratory status q4hr and prn Oxygen as ordered to maintain O_2 saturation >95% Incentive spirometer q2hr until fully ambulatory Intake and output every shift Assess voiding pattern every shift Dressing change and wound assessment BID and prn	Vital signs, neurovascular and cranial nerve assessment, O_2 saturation, and dressing and wound drainage assessment q4–8hr and prn Assess respiratory status q4–8hr Dressing change and wound assessment BID and prn Assess coping status and provide appropriate emotional support
Knowledge deficit	Review plan of care and importance of early mobilization Begin discharge teaching regarding wound care/dressing change, diet, and activity Review written discharge instructions with client and family Evaluate understanding of teaching	Complete discharge teaching to include wound care, diet, follow-up care and appointment, signs and symptoms to report, strategies to slow the progression of arteriosclerosis, activity, and medication: name, purpose, dose, frequency, route, food interactions, and side effects Provide client with written discharge instructions
Psychosocial	Assess level of anxiety Assess coping status of client and family Encourage verbalization of concerns Provide information and ongoing support and encouragement to client and family	Assess level of anxiety Encourage verbalization of concerns Provide information and ongoing support and encouragement to client and family

	Date _____ **2nd Day Postoperative**	Date _____ **3–4 Days Postoperative**
Diet	Diet per order or low-salt, low-saturated fat and low cholesterol diet as tolerated HOB up for meals Dietary consult for diet teaching	Diet per order or low-salt, low-saturated fat, and low cholesterol diet as tolerated Provide written copy of diet
Activity	Maintain safety precautions Fully ambulatory in room with required assistance Walk in hall 4 to 6 times with required assistance	Maintain safety precautions Fully ambulatory
Medications	Oral analgesics Intermittent IV device Antihypertensives as ordered Aspirin or anticoagulant therapy if ordered	Oral analgesics D/C IV device Other medications as ordered Aspirin or anticoagulant therapy if ordered
Transfer/ discharge plans	Review progress toward discharge goals Make appropriate referrals Finalize discharge plans	Finalize any home care arrangements Complete discharge instructions

Potential Client Variances
Carotid Endarterectomy

Possible Complications

- Cerebrovascular accident
- Hemorrhage

Health Conditions

- History of strokes
- Pre-existing heart disease, hypertension
- History of bleeding tendencies

Nursing Diagnoses

- Altered cerebral tissue perfusion
- Sensory perceptual alterations
- Self-care deficits
- Impaired verbal communication
- Risk for impaired swallowing

Discharge Teaching for Client Following
Carotid Endarterectomy

Activity
- Gradually return to usual level of activity by increasing activity each day. Alternate activity with rest periods. Avoid fatigue.
- No strenuous activity until okayed by physician.
- Avoid heavy housework, straining, and driving for the period designated by your physician.

Diet
- Eat a well-balanced diet, including all food groups. Maintain any recommended dietary restrictions.
- Drink 6–8 glasses of fluid each day.

Signs and Symptoms to Report
Notify physician if any of these symptoms occur:
- Increase in pain, redness, or swelling
- Sudden increase in wound drainage, especially if drainage has pus or a foul odor
- Chills or fever greater than 100F or 38C
- Symptoms similar to those experienced before the surgery

Follow-Up Care and General Health Care
- Schedule follow-up appointment with physician as directed.
- Do not smoke and avoid second-hand smoke.
- Discuss alcohol use with your physician.

Medications
- Review written list of medications, including dose, frequency, food interactions, and side effects.

Wound and Dressing Care
- Cleanse skin around incision daily with mild soap and water.
- If you require a dressing, change it daily and as often as necessary to keep dressing dry and clean.
- Remove dressing prior to showering and replace with a clean dressing afterward.
- Drainage, if present, should gradually decrease.
- If there is a marked increase in drainage, swelling, tenderness, fever, or if drainage is foul-smelling, notify physician.

Cataract Surgery

Expected length of stay: Less than 6 hours

	Date _____ **Preoperative**	Date _____ **By Discharge**
Daily outcomes	Client is prepared for eye surgery, including instillation of eye drops, presurgical scrub, NPO per order, IV infusion, and emptying bladder Client verbalizes ability to cope with fear and anxiety regarding surgery and potential loss of vision Client verbalizes understanding of preoperative teaching, including preoperative routine, intraoperative experience, and postoperative care Client remains oriented to time, place, person, and situation Client demonstrates the ability to compensate for sensory deficits	Client is afebrile Client is independent in self-care Client is fully ambulatory Client has resumed preadmission urine elimination pattern Client verbalizes/demonstrates home care instructions, including: 1) signs and symptoms of infection and hemorrhage, 2) instillation of eye drops, 3) avoiding activities that increase intraocular pressure, 4) maintaining eye shield, 5) aseptic technique when caring for eyes, and 6) follow-up care Client verbalizes control of pain with oral analgesics or nonpharmacological pain relief measures such as relaxation techniques Client tolerates usual diet Client verbalizes ability to cope with ongoing stressors Client demonstrates the ability to compensate for sensory deficits
Assessments, tests, and treatments	CBC Urinalysis Baseline physical assessment with a focus on mental status and sensory-perceptual needs Anesthesia consult Assess use of anticoagulants, aspirin, or nonsteroidal anti-inflammatory medications	Vital signs and O_2 saturation, neurovascular assessment, and dressing q15min × 4; q3 min × 4; q1hr × 4 and then q4hr and prn Monitor for complaints of sudden pain in eye accompanied with nausea, diaphoresis, or increased pulse rate, and report immediately Assess voiding—if unable to void, try suggestive voiding techniques or if still unable, catheterize prn
Knowledge deficit	Orient to room and surroundings Provide simple, brief instructions Include family in teaching Review preoperative preparation including hospital and surgical routines Reinforce preoperative teaching regarding specific postoperative care: lying on the nonoperative side, avoiding bending at the waist, requesting assistance with ambulation Instruct client not to touch eye Evaluate client understanding of teaching	Reorient to room and postoperative routine Review plan of care Include family in teaching Complete discharge teaching regarding using standardized teaching sheet and provide client with large print copy Evaluate client understanding of teaching

	Date _____ **Preoperative**	Date _____ **By Discharge**
Sensory/ perceptual	Assess level of consciousness on admission and prn Use dim lights, limit visitors, and provide rest periods Introduce self upon entering room Speak clearly and distinctly, facing the client and assess client's understanding Use large print teaching materials on off-white paper Minimize extraneous noise	Assess level of consciousness prn and prior to discharge Use dim lights, limit visitors, and provide rest periods Introduce self upon entering room Speak clearly and distinctly and assess client's understanding Use large print teaching materials on off-white paper
Psychosocial	Assess anxiety related to pending surgery Assess fears of the unknown related to surgery Encourage verbalization of concerns Provide information regarding the surgical experience	Assess level of anxiety Encourage verbalization of concerns Provide information and ongoing support and encouragement
Diet	NPO Baseline nutritional assessment	Offer liquids ad lib: if tolerated, advance to usual diet
Activity	OOB ad lib with assistance until premedicated for surgery Protect from injury by removing any potential hazards	Provide safety precautions Bathroom privileges with assistance after surgery and begin progressive ambulation with assistance to tolerance until fully ambulatory
Medications	Preoperative medications as ordered	Oral analgesics IV fluids until adequate po intake
Transfer/ discharge plans	Assess discharge plans and support system Assess client and family to plan for home care for first two weeks following surgery Make any appointment referrals Encourage family to remove hazards from home environment such as throw rugs, low furniture, and cords	Probable discharge within 2–6 hours of surgery Complete discharge home care teaching when fully awake and oriented and before discharge Include family/significant other in discharge teaching Provide a written copy of discharge instructions

Potential Client Variances
Cataract Surgery

Possible Complications
- Infection
- Hemorrhage

Health Conditions
- Pre-existing conditions related to mobility
- History of bleeding tendencies

Nursing Diagnoses
- Sensory/perceptual alterations
- Risk for injury
- Self-care deficits

Discharge Teaching for Client Following
Cataract Surgery

Activity

- Do not drive or operate hazardous equipment for period designated by your physician.
- Avoid heavy housework, straining, heavy lifting, and driving for the period designated by your physician.
- Take frequent rest periods.
- You may wash your hair when your physician permits this activity. Be sure to lean backward, not forward.

Diet

- For the first 24 hours, eat lightly as tolerated. Then eat a well-balanced diet including all food groups.
- Report nausea or vomiting.
- No alcohol for 24 hours.

Signs and Symptoms to Report

Notify physician if any of these symptoms occur:
- Pain or discomfort in eye
- Drainage from eye, especially if drainage has pus or a foul odor
- Chills, or fever greater than 100F or 38C

Follow-Up Care and General Health Care

- Schedule follow-up appointment with physician as directed.

Medications

- Review written list of medications, including dose, route, frequency, food interactions, and side effects.
- To administer eye medications, tilt your head back, gaze at the ceiling, and gently pull the lower lid down.
- Take eye medications to follow-up medical appointments.

Eye Care

- Wash hands before and after contact with eye.
- Do not rub eye, strain, bend with head below waist, or lift items over 10 pounds.
- Wear eye shield at night.
- Wear glasses during day and use sunglasses for comfort.

Cholecystectomy (Laparoscopic)

Expected length of stay: less than 24 hours

	Date _____ **Preoperative**	Date _____ **1st 24 Hours Following Surgery**
Daily outcomes	Client verbalizes understanding of preoperative teaching including, turning, coughing, deep breathing, incentive spirometer, mobilization, and pain management Client exhibits effective coping with preoperative preparation Client verbalizes understanding of procedure, indications for procedure, comparative risks, benefits and implications of various options	Client is afebrile Client has a clean, dry wound with edges well-approximated, healing by first intention Client manages pain with non-pharmacologic measures or oral medications Client is independent in self-care Client is fully ambulatory Client has resumed preadmission urine and bowel elimination pattern Client verbalizes/demonstrates home care instructions Client tolerates usual diet Client exhibits effective coping with ongoing stressors
Assessments, tests, and treatments	CBC Urinalysis Baseline physical assessment with a focus on respiratory status and gastrointestinal function Anesthesia consult	Vital signs and O_2 saturation, neurovascular assessment, dressing and wound drainage assessment q15min × 4; q30min × 4; q1hr × 4 and then q4hr and prn Assess lung sounds and gastrointestinal function q4hr and prn Intake and output every shift Assess voiding—if unable to void, try suggestive voiding techniques or, if still unable, catheterize q8hr or prn
Knowledge deficit	Orient to room and surroundings Include family in teaching Provide simple, brief instructions Review preoperative preparation including hospital and surgical routines Reinforce preoperative teaching regarding specific postoperative care: turning, coughing, deep breathing, incentive spirometer, mobilization, and pain management Evaluate understanding of teaching	Reorient to room and postoperative routine Include family in teaching Review plan of care and importance of early mobilization, as well as any activity restrictions Complete discharge teaching regarding wound care/dressing change, follow-up care, signs and symptoms to report, medications, and diet Evaluate understanding of teaching
Psychosocial	Assess anxiety related to pending surgery Assess fears of the unknown related to surgery Encourage verbalization of concerns Provide emotional support to client and family Minimize external stimuli (eg, noise, movement)	Assess level of anxiety Encourage verbalization of concerns Provide emotional support to client and family Provide information and ongoing support and encouragement
Diet	NPO Baseline nutritional assessment	Advance to clear liquids; if tolerated, advance to full liquids/soft diet morning following surgery

Cholecystectomy (Laparoscopic) *(continued)*

	Date _____ **Preoperative**	Date _____ **1st 24 Hours Following Surgery**
Activity	OOB ad lib until premedicated for surgery	Provide safety precautions Bathroom privileges with assistance evening after surgery Begin progressive ambulation as tolerated the morning following surgery until fully ambulatory
Medications	NPO except ordered medications	IM or oral analgesics Antibiotics if ordered IV fluids until adequate oral intake, then intermittent IV device Discontinue prior to discharge
Transfer/ discharge plans	Assess discharge plans and support system	Probable discharge within 24 hours of surgery Complete discharge home care teaching when fully awake and oriented and before discharge Provide a written copy of discharge instructions

Potential Client Variances
Cholecystectomy (Laparoscopic)

Possible Complications

- Hemorrhage
- Infection
- Peritonitis

Health Conditions

- Pre-existing respiratory problems
- Undernutrition

Nursing Diagnoses

- Ineffective breathing pattern
- Altered nutrition: less than body requirements
- Acute pain

Discharge Teaching for Client Following
Cholecystectomy (Laparoscopic)

Activity

- Gradually return to usual level of activity by increasing activity each day. Alternate activity with rest periods. Avoid fatigue.
- Avoid heavy housework, working, straining, heavy lifting, and driving for the period designated by your physician.

Diet

- Eat a well-balanced diet, including all food groups.
- Drink 6-8 glasses of fluids each day.

Signs and Symptoms to Report

Notify physician if any of these symptoms occur:
- Increase in pain, redness, or swelling
- Sudden increase in wound drainage, especially if drainage has pus or a foul odor
- Chills or fever greater than 100F or 38C
- Nausea, vomiting, or change in bowel habits

Follow-Up Care and General Health Care

- Schedule follow-up appointment with physician as directed.
- Avoid constipation; increasing fiber and fluids may help.

Medications

- Review written list of medications, including dose, route, frequency, food interactions, and side effects.

Wound and Dressing Care

- Cleanse skin around incisions daily with mild soap and water.
- Change dressings daily and as often as necessary to keep dressing dry and clean.
- Remove dressing prior to showering and replace with a clean dressing afterward.
- Drainage, if present, should gradually decrease.
- If there is a marked increase in drainage, swelling, tenderness, or fever, or if drainage is foul-smelling, notify physician.

Colon Resection

Expected length of stay: 6–7 days

	Date _____ **Preoperative**	Date _____ **1st 24 Hours Postoperative**	Date _____ **2nd–3rd Days Postoperative**
Daily outcomes	Client verbalizes understanding of preoperative teaching, including: turning, coughing, deep breathing, incentive spirometer, mobilization, possible tubes (nasogastric tube, IV, Foley catheter, penrose or other drains), and pain management Client demonstrates ability to cope Client verbalizes understanding of procedure Obtain informed consent	Client will: • have stable vital signs • have a clean, dry wound with edges well-approximated, healing by first intention • recover from anesthesia as evidenced by VS return to baseline, and being awake, alert, and oriented • verbalize understanding of and demonstrate cooperation with turning, coughing, deep breathing, and splinting • have lungs clear to auscultation • demonstrate ability to use PCA if in use • verbalize control of incisional pain • transfer out of bed with assistance 2–3 times • demonstrate ability to cope	Client will: • be afebrile and have stable vital signs • have a clean, dry wound with edges well-approximated, healing by first intention • have active bowel sounds • tolerate ordered diet without vomiting • demonstrate cooperation with turning, coughing, deep breathing, and splinting • ambulate 4 times • verbalize control of incisional pain • verbalize ability to cope • verbalize beginning understanding of home care instructions
Assessments, tests, and treatments	CBC Urinalysis Chest x-ray Baseline physical assessment with a focus on respiratory status and gastrointestinal function Assess and record the description, location, duration, and characteristics of client's pain Reduce or eliminate pain-producing factors, such as fear and anxiety	CBC Electrolytes Vital signs and O_2 saturation, neurovascular assessment, and dressing and wound drainage assessment q15min × 4; q30min × 4; q1hr × 4 and then q4hr and prn Assess respiratory status and gastrointestinal function q4hr and prn Incentive spirometer q2hr O_2 as indicated Intake and output every shift Assess patency of NG tube q2hr, noting volume q4–8hr Assess Foley catheter or voiding—if unable to void try suggestive voiding techniques or, if still unable, catheterize q8hr or prn	Vital signs and dressing and wound drainage assessment q4hr and prn Assess respiratory status and gastrointestinal function q4hr Incentive spirometer q2hr until fully ambulatory O_2 as indicated Intake and output every shift If still in place, assess patency and output of NG tube q4–8hr Assess voiding pattern every shift Using sterile asepsis, change dressing: assess wound healing and wound drainage Assess and record the description, location, duration, and characteristics of client's pain q4hr and prn Reduce or eliminate pain-producing factors, employ distraction or relaxation techniques, and offer back rubs

Colon Resection *(continued)*

	Date _____ **Preoperative**	Date _____ **1st 24 Hours Postoperative**	Date _____ **2nd–3rd Days Postoperative**
Assessments, tests, and treatments (continued)		Assess and record the description, location, duration, and characteristics of client's pain q2–4hr and prn Encourage verbalization of pain and discomfort Reduce or eliminate pain-producing factors and employ distraction or relaxation techniques Provide back rubs Encourage client to request analgesic or use PCA before pain becomes severe	
Knowledge deficit	Orient to room and surroundings Provide simple, brief instructions Review preoperative preparation including hospital and surgical routines Include family in teaching Discuss surgery and specific postoperative care: turning, coughing, deep breathing, splinting incision, incentive spirometer, mobilization, possible tubes (nasogastric tube [NG] and intravenous [IV]), and pain management (PCA, epidural, or prn medications) Instruct regarding distraction techniques, such as slow rhythmic breathing and guided imagery, to produce pain relief Instruct in relaxation techniques, such as tensing and relaxing muscle groups and rhythmic breathing Evaluate understanding of teaching	Reorient to room and postoperative routine Include family in teaching Review plan of care and importance of early mobilization Review importance of turning, coughing, deep breathing, splinting incision, incentive spirometer, mobilization, drainage tubes (Foley catheter and intravenous), and pain management (PCA, epidural, or prn medications) Evaluate understanding of teaching	Reinforce earlier teaching regarding ongoing care Include family in teaching Begin discharge teaching regarding wound care/dressing change Evaluate understanding of teaching
Psychosocial	Assess anxiety related to diagnosis and pending surgery Assess fears of the unknown related to surgery Encourage verbalization of concerns Provide information regarding surgical experience Minimize external stimuli (eg, noise, movement)	Assess level of anxiety Encourage verbalization of concerns Provide information and ongoing support and encouragement to client and family	Encourage verbalization of concerns Provide ongoing support and encouragement

➤

Colon Resection *(continued)*

	Date _____ **Preoperative**	Date _____ **1st 24 Hours Postoperative**	Date _____ **2nd–3rd Days Postoperative**
Diet	NPO Baseline nutritional and hydration assessment	NPO NG tube until return of bowel sounds	When NG tube removed, begin clear liquids to tolerance
Activity	Assess safety needs and provide appropriate measures Activity as ordered	Maintain safety precautions Assist to chair 2–3 times	Maintain safety precautions Ambulate 4 times with assistance
Medications	Preoperative medications as ordered	IV fluids IV antibiotics Analgesics as ordered	IV fluids IV antibiotics When ordered convert IV to intermittent IV device Analgesics as ordered
Transfer/ discharge plans	Assess discharge plans and support system Establish discharge goals with client and family	Review progress toward discharge goals with client and family Consult with social service regarding VNA and projected needs for home health care (if any)	Review progress toward discharge goals with client and family Make appropriate discharge referrals

	Date _____ **4th Day Postoperative**	Date _____ **5th Day Postoperative**	Date _____ **6th–7th Days Postoperative**
Daily outcomes	Client will: • be afebrile and have stable vital signs • have a clean, dry wound with edges well-approximated, healing by first intention • tolerate ordered diet without nausea or vomiting • ambulate 4–6 times • verbalize control of incisional pain • verbalize ability to cope • verbalize beginning understanding of home care instructions	Client will: • be afebrile and have stable vital signs • have a clean, dry wound with edges well-approximated, healing by first intention • tolerate ordered diet without nausea or vomiting • ambulate 4–6 times • verbalize control of incisional pain • verbalize ability to cope • verbalize understanding of home care instructions	Client is afebrile and has stable vital signs Client has a dry, clean wound with edges well-approximated, healing by first intention Client manages pain with nonpharmacologic measures and any ordered medications Client is independent in self-care Client is fully ambulatory Client has resumed preadmission urine and bowel elimination patterns Client verbalizes home care instructions Client tolerates usual diet Client verbalizes ability to cope with ongoing stressors

Colon Resection *(continued)*

	Date _____ **4th Day Postoperative**	Date _____ **5th Day Postoperative**	Date _____ **6th–7th Days Postoperative**
Assessments, tests, and treatments	Vital signs and dressing and wound drainage assessment q4hr and prn Incentive spirometer q2hr until fully ambulatory O_2 if indicated Intake and output every shift Assess voiding pattern every shift Assess respiratory status and gastrointestinal function q4–8hr Using sterile asepsis, change dressing: assess wound healing and wound drainage Assess and record description, location, duration, and characteristics of client's pain q4hr and prn Encourage client to employ distraction or relaxation techniques	Vital signs and dressing and wound drainage assessment q4hr and prn Assess respiratory status and gastrointestinal function q4–8 hr Remove dressing and assess wound healing and drainage Assess and record description, location, duration, and characteristics of client's pain q4hr and prn Encourage client to employ distraction or relaxation techniques	Vital signs and dressing and wound drainage assessment q4–8hr Assess respiratory status and gastrointestinal function Assess wound healing Assess and record description, location, duration, and characteristics of client's pain q4hr and prn Encourage client to employ distraction or relaxation techniques
Knowledge deficit	Include family in teaching Initiate discharge teaching regarding wound care, diet, and activity Review written discharge instructions with client and family Evaluate understanding of teaching	Continue discharge teaching to client and family regarding wound care, diet, signs and symptoms to report, medications, and activity Review written discharge instructions with client and family Evaluate understanding of teaching	Complete discharge teaching to include wound care, diet, follow-up care, signs and symptoms to report, activity, and medications: name, purpose, dose, frequency, route, dietary interactions, and side effects Provide client with written discharge instructions Evaluate understanding of teaching
Psychosocial	Encourage verbalization of concerns Provide ongoing support and encouragement	Encourage verbalization of concerns Provide ongoing support and encouragement	Encourage verbalization of concerns Provide ongoing support and encouragement
Diet	If tolerating clear liquids, advance to full liquids as tolerated	Advance diet to soft, regular diet as tolerated	Regular diet as tolerated
Activity	Ambulate independently at least 4 times Maintain safety precautions	Fully ambulatory Maintain safety precautions	Fully ambulatory
Medications	Analgesics as ordered Intermittent IV device for any IV medications—D/C when so ordered	Analgesics as ordered	Analgesics as ordered

➤

Colon Resection *(continued)*

	Date _____ **4th Day Postoperative**	Date _____ **5th Day Postoperative**	Date _____ **6th–7th Days Postoperative**
Transfer/ discharge plans	Continue to review progress toward discharge goals	Finalize discharge plans Continue to review progress toward discharge goals Finalize plans for home care if needed	Complete discharge instructions

Potential Client Variances
Colon Resection

Possible Complications

- Peritonitis
- Ileus
- Fluid and electrolyte disturbances

Health Conditions

- Undernutrition
- Pre-existing respiratory problems

Nursing Diagnoses

- Altered nutrition: less than body requirements
- Risk for infection
- Urinary retention

Discharge Teaching for Client Following
Colon Resection

Activity
- Gradually return to usual level of activity by increasing activity each day. Alternate activity with planned rest periods. Avoid fatigue.
- You may go up and down stairs as long as you feel comfortable.
- Avoid heavy housework, straining, heavy lifting, and driving for the period designated by your physician.
- Check with your physician regarding returning to work.

Diet
- Eat a well-balanced diet including fruits, vegetables, meats, milk products, and starches and bread.

Signs and Symptoms to Report
Notify physician if any of these symptoms occur:
- Increase in pain, redness, or swelling in wound
- Sudden increase in wound drainage, especially if drainage has pus or a foul odor.
- Chills, or fever greater than 100F or 38C
- Nausea, vomiting, or change in bowel habits

Follow-Up Care and General Health Care
- Schedule follow-up appointment with physician as directed.

Medications
- Review written list of medications, including dose, route, frequency, food interactions, and side effects.
- Avoid over-the-counter medications unless recommended by physician.

Wound and Dressing Care
- Cleanse skin around incision daily with mild soap and water.
- If dressing present, change it daily and as often as necessary to keep dressing dry and clean.
- Drainage, if present, should gradually decrease.
- If there is a marked increase in drainage, swelling, tenderness, fever, or if drainage is foul-smelling, notify physician.

Percutaneous Transluminal Coronary Angioplasty (PTCA)

Expected length of stay: 24–36 hours

	Date _____ **Pre-PTCA**	Date _____ **Post-PTCA**	Date _____ **Post Sheath Removal Until Discharge**
Daily outcomes	Client verbalizes understanding of pre-procedure teaching, including bed rest, safety precautions, groin prep, and pre-procedure sedation Client demonstrates ability to cope Client verbalizes understanding of procedure Obtain informed consent	Client will: • maintain stable vital signs, and be alert and oriented • have lungs clear to auscultation • have unlabored respirations and maintain oxygen saturation >95% • demonstrate cooperation with activity restrictions • tolerate ordered diet without nausea and vomiting • demonstrate ability to cope • verbalize/demonstrate beginning understanding of home care instructions	Client is afebrile Client has stable vital signs and B/P within specified range Client has lungs clear to auscultation and unlabored respiration with an oxygen saturation >95% Client manages pain with oral medications and/or non-pharmacologic measures Client is independent in self-care Client is fully ambulatory Client has resumed preadmission urine elimination pattern Client has a soft non-distended abdomen with active bowel sounds Client verbalizes ability to cope Client verbalizes/demonstrates home care instructions Client tolerates ordered diet without nausea or vomiting Client demonstrates ability to cope with ongoing stressors, including current illness
Assessments, tests, and treatments	Complete blood count Urinalysis PT/PTT Type and screen Chest x-ray EKG History and physical Vital signs and O_2 saturation, neurovascular and mental status O_2 via nasal canula to maintain oxygen saturation >95% Assess coping status of client and family Provide ongoing emotional support to client and family	Vital signs, CSM assessment, O_2 saturation and dressing and site assessment q15min × 4; q30min × 4; q1hr × 4; then q4hr and prn Continuous cardiac monitoring HOB <30 degrees Monitor for bleeding PTT if ordered prior to sheath removal Assess respiratory status q4hr and prn O_2 via nasal canula to maintain oxygen saturation >95% Follow sheath removal protocol	Vital signs, O_2 saturation, and dressing and site drainage assessment q4–8hr and prn Continuous cardiac monitoring Assess respiratory status q4–8hr Assess wound and apply dry sterile dressing every day and prn Encourage client to verbalize regarding any changes in appearance and functional ability Assist the client and family to identify any resources or strategies to cope with changes in appearance and functional ability

Percutaneous Transluminal Coronary Angioplasty *(continued)*

	Date _____ **Pre-PTCA**	Date _____ **Post-PTCA**	Date _____ **Post Sheath Removal Until Discharge**
Assessments, tests, and treatments (continued)	Allow for client's input regarding care	Assess coping status of client and family Encourage client and family to verbalize feelings regarding any changes in appearance and functional abilities Provide ongoing emotional support to client and family	Assess coping status and provide appropriate emotional support
Knowledge deficit	Orient to room and surroundings Provide simple, brief instructions Include family in teaching Review specific post-procedure care Evaluate understanding of teaching	Review plan of care, including activity restrictions Begin discharge teaching regarding site care, diet, and activity Review written discharge instructions with client and significant other Evaluate understanding of teaching	Complete discharge teaching to include site care, diet, follow-up care and appointment, signs and symptoms to report, strategies to slow the progression of arteriosclerosis, activity, and medication: name, purpose, dose, frequency, route, food interactions, and side effects Evaluate understanding of teaching
Diet	NPO Consider referral to dietician	Encourage fluids and advance to American Heart Association diet as tolerated	American Heart Association diet as tolerated
Activity	Assess safety needs and provide adequate precautions	Maintain safety precautions HOB <30 degrees Bed rest Extremity straight	Maintain safety precautions Continue activity restrictions until 6 hr after sheath removal After 6 hr, begin progressive ambulation with assistance
Medications	IV as ordered Pre-procedure meds as ordered	IV as ordered Manage chest pain per protocol	Oral analgesics D/C IV device Other medications as ordered
Transfer/ discharge plans	Establish discharge objectives with client and family Assess discharge needs and support system Consider consultation with cardiac rehab	Review progress toward discharge goals Begin home care instructions Make any referrals Finalize discharge plans	Finalize any home care arrangements Complete discharge instructions

Percutaneous Transluminal Coronary Angioplasty (PTCA) **121**

Potential Client Variances

Percutaneous Transluminal Coronary Angioplasty (PTCA)

Possible Complications

- Dysrhythmia
- Myocardial infarction
- Coronary occlusion or dissection
- Hemorrhage at insertion site

Health Conditions

- Diabetes
- Peripheral vascular disease
- Clotting disorders

Nursing Diagnoses

- Altered tissue perfusion: peripheral, cardiopulmonary
- Ineffective management of therapeutic regimen
- Ineffective individual/family coping

Discharge Teaching for Client Following

Percutaneous Transluminal Coronary Angioplasty (PTCA)

Activity

- Gradually return to usual level of activity by increasing activity each day. Alternate activity with rest periods. Avoid fatigue.
- No strenuous activity, driving, or return to work until okayed by physician (usually one week).
- Avoid heavy housework or straining for the period designated by your physician.
- Cardiac rehabilitation as directed.

Diet

- Follow low-fat, low-cholesterol diet. Drink plenty of fluids and eat a well-balanced diet including fruits, meat, vegetables, bread and starches, and milk products. Low-salt diet if so directed.

Signs and Symptoms to Report

Notify physician if any of these symptoms occur:
- Chills, or fever greater than 100F or 38C
- Chest pain or shortness of breath
- Worsening pain or discomfort or redness, swelling, drainage, or warmth at the PTCA insertion site
- Any unusual sensations or changes in temperature in the involved leg

Follow-Up Care and General Health Care

- Schedule follow-up appointment with physician as directed.
- Contact cardiac rehabilitation as directed.

Medications

- Review written list of medications, including dose, frequency, food interactions, and side effects.
- Avoid over-the-counter medications unless recommended by physician.
- Ask your physician about flu and pneumonia vaccines.

Wound and Dressing Care

- Shower daily and wash insertion site with soap and water.
- Wear comfortable, non-constrictive clothing until the insertion site is healed and non-tender.

Coronary Artery Bypass Surgery

Expected length of stay: 5–6 days

	Date _____ **Preoperative**	Date _____ **1st 12–24 Hours Postoperative**	Date _____ **2nd Day Postoperative**
Daily outcomes	Client verbalizes understanding of preoperative teaching, including: ventilator, turning, coughing, and deep breathing, mobilization, O_2 therapy, chest tubes, IV therapy, Foley catheter, cardiac monitoring, and pain management Client demonstrates ability to cope Client verbalizes understanding of procedures Obtain informed consent	Client will: • have stable hemodynamic measurements • maintain adequate cardiac output • have equal and bilateral peripheral pulses • maintain urine output >30 mL/hr • respond adequately to diuretic therapy • maintain an effective breathing pattern • have patent chest tubes • recover from anesthesia as evidenced by VS return to baseline and response to stimuli • have a clean wound with edges well-approximated, healing by first intention • when extubated, demonstrate an effective breathing pattern • verbalize understanding of and demonstrate cooperation with turning, deep breathing, coughing, and splinting • verbalize understanding and demonstrate cooperation with sternotomy precautions • verbalize control of incisional pain with ordered medications • demonstrate ability to cope	Client will: • have stable vital signs, stable cardiac rhythm, and be awake, alert, and oriented • maintain an adequate cardiac output and effective breathing pattern • maintain urine output >30 mL/hr • respond adequately to diuretics • have a clean wound with edges well-approximated, healing by first intention • demonstrate cooperation with turning, deep breathing, and splinting • have patent chest tubes (if not removed) • tolerate ordered diet without nausea or vomiting • demonstrate cooperation with sternotomy precautions • verbalize control of incisional pain • ambulate 2–3 times/day as tolerated • demonstrate ability to cope • tolerate activity level without dyspnea, shortness of breath, or chest pain

Assessments, tests, and treatments	CBC
	Urinalysis
	EKG
	CXR
	Chemistries
	Electrolytes
	Type and crossmatch
	Baseline physical assessment with focus on respiratory and renal status
	Preoperative O_2 saturation
		On admission to unit:
		  Portable chest x-ray
		  EKG
		  CBC
		  K^+
		Vital signs and O_2 saturation, neurovascular assessment, and dressing assessment per guideline for care
		Head to toe assessment q1-2hr and prn
		Ventilator care and weaning per protocol
			Vital signs and O_2 saturation, neurovascular assessment, dressing assessment q2–4hr and prn
			Head to toe assessment q2-4hr and prn
			Intake and output q4–8hr
			Foley catheter
			K^+
			Incentive spirometer q2hr
			O_2 as indicated
			Assess calves for redness, tenderness, swelling, heat, edema every shift

	Date _____ **Preoperative**	Date _____ **1st 12–24 Hours Postoperative**	Date _____ **2nd Day Postoperative**
Assessments, tests, and treatments (continued)		ABGs prn Cardiac monitoring Hemodynamic monitoring per guidelines for care Initiate weaning protocol when ABG stable, then oxygen via face mask Chest tubes to 10–20 cm of H_2O pressure Foley catheter to constant drainage Assess peripheral pulses q1–2hr and prn ACE wraps to lower legs—remove and replace every shift Intake and output q1hr Transfuse as ordered Maintain sterile dressing—reinforce prn D/C A line before transfer to step-down	ACE wraps—remove and replace every shift Maintain dry, sterile dressing—reinforce prn Assess wound and change dressing per MD order Cardiac monitoring Weight Epicardial wire care per protocol
Knowledge deficit	Orient to room and surroundings Provide simple, brief instructions Preoperative teaching including hospital and surgical routines: ventilator, TCDB, mobilization, O_2 therapy, chest tubes, IV therapy, Foley catheter, telemetry, and pain management	Orient patient and family to room and postoperative routine Include family in teaching Review plan of care When extubated, review importance of deep breathing, coughing, splinting incision, incentive spirometer, mobilization, drainage or intravenous tubes, sternotomy precautions, and pain management Prepare for transfer to stepdown unit Evaluate understanding of teaching	Review importance of early progressive exercise Review plan of care with client and family Reinforce sternotomy precautions and safety measures Evaluate understanding of teaching
Diet	Baseline nutritional and hydration assessment	NPO	If clear liquids are tolerated, advance to full liquids, then to American Heart Association (AHA) diet as tolerated
Activity	Assess safety needs and provide appropriate measures	Bed rest/sternotomy precautions Turn, cough, and take deep breath q2hr ROM every shift Assess safety needs and maintain appropriate precautions	Maintain safety and sternotomy precautions TCDB q1–2hr Assist out of bed 2–3 times Begin ambulation per physical therapy protocol

	Date _____ **Preoperative**	Date _____ **1st 12–24 Hours** **Postoperative**	Date _____ **2nd Day Postoperative**
Psychosocial	Assess potential for post-op confusion Assess anxiety regarding impending surgery Assess fear of unknown related to surgery Offer emotional support Encourage verbalization of concerns Include family in teaching and provide support Minimize external stimuli (noise and movement)	Assess level of anxiety Provide information and ongoing support and encouragement to client and family	Assess level of anxiety Encourage verbalization of concerns Provide information and ongoing support and encouragement to client and family
Medications	Preoperative medications as ordered per anesthesia	Analgesics as ordered IV antibiotics IV fluids per protocol IV—KCL & magnesium as ordered Vasoactive IV meds as ordered/per protocol Diuretics as ordered Routine meds as ordered	Analgesics as ordered Stool softener Initiate aspirin therapy as ordered SC heparin IV fluid per protocol IV—KCL as ordered Diuretics as ordered Routine meds as ordered
Transfer/ discharge plans	Assess potential discharge needs and support system Establish discharge goals with client and family	Home assessment if not previously completed Consult with social service regarding projected needs for home health care; including home health aides, visiting nurse, physical and occupational therapy Establish discharge objectives with client and family	Review with client and significant others discharge objectives regarding activity and home care Consult and collaborate with cardiac rehab and physical therapy Complete discharge planning

	Date _____ **3rd Day Postoperative**	Date _____ **4th Day Postoperative**
Daily outcomes	Client will: • be afebrile, with stable vital signs • have stable cardiac rhythm • have lungs clear to auscultation • have a clean wound with edges well-approximated, healing by first intention • have stable vital signs	Client will: • be afebrile, have stable vital signs, stable cardiac rhythm, and be awake, alert and oriented • have a clean wound with edges well-approximated, healing by first intention

➤

	Date _____ **3rd Day Postoperative**	Date _____ **4th Day Postoperative**
Daily outcomes (continued)	• demonstrate cooperation with turning, deep breathing, and splinting • tolerate ordered diet without nausea or vomiting • demonstrate cooperation with sternotomy precautions • verbalize control of incisional pain • ambulate 50–100 feet 3 or 4 times • demonstrate ability to cope • tolerate activity level without dyspnea, shortness of breath, or chest pain	• demonstrate cooperation with turning, deep breathing, coughing, and splinting • tolerate ordered diet without nausea and vomiting • demonstrate cooperation with sternotomy precautions • verbalize control of incisional pain • ambulate 150–200 feet 4 times • demonstrate ability to cope • tolerate activity level without dyspnea, shortness of breath, or chest pain
Assessments, tests, *and treatments*	Vital signs and O_2 saturation, neurovascular assessment, and dressing assessment q4hr Head to toe assessment q4hr and prn Intake and output every shift Remove chest dressings and paint incisions with betadine BID Rewrap aces on legs BID and prn Incentive spirometer q2hr O_2 as indicated Assess calves for redness, tenderness, swelling, heat, and edema every shift TED stockings—remove and replace every shift day and prn D/C chest tubes Cardiac monitoring Weight Epicardial wire care per protocol D/C Foley and assess voiding D/C oxygen when O_2 saturation >95% on room air K^+	EKG/CXR Serum K^+ and CBC Vital signs and O_2 saturation q4hr and prn Head to toe assessment q4hr and prn Change dressings every day and prn Assess wound healing BID TED stockings—remove and replace every shift Assess calves for redness, tenderness, swelling, heat, and edema every shift Intake and output every shift; assess urine output—notify MD of inbalance Weight—notify MD of weight gain Epicardial wire care D/C oxygen if O_2 saturation >92% D/C cardiac monitoring if indicated
Knowledge deficit	Review plan of care Include family in teaching Initiate discharge teaching regarding wound care, home exercise program, and diet Cardiac teaching Evaluate understanding of teaching	Review plan of care Include family in teaching Continue discharge teaching regarding wound care, activity, and diet Cardiac teaching with family Evaluate understanding of teaching

	Date _____ **3rd Day Postoperative**	Date _____ **4th Day Postoperative**
Diet	AHA diet as tolerated Encourage high-fiber diet, rich in Vitamin C Dietary consult for dietary instruction	AHA diet as tolerated Encourage high fiber diet, rich in Vitamin C
Activity	Maintain safety and sternotomy precautions TCDB q2hr Assist out of bed 2–3 times Begin ambulation per physical therapy protocol (50–100 feet)	Encourage self-care to tolerance Ambulate 150–200 feet qid
Psychosocial	Assess level of anxiety Encourage verbalization of concerns Provide information and ongoing support and encouragement to client and family	Encourage verbalization of concerns Provide ongoing support and encouragement to client and family
Medications	Oral analgesics Stool softener Diuretics as ordered Aspirin therapy SC heparin Intermittent IV device Routine meds as ordered	Oral analgesics Stool softener Aspirin therapy SC heparin (D/C per order) Routine meds as ordered D/C intermittent IV device if off telemetry Coumadin therapy if ordered
Transfer/ discharge plans	Review with patient and significant others progress toward discharge objectives Collaborate with physical therapy Make appropriate referrals	Review with client and family discharge objectives regarding activity and home care Collaborate with cardiac rehab and physical therapy

	Date _____ **5th Day Postoperative**	Date _____ **6th Day Postoperative**
Daily outcomes	Client will: • be afebrile, have stable vital signs, stable cardiac rhythm, and be awake, alert, and oriented • have a clean wound with edges well-approximated, healing by first intention	Client is afebrile Client is alert and oriented Client has a dry, clean wound with edges well-approximated, healing by first intention Client has stable vital signs and stable rhythm pattern Client manages pain with non-pharmacologic measures and ordered medications

Coronary Artery Bypass Surgery *(continued)*

	Date _____ **5th Day Postoperative**	Date _____ **6th Day Postoperative**
Daily outcomes (continued)	• demonstrate cooperation with turning, coughing, deep breathing, and splinting • tolerate ordered diet without nausea and vomiting • verbalize control of incisional pain • ambulate 150–300 feet 4 times • tolerate activity level without dyspnea, shortness of breath, or chest pain • demonstrates ability to cope	Client is independent in self-care Client ambulates 300–500 feet qid Client has resumed preadmission urine and bowel elimination pattern Client verbalizes/demonstrates home care instructions Client tolerates AHA diet Client demonstrates ability to cope with ongoing stressors
Assessments, tests, and treatments	Hemoglobin and hematocrit Vital signs q4hr and prn Head to toe assessment Remove dressings Assess wound healing Weight D/C epicardial pacing wires	Vital signs every shift Head to toe assessment q4-8hr and prn Assess wound healing Weight Assess pacing wire site
Knowledge deficit	Review plan of care with client and family Continue discharge teaching regarding wound care, activity, and diet Review safety measures for transfers and ambulation for home care Cardiac teaching Evaluate understanding of teaching	Client and family verbalizes understanding of discharge teaching, including wound care, activity level and exercise program, safety measures, diet, signs and symptoms to report, follow-up care and MD appointment, cardiac rehab, medications: name, purpose, dose, frequency, route, dietary interactions, and side effects, and home care arrangements Evaluate understanding of teaching
Diet	AHA diet as tolerated Encourage high-fiber diet, rich in vitamin C	AHA diet as tolerated Encourage high-fiber diet, rich in vitamin C
Activity	Ambulate 150–300 feet qid and stair climbing per physical therapy Shower	Ambulate 300–500 feet qid Shower
Psychosocial	Encourage verbalization of concerns Provide ongoing support and encouragement to client and family	Encourage verbalization of concerns Provide ongoing support and encouragement to client and family

Coronary Artery Bypass Surgery *(continued)*

	Date _____ **5th Day Postoperative**	Date _____ **6th Day Postoperative**

Medications	Oral analgesics
	Stool softener
	Laxative if no BM in 3 days
	Aspirin or coumadin therapy as
	   ordered
	Routine meds as ordered
		Oral analgesics
		Stool softener
		Aspirin or coumadin therapy as
		   ordered
		Routine meds as ordered

*Transfer/
discharge plans*
	Review with client and family dis-
	   charge objectives regarding
	   activity and home care
	Collaborate with cardiac rehab
	   and physical therapy
	Complete referrals for home
	   health care; including home
	   health aides, visiting nurse,
	   physical therapy, and cardiac
	   rehab
		Discharge with referrals for home
		   health care and cardiac rehab

Potential Client Variances
Coronary Artery Bypass Surgery

Possible Complications

- Myocardial infarction
- Dysrhythmias
- Heart failure
- Cardiac tamponade
- Pneumothorax, hemothorax
- Altered cerebral or renal tissue perfusion
- Pleural effusion
- Infection
- Non-union of sternum

Health Conditions

- Diabetes
- Recent myocardial infarction
- History of strokes

- Altered mental status
- Pre-existing respiratory disease
- Smoker
- Congestive heart failure
- Hypertension

Nursing Diagnoses

- Decreased cardiac output
- Fluid volume deficit or excess
- Risk for injury
- Activity tolerance
- Sensory/perceptual alterations
- Altered cerebral tissue perfusion
- Ineffective individual and/or family coping

Discharge Teaching for Client Following
Coronary Artery Bypass Surgery

Activity

- Gradually return to usual level of activity by increasing activity each day. Alternate activity with planned rest periods. Avoid fatigue.
- Continue exercise program as instructed by physical therapist.
- Avoid sitting or standing for long periods.
- Do not cross your legs.
- No strenuous activity until okayed by physician.
- Avoid heavy housework, straining, and driving for the period designated by your physician.

Diet

- Eat a well-balanced diet including all food groups. Continue any recommended dietary restrictions (usually low fat, low cholesterol, and low sodium).

Signs and Symptoms to Report

Notify physician if any of these symptoms occur:
- Increase in pain, redness, or swelling
- Sudden increase in wound drainage, especially if drainage has a foul odor.
- Chills, or fever greater than 100F or 38C
- Chest pain, dyspnea, shortness of breath, weight gain, or decrease in exercise tolerance

Follow-Up Care and General Health Care

- Schedule follow-up appointment with physician as directed.
- Schedule follow-up laboratory work as directed.
- Do not smoke, and avoid second-hand smoke.
- Discuss alcohol use with your physician.
- Begin cardiac rehabilitation program as directed.

Medications

- Review written list of medications, including dose, frequency, food interactions, and side effects.

Wound and Dressing Care

- Cleanse skin around incision daily with mild soap and water.
- If dressing present, change it daily and as often as necessary to keep dressing dry and clean.
- Remove dressing prior to showering and replace with a clean dressing afterward.
- Drainage, if present, should gradually decrease.
- If there is a marked increase in drainage, swelling, tenderness, fever, or if drainage is foul-smelling, notify physician.

Craniotomy for Brain Tumor

Expected length of stay: 3–4 days

	Date _____ **1st 24 Hours Postoperative**	Date _____ **2nd Day Postoperative**	Date _____ **3rd–4th Days Postoperative**
Daily outcomes	Client will: • maintain adequate cerebral blood flow as evidenced by stable vital signs, being alert and oriented, and maintaining usual sensory and motor function • maintain cranial nerve function • have stable vital signs and B/P within specified range • have lungs clear to auscultation • have unlabored respirations and maintain oxygen saturation > 95% • have clean, dry dressing • recover from anesthesia • verbalize understanding and demonstrate cooperation with turning and deep breathing • tolerate ordered diet without nausea and vomiting • verbalize control of incisional pain with ordered medications • demonstrate ability to cope	Client will: • maintain adequate cerebral blood flow as evidenced by stable vital signs, being alert and oriented, and maintaining usual sensory and motor function • maintain cranial nerve function • have stable vital signs and B/P within specified range • have lungs clear to auscultation • have unlabored respirations and maintain oxygen saturation > 95% • have clean, dry wound with edges well-approximated, healing by first intention • demonstrate cooperation with turning and deep breathing • tolerate ordered diet without nausea and vomiting • ambulate 4 times per day in hallway • verbalize control of incisional pain • demonstrate ability to cope • verbalize/demonstrate beginning understanding of home care instructions	Client is afebrile Client maintains adequate cerebral blood flow as evidenced by stable vital signs, being alert and oriented, and maintaining usual sensory and motor function Client maintains cranial nerve function Client has stable vital signs and B/P within specified range Client has lungs clear to auscultation and unlabored respiration with an oxygen saturation > 95% Client has clean, dry wound with edges well-approximated, healing by first intention Client manages pain with oral medications and/or non-pharmacologic measures Client is independent in self-care Client is fully ambulatory Client has resumed preadmission urine and bowel elimination pattern Client verbalizes ability to cope with changes and body image and utilizes strategies to cope with shaved scalp, scars, indentations, and any neurologic deficits Client verbalizes/demonstrates home care instructions Client tolerates ordered diet without nausea or vomiting Client demonstrates ability to cope with ongoing stressors including current illness and any neurologic deficits

➤

Craniotomy for Brain Tumor *(continued)*

	Date _____ **1st 24 Hours Postoperative**	Date _____ **2nd Day Postoperative**	Date _____ **3rd–4th Days Postoperative**
Assessments, tests, and treatments	Vital signs and O_2 saturation, neurovascular and mental status assessment, and dressing and wound drainage assessment q15min × 4; q30min × 4; q1hr × 24 and prn Ventilator care and weaning per protocol ABGs as indicated Cardiac monitoring Head of the bed up 30–45 degrees Avoid flexion, extension, and rotation of head and neck Monitor for seizures and protect from injury ICP monitoring per clinical protocol Maintain patency of any drains Assess cranial nerve function q2–4hr and prn Monitor for bleeding, cerebral edema and/or cerebral ischemia Incentive spirometer q2hr Intake and output every shift Foley catheter Assess coping status of client and family Provide ongoing emotional support to client and family Allow for client's input regarding care When extubated, administer oxygen as ordered to maintain O_2 saturation >92%	Vital signs, neurovascular and cranial nerve assessment, O_2 saturation and dressing and wound drainage assessment q2–4hr and prn Head of the bed up 30–45 degrees Avoid flexion, extension, and rotation of head and neck Monitor for seizures and protect from injury Monitor for bleeding, cerebral edema and/or cerebral ischemia Assess respiratory status q4hr and prn Incentive spirometer q2hr until fully ambulatory Intake and output every shift O_2 as indicated Remove catheter and assess voiding—if unable to void, try suggestive voiding techniques or, if still unable, catheterize q8hr or prn Dressing change BID and prn Assess coping status of client and family Encourage client and family to verbalize feelings regarding any changes in appearance and functional abilities Provide ongoing emotional support to client and family	Vital signs, neurovascular and cranial nerve assessment, O_2 saturation, and dressing and wound drainage assessment q4–8hr and prn Assess respiratory status q4–8hr Assess wound and apply dry sterile dressing every day and prn Encourage client to verbalize regarding any changes in appearance and functional ability Assist client and family to identify any resources or strategies to cope with changes in appearance and functional ability Assess coping status and provide appropriate emotional support Provide ongoing emotional support to client and family
Knowledge deficit	Orient to room and surroundings Provide simple, brief instructions Include family in teaching Review specific postoperative care: turning, deep breathing, incentive spirometer, mobilization, intravenous, pain management (prn medications) Instruct client regarding the importance of supporting head and neck during position changes Evaluate understanding of teaching	Review plan of care and importance of early mobilization Begin discharge teaching regarding wound care/dressing change, diet, and activity Review written discharge instructions with client and family Evaluate understanding of teaching	Complete discharge teaching to include wound care, diet, follow-up care and appointment, signs and symptoms to report, activity, and medication: name, purpose, dose, frequency, route, food interactions, and side effects Provide client with written discharge instructions regarding home care Evaluate understanding of teaching

Craniotomy for Brain Tumor *(continued)*

	Date _____ 1st 24 Hours Postoperative	Date _____ 2nd Day Postoperative	Date _____ 3rd–4th Days Postoperative
Diet	Prior to offering fluids, assess return of gag reflex and ability to chew and swallow HOB up for meals Maintain fluid restriction When fully awake clear liquids as tolerated	Full liquids to diet as tolerated Maintain fluid restriction HOB up for meals	Diet as tolerated Maintain fluid restriction HOB up for meals
Activity	Assess safety needs and provide adequate precautions HOB up 30 degrees, support head and neck when changing positions Dangle/chair evening of surgery if stable	Maintain safety precautions Fully ambulatory in room with required assistance Walk in hall 4–6 times with required assistance	Maintain safety precautions Fully ambulatory
Medications	IV fluids Antiepilepsy medications as ordered Glucocorticosteroids as ordered Diuretics as ordered Analgesics as ordered H_2-receptor antagonists as ordered Stool softeners, antitussives, and antiemetics as ordered Antihypertensives as ordered	Intermittent IV device Antiepilepsy medications as ordered Glucocorticosteroids as ordered Diuretics as ordered Analgesics as ordered H_2-receptor antagonists as ordered Stool softeners, antitussives, and antiemetics as ordered	D/C IV device Antiepilepsy medications as ordered Glucocorticosteroids as ordered Diuretics as ordered Analgesics as ordered Other medications as ordered
Transfer/ discharge plans	Establish discharge objectives with client and family Determine discharge needs and assess support system Begin home care instructions	Review progress toward discharge goals Make appropriate referrals Finalize discharge plans	Finalize any home care arrangements Complete discharge instructions

Potential Client Variances
Craniotomy for Brain Tumor

Possible Complications

- Increased intracranial pressure
- Hemorrhage or infection
- Altered cerebral tissue perfusion
- Seizures
- Diabetes insipidus

Health Conditions

- Pre-existing neurologic or sensory/perceptual problems
- Pre-existing respiratory problems

Nursing Diagnoses

- Acute pain/headache
- Risk for infection
- Self-concept disturbance

Discharge Teaching for Client Following
Craniotomy for Brain Tumor

Activity
- Gradually return to usual level of activity by increasing activity each day. Alternate activity with rest periods. Avoid fatigue.
- No strenuous activity until okayed by physician.
- Avoid heavy housework, straining, and driving for the period designated by your physician.

Diet
- Eat a well-balanced diet, including all food groups. Maintain any recommended dietary prescription.
- Drink 6–8 glasses of fluid each day.

Signs and Symptoms to Support
Notify physician if any of these symptoms occur:
- Increase in pain, redness, or swelling
- Headaches, seizures, or nausea
- Sudden increase in wound drainage, especially if drainage has pus or has a foul odor
- Chills, or fever greater than 100F or 38C

Follow-Up Care and General Health Care
- Schedule follow-up appointment with physician as directed.
- Discuss alcohol use with your physician.

Medications
- Review written list of medications, including dose, frequency, food interactions, and side effects.

Wound and Dressing Care
- Cleanse skin around incision daily with mild soap and water.
- If dressing present, change it daily and as often as necessary to keep dressing dry and clean.
- Remove dressing prior to showering and replace with a clean dressing afterward.
- Drainage, if present, should gradually decrease.
- If there is a marked increase in drainage, swelling, tenderness, or fever, or if drainage is foul-smelling, notify physician.

Cystectomy with Ileal Conduit

Expected length of stay: 6–7 day

	Date _____ **Preoperative**	Date _____ **1st 24 Hours Postoperative**	Date _____ **2nd-3rd Days Postoperative**
Daily outcomes	Client verbalizes understanding of preoperative teaching, including: turning, coughing, deep breathing, incentive spirometer, mobilization, possible tubes (nasogastric tube, IV, penrose or other drains), urostomy, and pain management Client demonstrates ability to cope Client verbalizes understanding of procedure Obtain informed consent	Client will: • have stable vital signs • have a clean, dry wound with edges well-approximated, healing by first intention • recover from anesthesia as evidenced by VS return to baseline and being awake, alert, and oriented • verbalize understanding and demonstrate cooperation with turning, coughing, deep breathing and splinting • have lungs clear to auscultation • have urine output >30 mL/hr and patent urostomy • verbalize understanding of PCA/epidural if in use • verbalize control of incisional pain • transfer out of bed with assistance 2–3 times • demonstrate ability to cope	Client will: • be afebrile • have a clean, dry wound with edges well-approximated, healing by first intention • have intact, non-reddened peristomal skin • have active bowel sounds • tolerate ordered diet without vomiting • have urine output >30mL/hr and patent urostomy • demonstrate cooperation with turning, coughing, deep breathing and splinting • ambulate 4 times • verbalize control of incisional pain • verbalize ability to cope • verbalize beginning understanding of home care instructions including self-management of urostomy
Assessments, tests, and treatments	CBC Urinalysis Chest x-ray Baseline physical assessment with a focus on respiratory status and gastrointestinal function Assess and record the description, location, duration, and characteristics of client's pain Reduce or eliminate pain-producing factors, such as fear and anxiety	CBC Electrolytes Vital signs and O_2 saturation, neurovascular assessment, and dressing and wound drainage assessment q15min × 4; q30min × 4; q1hr × 4 and then q4hr and prn Assess respiratory status and gastrointestinal function q4hr and prn Incentive spirometer q2hr O_2 as indicated Intake and output every shift Assess patency of NG tube q2 hr, noting volume q2hr and prn Assess urinary output from urostomy q1–2hr and prn	Vital signs and dressing and wound drainage assessment q4hr Assess respiratory status and gastrointestinal function q4hr Incentive spirometer q2hr until fully ambulatory O_2 as indicated Intake and output every shift If still in place, assess patency and output of NG tube q4hr Assess urinary output q2–4hr Using sterile asepsis, change dressing: assess wound healing and wound drainage Assess and record the description, location, duration, and characteristics of client's pain q4hr and prn

➤

Cystectomy with Ileal Conduit *(continued)*

	Date _____ **Preoperative**	Date _____ **1st 24 Hours Postoperative**	Date _____ **2nd-3rd Days Postoperative**
Assessments, tests, and treatments (continued)		Assess and record the description, location, duration, and characteristics of client's pain q2–4hr and prn Encourage verbalization of pain and discomfort Reduce or eliminate pain-producing factors and employ distraction or relaxation techniques Provide back rubs Encourage client to request analgesic or use PCA (if in use) before pain becomes severe Assess effectiveness of pain relief measures Assess stoma for edema, cyanosis, and bleeding Assess peristomal skin for erythema, integrity, or irritation Assess appliance for proper fit	Reduce or eliminate pain-producing factors, employ distraction or relaxation techniques, and offer back rubs Assess effectiveness of pain relief measures Assess stoma for edema, cyanosis, and bleeding Assess appliance for proper fit Assess peristomal skin for erythema, integrity, or irritation
Knowledge deficit	Orient to room and surroundings Provide simple, brief instructions Review preoperative preparation including hospital and surgical routines Include family in teaching Discuss surgery and specific postoperative care: turning, coughing, deep breathing, splinting incision, incentive spirometer, mobilization, possible tubes (nasogastric [NG] and intravenous [IV]), and pain management (PCA , epidural, or prn medications) Instruct regarding distraction techniques, such as slow rhythmic breathing and guided imagery, to produce pain relief Instruct in relaxation techniques, such as tensing and relaxing muscle groups and rhythmic breathing Evaluate understanding of teaching	Reorient to room and postoperative routine Include family in teaching Review plan of care and importance of early mobilization Review importance of turning, coughing, deep breathing, splinting incision, incentive spirometer, mobilization, drainage and intravenous tubes, and pain management (PCA, epidural, or prn medications) Evaluate understanding of teaching	Reinforce earlier teaching regarding ongoing care Include family in teaching Begin discharge teaching regarding wound care/dressing change and care of stoma and skin, including application of an appliance, and signs and symptoms of urinary tract infection Evaluate understanding of teaching

Cystectomy with Ileal Conduit *(continued)*

	Date _____ **Preoperative**	Date _____ **1st 24 Hours Postoperative**	Date _____ **2nd–3rd Days Postoperative**
Psychosocial	Assess anxiety related to diagnosis and pending surgery Assess fears of the unknown related to surgery Encourage verbalization of concerns Minimize external stimuli (e.g. noise, movement) Offer emotional support	Assess level of anxiety Encourage verbalization of concerns Provide information and ongoing support and encouragement to client and family Offer emotional support	Assess level of anxiety Encourage verbalization of concerns Provide ongoing support and encouragement Offer emotional support
Diet	NPO Baseline nutritional and hydration assessment	NPO NG tube until return of bowel sounds	When NG tube removed, begin clear liquids to tolerance
Activity	Assess safety needs and provide appropriate measures Activity as ordered	Maintain safety precautions Assist to chair 2–3 times	Maintain safety precautions Ambulate 4 times with assistance
Medications	Preoperative medications as ordered	IV fluids IV antibiotics Analgesics as ordered	IV fluids IV antibiotics When ordered, convert IV to intermittent IV device Analgesics as ordered
Transfer/ discharge plans	Assess potential discharge needs and support system Establish discharge goals with client and family	Review progress toward discharge goals with client and family Consult with social service regarding VNA and projected needs for home health care (if any)	Review progress toward discharge goals with client and family Make appropriate discharge referrals

	Date _____ **4th Day Postoperative**	Date _____ **5th Day Postoperative**	Date _____ **6th Day Postoperative**
Daily outcomes	Client will: • be afebrile and have stable vital signs • have a clean, dry wound with edges well-approximated, healing by first intention • have intact, non-reddened peristomal skin • tolerate ordered diet without nausea or vomiting • maintain urine output >30 mL/hr and patent urostomy • ambulate 4–6 times • verbalize control of incisional pain	Client will: • be afebrile and have stable vital signs • have a clean, dry wound with edges well-approximated, healing by first intention • have intact, non-reddened peristomal skin • tolerate ordered diet without nausea or vomiting • maintain urine output >30 mL/hr and patent urostomy • ambulate 4–6 times • verbalize control of incisional pain	Client is afebrile and has stable vital signs Client has a clean, dry wound with edges well-approximated, healing by first intention Peristomal skin remains intact and without redness Client manages pain with non-pharmacologic measures and any ordered medications Client is independent in self-care Client is fully ambulatory Client has resumed preadmission bowel elimination pattern

➤

Cystectomy with Ileal Conduit *(continued)*

	Date _____ **4th Day Postoperative**	Date _____ **5th Day Postoperative**	Date _____ **6th Day Postoperative**
Daily outcomes *(continued)*	• verbalize ability to cope • verbalize beginning understanding of home care instructions • verbalize/demonstrate understanding of self-management of urostomy	• verbalize ability to cope • verbalize beginning understanding of home care instructions • safely and correctly demonstrate self-management of urostomy	Client has a patent urostomy and urine remains free of infection Client verbalizes home care instructions, including self-managment of urostomy Client tolerates usual diet Client verbalizes ability to cope with ongoing stressors
Assessments, tests, and treatments	Vital signs and dressing and wound drainage assessment q4hr and prn Incentive spirometer q2hr until fully ambulatory Intake and output every shift Assess urinary output q4hr and prn Assess respiratory status and gastrointestinal function q4–8hr Using sterile asepsis, change dressing, assess wound healing and wound drainage Assess and record description, location, duration, and characteristics of client's pain q4hr and prn Encourage client to employ distraction or relaxation techniques	Vital signs and dressing and wound drainage assessment q4hr and prn Assess respiratory status and gastrointestinal function q4–8hr Assess urinary output q4hr and prn Remove dressing and assess wound healing and drainage Assess and record description, location, duration, and characteristics of client's pain q4hr and prn Encourage client to employ distraction or relaxation techniques	Vital signs and dressing and wound drainage assessment q4–8hr Assess respiratory status and gastrointestinal function Assess wound healing Assess urinary output Assess and record description, location, duration, and characteristics of client's pain q4hr and prn Encourage client to employ distraction or relaxation techniques
Knowledge deficit	Include family in teaching Initiate discharge teaching regarding wound care, diet, and activity Continue teaching related to stoma care including care of stoma, peristomal skin, and application of appliance Review written discharge instructions with client and family Evaluate understanding of teaching	Continue discharge teaching to client and family regarding wound care, diet, signs and symptoms to report, medications, and activity Continue teaching related to stoma care including care of stoma, peristomal skin, and application of appliance Review written discharge instructions with client and family Evaluate understanding of teaching	Complete discharge teaching to include wound care, diet, follow-up care, signs and symptoms to report, activity, and medications: name, purpose, dose, frequency, route, dietary interactions, and side effects Complete teaching related to stoma care Provide client with written discharge instructions Refer any knowledge deficits to appropriate community resources Evaluate understanding of teaching

Cystectomy with Ileal Conduit *(continued)*

	Date _____ **4th Day Postoperative**	Date _____ **5th Day Postoperative**	Date _____ **6th Day Postoperative**
Psychosocial	Encourage verbalization of concerns Provide ongoing support and encouragement	Encourage verbalization of concerns Provide ongoing support and encouragement	Encourage verbalization of concerns Provide ongoing support and encouragement
Diet	If tolerating clear liquids, advance to full liquids as tolerated	Advance diet to soft, regular diet as tolerated	Regular diet as tolerated
Activity	Ambulate independently at least 4 times Maintain safety precautions	Fully ambulatory Maintain safety precautions	Fully ambulatory
Medications	Oral analgesics as ordered Intermittent IV device for any IV medications—D/C when so ordered	Provide oral analgesics	Provide oral analgesics
Transfer/ discharge plans	Continue to review progress toward discharge goals	Finalize discharge plans Continue to review progress toward discharge goals Finalize plans for home care if needed	Complete discharge instructions

Potential Client Variances
Cystectomy with Ileal Conduit

Possible Complications

- Peritonitis
- Infection
- Hemorrhage

Health Conditions

- Diabetes
- Pre-existing renal disease
- Pre-existing respiratory disease

Nursing Diagnoses

- Body image disturbance
- Self-care deficits
- Impaired skin integrity
- Ineffective individual coping

Discharge Teaching for Client Following
Cystectomy with Ileal Conduit

Activity

- Gradually return to usual level of activity by increasing activity each day. Alternate activity with rest periods. Avoid fatigue and plan rest periods throughout the day.
- You may go up and down stairs.
- Avoid heavy housework, straining, heavy lifting, and driving for the period designated by your physician.
- You may shower with your pouch on.

Diet

- Eat a well-balanced diet, including all food groups.
- Report nausea, vomiting, or change in bowel habits.
- Drink 6–8 glasses of fluid each day.

Signs and Symptoms to Report

Notify physician if any of these symptoms occur:
- Increase in pain or any redness or swelling in wound
- Sudden increase in wound drainage, especially if drainage has pus or a foul odor
- Report redness or skin breakdown around stoma
- Report foul-smelling urine
- Chills, or fever greater than 100F or 38C

Follow-Up Care and General Health Care

- Schedule follow-up appointment with physician as directed
- Refer to local support group

Medications

- Review written list of medications, including dose, route, frequency, food interactions, and side effects.
- Avoid alcohol if taking medication.

Wound and Dressing Care

- Cleanse skin around incision daily with mild soap and water.
- If dressing present, change it daily and as often as necessary to keep dressing dry and clean.
- Remove dressing prior to showering and replace with a clean dressing afterward.
- Drainage, if present, should gradually decrease.
- If there is a marked increase in drainage, swelling, tenderness, or fever, or if drainage is foul-smelling, notify physician.

Stoma Care

- Drain your drainage bag when it is one-half full.
- Plan to change your drainage system every 3 to 5 days. If there is evidence of leakage before this time, be sure to change the system.
- Before changing the system, gather your supplies and prepare the pouch.
- Remove the old bag from around the stoma and discard the old bag.
- Place a tampon or gauze wick over the stoma to help keep urine from leaking from the stoma. Cleanse the skin around the stoma with warm water and skin cleanser. Rinse the skin well and pat it dry. Carefully inspect the skin around the stoma for any signs of irritation, chafing, or rash. Check the skin every time you change the bag. If there is redness or skin breakdown, notify your ostomy nurse or physician.
- Wipe the skin around the stoma with the skin gel protective wipe. Allow it to dry thoroughly.
- Apply the pouch over the stoma and press it firmly into place. Make sure the adhesive is sealed firmly around the stoma and smooth the tape around the edges.
- Report any significant changes in the character, quality, or quantity of urine output.

Femoral Popliteal Bypass Graft

Expected length of stay: 3–4 days

	Date _____ **Preoperative**	Date _____ **1st 24 Hours Postoperative**
Daily outcomes	Client verbalizes understanding of preoperative teaching, including turning, coughing, and deep breathing, IV therapy, mobilization, O_2 therapy and pain management Client demonstrates ability to cope Client verbalizes understanding of procedure Obtain informed consent	Client will: • maintain adequate circulation to affected extremity(ies) as evidenced by capillary refill less than 3 seconds, pink and warm extremity, palpable, distal pulses (or pulses by Doppler), and adequate sensation and motion • have clean, dry dressing • recover from anesthesia as evidenced by VS return to baseline, and being awake, alert, and oriented • verbalize understanding and demonstrate cooperation with turning, deep breathing, coughing, and splinting • tolerate ordered diet without nausea and vomiting • verbalize control of incisional pain with ordered medications • demonstrate cooperation with measures to prevent compromised blood flow • demonstrate ability to cope
Assessments, tests, and treatments	CBC Urinalysis CXR EKG Baseline physical assessment with focus on respiratory, cardiovascular, and renal function	Vital signs and O_2 saturation, neurovascular assessment, and dressing and wound drainage assessment q15min × 4; q30min × 4; q1hr × 4 and then q4hr and prn Peripheral CSM assessment q1hr and prn Report diminished or absent pulse stat Report signs or symptoms of diminished peripheral blood flow immediately Monitor for compartment syndrome or nerve damage Head to toe assessment q4hr and prn Incentive spirometer q2hr O_2 if indicated Intake and output every shift Assess voiding — if unable to void, try suggestive voiding techniques or, if still unable, catheterize q8hr or prn Minimize stressful situations Maintain comfortable room temperature and avoid chilling

➤

	Date _____ **Preoperative**	Date _____ **1st 24 Hours Postoperative**
Knowledge deficit	Orient to room and surroundings Provide simple, brief instructions Preoperative teaching to include: turning, coughing, and deep breathing, IV therapy, mobilization, O$_2$ therapy, and PCA/epidural for pain management Evaluate understanding of teaching	Orient to room and surroundings Provide simple, brief instructions Include family in teaching Review specific postoperative care: turning, coughing, deep breathing, incentive spirometer, mobilization, intravenous, and pain management (epidural, PCA, or prn medications) Instruct client not to compromise blood flow by crossing legs or flexing hips at 90 degrees for prolonged periods Evaluate understanding of teaching
Psychosocial	Assess anxiety regarding impending surgery Assess fear of unknown related to surgery Offer emotional support Encourage verbalization of concerns Minimize external stimuli (noise, movement)	Assess level of anxiety Assess coping status of client and family Provide information and ongoing support and encouragement to client and family
Diet	NPO Baseline nutritional and hydration assessment	Clear fluids to ordered diet as tolerated
Activity	Assess potential safety needs and provide appropriate safety measures	Assess safety needs and provide appropriate precautions Do not gatch bed Bedrest until AM then ambulate with assistance Active foot and leg exercises q1–2hr while awake Bed cradle over lower extremities
Medications	Preoperative medications per anesthesia IV fluids as ordered	Analgesics as ordered IV antibiotics if ordered IV fluids as ordered Routine meds as ordered
Transfer/ discharge plans	Assess potential discharge needs and support system Establish discharge goals with client and family	Establish discharge goals with client and family Determine possible discharge needs and support system with client and family Begin home care instructions

Femoral Popliteal Bypass Graft *(continued)*

	Date _____ **2nd Day Postoperative**	Date _____ **3rd–4th Days Postoperative**
Daily outcomes	Client will: • maintain adequate circulation to affected extremity(ies) as evidenced by capillary refill less than 3 seconds, pink, warm extremity, palpable, distal pulses (or pulses by Doppler), and adequate sensation and motion • have stable vital signs • have clean, dry wound with edges well-approximated, healing by first intention • demonstrate cooperation with turning, deep breathing, coughing, and splinting • tolerate ordered diet without nausea and vomiting • ambulate 4 times per day in hallway • verbalize control of incisional pain with ordered medications • demonstrate ability to cope • verbalize/demonstrate beginning understanding of home care instructions	Client is afebrile, with stable vital signs Client has adequate and stable circulation to affected extremity Client has clean, dry wound with edges well-approximated, healing by first intention Client manages pain with oral medications and/or non–pharmacologic measures Client is independent in self–care Client is fully ambulatory Client has resumed preadmission urine and bowel elimination patterns Client verbalizes home care instructions Client tolerates ordered diet Client demonstrates ability to cope with ongoing stressors Client verbalizes/demonstrates knowledge of discharge instructions and home care routines, including strategies to enhance circulation and prevent worsening arteriosclerosis
Assessments, tests, and treatments	Vital signs and dressing and wound drainage assessment q4hr and prn Peripheral CSM assessment q1–2hr and prn Report diminished or absent pulse stat Immediately report signs or symptoms of diminished peripheral blood flow Monitor for compartment syndrome or nerve damage Head to toe assessment q4hr Incentive spirometer q2hr until fully ambulatory Intake and output every shift Assess voiding pattern every shift Assess wound and change dressing BID Minimize stressful situations Maintain comfortable room temperature and avoid chilling	Vital signs, dressing, and wound drainage assessment q4–8hr Peripheral CSM assessment q2–4hr and prn Report absent or diminished pulse stat Immediately report signs or symptoms of diminished peripheral blood flow Monitor for compartment syndrome or nerve damage Head to toe assessment q4–8hr Assess wounds and apply dry sterile dressing every day and prn Minimize stressful situations Maintain comfortable room temperature and avoid chilling
Knowledge deficit	Review plan of care and importance of early mobilization Include family in teaching Begin discharge teaching regarding wound care/dressing change, diet, and activity Review written discharge instructions with client and family Review precautions to minimize the compromise of blood flow Evaluate understanding of teaching	Complete discharge teaching to include wound care, diet, follow-up care, signs and symptoms to report, activity, and medication: name, purpose, dose, frequency, route, food interactions, and side effects Include family in teaching Provide client with written discharge instructions Evaluate understanding of teaching

➤

	Date _____ **2nd Day Postoperative**	Date _____ **3rd–4th Days Postoperative**
Psychosocial	Assess level of anxiety Assess coping status of client and family Encourage verbalization of concerns Provide ongoing support and encouragement to client and family	Assess level of anxiety Assess coping status of client and family Encourage verbalization of concerns Provide ongoing support and encouragement to client and family
Diet	Diet as ordered or low-salt, low-fat and low-cholesterol diet as tolerated Dietary consult for teaching	Diet as ordered or low-salt, low-fat and low-cholesterol diet as tolerated Provide client written copy of diet
Activity	Maintain safety precautions Fully ambulatory in room No prolonged sitting Walk in hall 4–6 times per day Active foot and leg exercises q1–2hr while awake Bed cradle over lower extremities	Maintain safety precautions Fully ambulatory Active foot and leg exercises q1–2hr while awake Bed cradle over lower extremities
Medications	D/C epidural Analgesics as ordered IV antibiotics if ordered Intermittent IV device Routine meds as ordered	Oral analgesics D/C IV device Routine meds as ordered
Transfer/ discharge plans	Review progress toward discharge goals Finalize discharge plans Make referrals for home care	Complete discharge instructions Finalize any arrangements for home care

Potential Client Variances
Femoral Popliteal Bypass Graft

Possible Complications
- Compartment syndrome
- Graft occlusion
- Saphenous nerve damage
- Hemorrhage

Health Conditions
- Diabetes
- Pre-existing tissue damage
- Smoker
- Advanced peripheral vascular disease
- Clotting disorders
- Pre-existing respiratory or cardiac disorders

Nursing Diagnoses
- Acute pain
- Risk for infection

Discharge Teaching for Client Following
Femoral Popliteal Bypass Graft

Activity

- Gradually return to usual level of activity by increasing activity each day. Alternate activity with rest periods. Avoid fatigue.
- No sitting or standing for long periods.
- Do not cross your legs.
- No strenuous activity until okayed by physician.
- Avoid heavy housework, straining, and driving for the period designated by your physician.

Diet

- Eat a well-balanced diet, including all food groups. Maintain any recommended dietary prescription.
- Drink 6–8 glasses of fluid each day.

Signs and Symptoms to Report

Notify physician if any of these symptoms occur:

- Increase in pain, redness, or swelling
- Sudden increase in wound drainage, especially if drainage has pus or a foul odor
- Chills, or fever greater than 100F or 38C
- Pain in your legs with or without numbness or tingling
- Calf pain when walking
- Cool feet or legs
- Pale or dusky-colored feet

Follow-Up Care and General Health Care

- Schedule follow-up appointment with physician as directed.
- Do not smoke, and avoid second-hand smoke.
- Discuss alcohol use with your physician.
- Do not wear restrictive or tight clothing.
- Avoid extremes of cold and heat.
- Keep your lower legs and feet warm.
- Avoid the use of artificial heating devices such as heating pads and hot water bottles.

Medications

- Review written list of medications, including dose, frequency, food interactions, and side effects.

Wound and Dressing Care

- Cleanse skin around incision daily with mild soap and water.
- If dressing present, change it daily and as often as necessary to keep dressing dry and clean.
- Remove dressing prior to showering and replace with a clean dressing afterward.
- Drainage, if present, should gradually decrease.
- If there is a marked increase in drainage, swelling, tenderness, or fever, or if drainage is foul-smelling, notify physician.

Critical Pathway for Client Following

Partial Gastrectomy

Expected length of stay: 5–7 days

	Date _____ **Preoperative**	Date _____ **1st Day Postoperative**	Date _____ **2nd–3rd Days Postoperative**
Daily outcomes	Client verbalizes understanding of preoperative teaching, including: turning, coughing, deep breathing, incentive spirometer, mobilization, nasogastric tube, possible other tubes, and pain management Client demonstrates ability to cope Client verbalizes understanding of procedures Obtain informed consent	Client will: • have stable vital signs • have a clean, dry wound with edges well-approximated, healing by first intention • recover from anesthesia as evidenced by: VS return to baseline, and being awake, alert, and oriented • verbalize understanding and demonstrate cooperation with turning, coughing, deep breathing and splinting • demonstrate ability to use PCA • verbalize control of incisional pain • be up to chair 2–3 times • demonstrate ability to cope	Client will: • have stable vital signs • have a clean, dry wound with edges well-approximated, healing by first intention • demonstrate cooperation with turning, coughing, deep breathing and splinting • ambulate 3–4 times • verbalize control of incisional pain • demonstrate ability to cope • verbalize beginning understanding of home care instructions
Assessments, tests, and treatments	CBC Urinalysis Chest x-ray Baseline physical assessment with a focus on respiratory status and gastrointestinal function Assess and record the description, location, duration, and characteristics of client's pain Instruct in relaxation and distraction techniques as an adjunct to pain medications	CBC Electrolytes Vital signs and O_2 saturation, neurovascular assessment, and dressing and wound drainage assessment q15min × 4; q30min × 4; q1hr × 4 and then q4hr and prn Assess respiratory status and gastrointestinal function q4hr and prn Incentive spirometer q2hr O_2 as indicated Intake and output every shift Assess patency of NG tube q2hr and prn, noting volume q2hr Report any nausea or vomiting Do not irrigate NG tube without MD order Assess voiding — if unable to void, try suggestive voiding techniques or, if still unable, catheterize q8hr or prn Assess and record the description, location, duration, and characteristics of client's pain q2–4hr and prn	Vital signs and dressing and wound drainage assessment q4hr and prn Assess respiratory status and gastrointestinal function q4hr Incentive spirometer q2hr until fully ambulatory O_2 as indicated Intake and output every shift Assess patency and output of NG tube q4–8hr Do not irrigate NG tube without MD order D/C NG tube when ordered Assess voiding pattern every shift Using sterile asepsis, change dressing: assess wound healing and wound drainage Assess and record the description, location, duration, and characteristics of client's pain q4hr and prn Reduce or eliminate pain-producing factors, employ distraction or relaxation techniques, and offer back rubs

Partial Gastrectomy *(continued)*

	Date _____ **Preoperative**	Date _____ **1st Day Postoperative**	Date _____ **2nd–3rd Days Postoperative**
Assessments, tests, and treatments (continued)		Encourage verbalization of pain and discomfort Reduce or eliminate pain-producing factors and employ distraction or relaxation techniques Provide back rubs	
Knowledge deficit	Orient to room and surroundings Provide simple, brief instructions Review preoperative preparation including hospital and surgical routines Discuss surgery and specific postoperative care: turning, coughing, deep breathing, splinting incision, incentive spirometer, mobilization, possible tubes (nasogastric [NG] and intravenous [IV]), and pain management (PCA or prn medications) Include family in teaching Evaluate understanding of teaching	Reorient to room and postoperative routine Review plan of care and importance of early mobilization Review importance of turning, coughing, deep breathing, splinting incision, incentive spirometer, mobilization, possible tubes (nasogastric [NG] and intravenous [IV]), pain management (PCA or prn medications) Include family in teaching Evaluate understanding of teaching	Reinforce earlier teaching regarding ongoing care Begin discharge teaching regarding wound care/dressing change Include family in teaching Evaluate understanding of teaching
Psychosocial	Assess anxiety related to diagnosis and pending surgery Assess fears of the unknown and surgery Encourage verbalization of concerns Offer emotional support Provide information regarding surgical experience Provide support to family Minimize external stimuli (eg, noise, movement)	Assess level of anxiety Encourage verbalization of concerns Provide information and ongoing support and encouragement to client and family	Encourage verbalization of concerns Provide information and ongoing support and encouragement to client and family
Diet	NPO Baseline nutritional assessment	NPO NG tube until return of bowel sounds	NPO NG tube until return of bowel sounds
Activity	Assess safety needs and provide safety precautions Activity as tolerated	Maintain safety precautions Bathroom privileges with assistance Assist to chair 2–3 times	Maintain safety precautions Ambulate 3–4 times with assistance

➤

Partial Gastrectomy *(continued)*

	Date _____ **Preoperative**	Date _____ **1st Day Postoperative**	Date _____ **2nd–3rd Days Postoperative**
Medications	Administer prescribed preopera-tive medications as ordered	Administer prescribed analgesics and record response Encourage client to request analgesic or use PCA before pain becomes severe IV antibiotics IV fluids TPN if ordered IV H$_2$– receptor antagonists if ordered	Administer prescribed analgesics and record response Encourage client to request analgesic or use PCA before pain becomes severe IV antibiotics IV fluids TPN if ordered IV H$_2$–receptor antagonists
Transfer/ discharge plans	Assess potential discharge needs and suport system Establish discharge goals with client and family	Review progress toward discharge goals with client and family Consult with social service regarding projected needs for home health care (if any)	Review progress toward discharge goals with client and family

	Date _____ **4th Day Postoperative**	Date _____ **5th Day Postoperative**	Date _____ **6th–7th Day Postoperative**
Daily outcomes	Client will: • be afebrile and have stable vital signs • have a clean, dry wound with edges well-approximated, heal-ing by first intention • tolerate clear liquids without nausea or vomiting • ambulate independently 4–6 times • verbalize control of incisional pain • demonstrate ability to cope • verbalize understanding of home care instructions	Client will: • be afebrile and have stable vital signs • have a clean, dry wound with edges well-approximated, heal-ing by first intention • tolerate ordered diet without nausea or vomiting • be fully ambulatory • verbalize control of incisional pain • demonstrate ability to cope • verbalize understanding of home care instructions	Client is afebrile and has stable vital signs Client has a clean, dry wound with edges well-approximated, heal-ing by first intention Client manages pain with non-pharmacologic measures Client is independent in self-care Client is fully ambulatory Client has resumed preadmission urine and bowel elimination pattern and remains free of diarrhea Client verbalizes home care instructions Client tolerates ordered diet Client remains free of dumping syndrome and afferent loop syndrome Client demonstrates ability to cope with ongoing stressors

Partial Gastrectomy *(continued)*

	Date _____ **4th Day Postoperative**	Date _____ **5th Day Postoperative**	Date _____ **6th–7th Days Postoperative**
Assessments, tests, and treatments	Vital signs and dressing and wound drainage assessment q4hr and prn Incentive spirometer q2hr until fully ambulatory Intake and output every shift Assess voiding pattern every shift Assess respiratory status and gastrointestinal function q4–8hrs Using sterile asepsis, change dressing: assess wound healing and wound drainage Assess and record description, location, duration, and characteristics of client's pain q4hr and prn Encourage client to employ distraction or relaxation techniques	Vital signs and dressing and wound drainage assessment q4hr and prn Assess respiratory status and gastrointestinal function Using sterile technique, change dressing and assess wound healing and drainage Assess and record description, location, duration, and characteristics of client's pain q4hr and prn Encourage client to employ distraction or relaxation techniques	Vital signs and dressing and wound drainage assessment q4hr Assess respiratory status and gastrointestinal function Remove dressing and assess wound healing Assess and record description, location, duration, and characteristics of client's pain q4hr and prn Encourage client to employ distraction or relaxation techniques
Knowledge deficit	Initiate discharge teaching regarding wound care, diet, and activity Review written discharge instructions with client and family Evaluate understanding of teaching	Continue discharge teaching regarding wound care, diet, signs and symptoms to report, medications, and activity Review interventions to minimize recurrence of peptic ulcer disease (if appropriate) Review written discharge instructions with client and family Evaluate understanding of teaching	Complete discharge teaching to include wound care, diet, follow-up care, signs and symptoms to report, activity, and medications: dose, frequency, route, food interactions, and side effects Review strategies to prevent dumping syndrome, the importance of adequate nutrition, and the necessity of follow-up care and laboratory work to monitor for pernicious anemia Provide client with written discharge instructions
Psychosocial	Encourage verbalization of concerns Provide ongoing support and encouragement	Encourage verbalization of concerns Provide ongoing support and encouragement	Encourage verbalization of concerns Provide ongoing support and encouragement
Diet	If NG tube removed and bowel sounds present, begin ordered diet (clear liquids) in small amounts Avoid simple carbohydrates	Advance to full liquid diet in small amounts throughout the day if tolerated Visit with dietitian for meal planning at home	Advance to soft diet if tolerated Offer small, frequent feedings Instruct client in the importance of drinking fluids between meals Instruct client to chew food well and eat slowly
Activity	Ambulate independently at least 4–6 times per day	Fully ambulatory	Fully ambulatory

	Date _____ **4th Day Postoperative**	Date _____ **5th Day Postoperative**	Date _____ **6th–7th Days Postoperative**
Medications	Provide ordered analgesics Intermittent IV device IV medications as ordered	Provide oral analgesics D/C intermittent IV device	Oral medications as ordered
Transfer/ discharge plans	Continue to review progress toward discharge goals	Finalize discharge plans Continue to review progress toward discharge goals Finalize plans for home care if needed	Complete discharge instructions

Potential Client Variances
Partial Gastrectomy

Possible Complications

- Peritonitis
- Dumping syndrome
- Afferent loop syndrome

Health Conditions

- Undernutrition
- Impaired physical mobility
- Anemia
- Pre-existing respiratory problems

Nursing Diagnoses

- Altered nutrition: less than body requirements
- Ineffective individual coping

Discharge Teaching for Client Following
Partial Gastrectomy

Activity
- Gradually return to usual level of activity by increasing activity each day. Alternate activity with rest periods. Avoid fatigue.
- You may go up and down stairs if you experience no discomfort.
- Avoid heavy housework, straining, heavy lifting, and driving for the period designated by your physician.
- You may shower.
- Return to work following physician approval.

Diet
- Follow diet instructions given by dietitian. Avoid foods that are spicy or gas-producing.
- If you experience discomfort during meals, decrease the amount of food consumed.
- Eat frequent, small meals.
- Avoid stress during and after meals.
- Rest after meals.
- Drink fluids between meals

Signs and Symptoms to Report
Notify physician if any of these symptoms occur:
- Pain, abdominal distension, nausea, vomiting, or diarrhea
- Increase in pain, redness, or swelling in your incision
- Sudden increase in wound drainage, especially if drainage has pus or a foul odor
- Chills, or fever greater than 100F or 38C

Follow-Up Care and General Health Care
- Schedule follow-up appointment with physician as directed.
- Check your weight weekly. Report weight gain or weight loss of more than 2–3 lb/week.
- Avoid constipation and straining. Check with your physician about using laxatives.

Medications
- Review written list of medications, including dose, route, frequency, food interactions, and side effects.

Wound and Dressing Care
- Cleanse skin around incision daily with mild soap and water.
- If dressing present, change it daily and as often as necessary to keep dressing dry and clean.
- Remove dressing prior to showering and replace with a clean dressing afterward.
- Drainage, if present, should gradually decrease.
- If there is a marked increase in drainage, swelling, tenderness, or fever, or if drainage is foul-smelling, notify physician.

Laparoscopic Hernia Repair

Expected length of stay: less than 24 hours

	Date _____ **Preoperative**	Date _____ **1st 24 Hours Postoperative**
Daily outcomes	Client verbalizes understanding of preoperative teaching, including: turning, deep breathing, incentive spirometer, mobilization, and pain management Client verbalizes understanding of procedures Client verbalizes ability to cope Obtain informed consent	Client is afebrile and has stable vital signs Client has a clean, dry wound with edges well-approximated, healing by first intention Client manages pain with non-pharmacologic measures or oral medications Client is independent in self-care Client is fully ambulatory Client has resumed preadmission urine and bowel elimination pattern Client verbalizes home care instructions Client tolerates usual diet Client verbalizes ability to cope with ongoing stressors
Assessments, tests, and treatments	CBC Urinalysis Baseline physical assessment with a focus on respiratory status and gastrointestinal function Anesthesia consult	Vital signs and O_2 saturation, neurovascular assessment, and dressing and wound drainage assessment q15min × 4; q30min × 4; q1hr × 4 and then q4hr and prn Assess lung sounds and gastrointestinal function q4hr and prn Intake and output every shift Assess voiding — if unable to void, try suggestive voiding techniques or, if still unable, catheterize q8hr or prn
Knowledge deficit	Orient to room and surroundings Provide simple, brief instructions Review preoperative preparation including hospital and surgical routines Reinforce preoperative teaching regarding specific postoperative care: turning, coughing, deep breathing, incentive spirometer, mobilization, and pain management Evaluate understanding of teaching	Reorient to room and postoperative routine Review plan of care and importance of early mobilization Begin discharge teaching regarding wound care/dressing change, diet, follow-up care, signs and symptoms to report, and activity Prior to discharge, review medications: name, purpose, dose, frequency, route, dietary interactions, and side effects Prior to discharge, reinforce teaching regarding wound care/dressing change, diet, follow-up care, signs and symptoms to report, and activity Evaluate understanding of teaching
Psychosocial	Assess anxiety related to pending surgery Assess fears of the unknown related to surgery Encourage verbalization of concerns Provide information regarding surgical experience Minimize external stimuli (eg, noise, movement)	Assess level of anxiety Encourage verbalization of concerns Provide information and ongoing support and encouragement

	Date _____ **Preoperative**	Date _____ **1st 24 Hours Postoperative**
Diet	NPO Baseline nutritional assessment	Advance to clear liquids; if tolerated, advance to full liquids/soft diet morning following surgery
Activity	OOB ad lib until premedicated for surgery	Provide safety precautions Bathroom privileges with assistance evening after surgery and begin progressive ambulation as tolerated the morning following surgery until fully ambulatory
Medications	NPO except ordered medications	IM or oral analgesics Antibiotics if ordered IV fluids until adequate oral intake; then intermittent IV device Discontinue prior to discharge
Transfer/ discharge plans	Assess discharge plans and support system	Probable discharge within 24 hours of surgery Complete discharge home care teaching when fully awake and oriented and before discharge Provide a written copy of discharge instructions

Potential Client Variances
Laparoscopic Hernia Repair

Possible Complications
- Infection
- Recurrence of herniation

Health Conditions
- Respiratory problems

Nursing Diagnoses
- Urinary retention
- Constipation
- Altered sexuality patterns

Discharge Teaching for Client Following
Laparoscopic Hernia Repair

Activity
- Gradually return to usual level of activity by increasing activity each day. Alternate activity with rest periods. Avoid fatigue.
- You may go up and down stairs.
- Avoid heavy housework, straining, heavy lifting, and driving for the period designated by your physician.

Diet
- Eat a well balanced diet, including all food groups.
- Include foods high in fiber, such as fresh fruits, vegetables, and whole grain breads and cereals.
- Report nausea, vomiting, or change in bowel habits.
- Prevent constipation and avoid straining for a bowel movement.
- Drink 6–8 glasses of fluid each day.

Signs and Symptoms to Report
Notify physician if these symptoms occur:
- Increase in pain or any redness or swelling in wound
- Sudden increase in wound drainage, especially if drainage has pus or a foul odor
- Constipation
- Chills, or fever greater than 100°F or 38°C
- Nausea, vomiting, or change in bowel habits

Follow-Up Care and General Health Care
- Schedule follow-up appointment with physician as directed.
- Bend at the knees to lift anything. No heavy lifting until okayed by physician. Use good body mechanics when lifting or moving.

Medications
- Review written list of medications including dose, route, frequency, food interactions, and side effects.
- Avoid alcohol if taking medication.

Wound and Dressing Care
- Cleanse skin around incision daily with mild soap and water.
- If dressing present, change it daily and as often as necessary to keep dressing dry and clean.
- Remove dressing prior to showering and replace with a clean dressing afterward.
- Drainage, if present, should gradually decrease.
- If there is a marked increase in drainage, swelling, tenderness, or fever, or if drainage is foul-smelling, notify physician.

Fractured Hip with Prosthesis or Internal Fixation

Expected length of stay: 6–7 days

	Date _____ **Preoperative**	Date _____ **1st Postoperative Day**	Date _____ **2nd Postoperative Day**
Daily outcomes	Client will have adequate CSMs Client will verbalize understanding of preoperative teaching, including: turning, coughing, and deep breathing, mobilization, IV therapy, and pain management Client will verbalize understanding of procedures Client exhibits effective coping Client verbalizes indications for procedure, comparative risks, and benefits	Client will: • have adequate CSMs and stable vital signs • have a clean, dry dressing • recover from anesthesia as evidenced by VS return to baseline, and being awake, alert, and oriented • verbalize understanding of and demonstrate cooperation with turning, coughing, and deep breathing • have clear breath sounds and use incentive spirometer q2hr while awake • maintain urine output >30 mL/hr • have active bowel sounds • tolerate ordered diet without nausea or vomiting • demonstrate cooperation with mobility restrictions and safety measures • demonstrate ability to use PCA • verbalize control of incisional pain • pivot to chair with 2 assists, morning after surgery • exhibit effective coping • remain free of infection and injury	Client will: • have adequate CSMs and stable vital signs • have a clean wound with edges well-approximated, healing by first intention • remain alert and oriented • verbalize understanding of and demonstrate cooperation with turning, coughing, and deep breathing • have clear breath sounds and use incentive spirometer q2hr while awake • maintain urine output >30 mL/hr • have active bowel sounds • tolerate ordered diet without nausea or vomiting • demonstrate cooperation with mobility restrictions and safety measures • demonstrate ability to use PCA • verbalize control of incisional pain • participate in progressive mobility program • exhibit effective coping • remain free of infection and injury

➤

Fractured Hip with Prosthesis or Internal Fixation *(continued)*

	Date _____ **Preoperative**	Date _____ **1st Postoperative Day**	Date _____ **2nd Postoperative Day**
Assessments, tests, and treatments	CBC Chem profile Type and crossmatch Urinalysis CXR EKG Baseline physical assessment Vital signs on admission and q1hr until stable then q4hr and prn Neurovascular assessment q15min × 4; q30min × 4; q1hr × 4; then q4hr and prn Apply Buck's traction as ordered Intake and output every shift Assess voiding—catheterize q8hr and prn	Prothrombin time Vital signs and O$_2$ saturation, neurovascular assessment, and dressing and hemovac assessment q15min x 4; q30min × 4; q1hr × 4; q4hr × 24 hr and prn Incentive spirometer q2hr Oxygen as indicated to maintain O$_2$ saturation >96% Assess calves for redness, tenderness, swelling, heat, and edema every shift TED stockings—remove and replace every shift Intake and output every shift Empty hemovac q4–8hr and prn Assess voiding—catheterize q8hr or prn if unable to void Transfuse as ordered	Hemoglobin and hematocrit Prothrombin time Vital signs and O$_2$ saturation, neurovascular assessment, and dressing and hemovac assessment q4hr and prn Intake and output every shift Empty hemovac q8hr and prn Assess voiding—catheterize q8hr or prn if unable to void Incentive spirometer q2hr Oxygen as indicated to maintain O$_2$ saturation > 96% Assess calves for redness, tenderness, swelling, heat, and edema every shift TED stockings—remove and replace every shift
Knowledge deficit	Orient to room and surroundings Review plan of care and importance of early mobilization Review importance of coughing, deep breathing, incentive spirometer, mobilization, any intravenous or drainage tubes, and pain management Evaluate understanding of teaching	Orient to room and postoperative routine, including hip precautions Evaluate understanding of teaching	Review importance of early progressive exercise Review plan of care Reinforce hip precautions and safety measures for transfers and ambulation Evaluate understanding of teaching
Diet	NPO prior to surgery	Clear liquids as tolerated	If clear liquids are tolerated, advance to full to regular diet as tolerated Encourage oral fluids
Activity	Assess safety needs and provide appropriate measures Bed rest with Buck's traction	Use abductor pillow when supine and with turning Turn, cough, and deep breathe q2hr Encourage muscle strengthening exercises: quadriceps, gluteal sets, plantar flexion and leg lifts q2hr	Continue Day 1 activities Pivot to chair with 2 assists on affected side 3 times; steps as tolerated Weightbearing per physical therapy

Fractured Hip with Prosthesis or Internal Fixation *(continued)*

	Date _____ **Preoperative**	Date _____ **1st Postoperative Day**	Date _____ **2nd Postoperative Day**
Psychosocial	Assess mental status every shift and prn Assess potential for post–op confusion Assess anxiety regarding impending surgery Offer emotional support and encourage verbalization of concerns Include family in teaching and provide support Minimize external stimuli	Assess mental status every shift and prn Assess level of anxiety Provide information and ongoing support and encouragement to client and family	Assess mental status every shift and prn Assess level of anxiety Encourage verbalization of concerns Provide information and ongoing support and encouragement to client and family
Medications	Preoperative medications as ordered per anesthesia Routine medications as ordered	Analgesics (PCA/IV) IV antibiotics Stool softener BID prn Evening following surgery: initiate aspirin or coumadin therapy IV fluids	Analgesics (PCA/IV) IV antibiotics Stool softener BID prn Laxative if no BM in 3 days Coumadin or aspirin therapyas ordered IV fluids or IV—KVO
Transfer/ discharge plans	Assess potential discharge needs and support system Establish discharge goals with client and family	Home assessment if not previously completed Consult with physical therapy	Review with client and family discharge objectives regarding activity and home care Collaborate with physical therapy Consult with social service regarding projected needs for home health care; including home health aides, visiting nurse, and physical and occupational therapy

➤

Fractured Hip with Prosthesis or Internal Fixation *(continued)*

	Date _____ **3rd Postoperative Day**	Date _____ **4th Postoperative Day**
Daily outcomes	Client will: • have adequate CSMs and stable vital signs • have a clean wound with edges well-approximated, healing by first intention • remain alert and oriented • verbalize understanding of and demonstrate cooperation with turning, coughing, and deep breathing • have clear breath sounds and use incentive spirometer q2hr while awake • maintain urine output >30 mL/hr • have active bowel sounds • tolerate ordered diet without nausea or vomiting • demonstrate cooperation with mobility restrictions and safety measures • verbalize control of incisional pain • begin gait training in room with assistive device per physical therapy • exhibit effective coping • remain free of infection and injury	Client will: • have adequate CSMs and stable vital signs • have a clean wound with edges well-approximated, healing by first intention • remain alert and oriented • verbalize understanding of and demonstrate cooperation with turning, coughing, and deep breathing • have clear breath sounds and use incentive spirometer q2hr while awake • maintain urine output >30 mL/hr • have active bowel sounds • tolerate ordered diet without nausea or vomiting • demonstrate cooperation with mobility restrictions and safety measures • verbalize control of incisional pain • participate in progressive gait training program • exhibit effective coping • remain free of infection and injury
Assessments, tests, and treatments	Prothrombin time Vital signs and O_2 saturation, neurovascular assessment, and dressing assessment q4hr and prn Intake and output every shift Hemovac removed if drainage less than 30 mL/shift Change dressing and assess wound healing Incentive spirometer q2hr while awake O_2 if indicated Assess calves for redness, tenderness, swelling, heat, and edema every shift TED stockings—remove and replace every shift	Prothrombin time Vital signs BID CSMs q4hr and prn Change dressing Assess wound healing TED stockings—remove and replace every shift Assess calves for redness, tenderness, swelling, heat, and edema every shift Intake and output every shift—assess urine output

Fractured Hip with Prosthesis or Internal Fixation *(continued)*

	Date _____ **3rd Postoperative Day**	Date _____ **4th Postoperative Day**
Knowledge deficit	Review plan of care Initiate discharge teaching regarding wound care, activity, and diet Evaluate understanding of teaching	Review plan of care Initiate discharge teaching regarding wound care, activity, and diet Evaluate understanding of teaching
Diet	Regular diet as tolerated Encourage oral fluids to 2000 mL/ day Encourage high-fiber diet, rich in vitamin C and iron and high in protein	Regular diet as tolerated Encourage oral fluids to 2000 mL/ day Encourage high-fiber diet, rich in vitamin C and iron and high in protein
Activity	Continue Day 1 activities Ambulate 10 feet with walker 3 to 4 times (Weightbearing per physical therapy)	Continue Day 1 activities Ambulate 20–30 feet qid (Weightbearing and assistive devices per physical therapy)
Psychosocial	Assess mental status every shift and prn Assess level of anxiety Encourage verbalization of concerns Provide information and ongoing support and encouragement to client and family	Assess level of anxiety Encourage verbalization of ongoing concerns Provide information and ongoing support and encouragement to client and family
Medications	D/C antibiotics D/C PCA and/or wean to oral analgesics Stool softener BID prn Coumadin or aspirin therapy as ordered Intermittent IV device if needed	Oral analgesics Stool softener BID prn Aspirin or coumadin therapy D/C intermittent IV device
Transfer/ discharge plans	Review with patient and family progress toward discharge objectives Evaluate and discuss need for referral to skilled care or rehab facility Collaborate with physical therapy	Review with client and family discharge objectives regarding activity and home care Collaborate with physical therapy Complete referrals for rehab facility or skilled care, if indicated

➤

Fractured Hip with Prosthesis or Internal Fixation *(continued)*

	Date _____ **5th Postoperative Day**	Date _____ **6th Postoperative Day**
Daily outcomes	Client will: • have adequate CSMs and stable vital signs • have a clean wound with edges well-approximated, healing by first intention • remain alert and oriented • verbalize understanding and demonstrate cooperation with turning, coughing, and deep breathing • have clear breath sounds and use incentive spirometer q 2 hr while awake • maintain urine output >30 mL/hr • have active bowel sounds • tolerate ordered diet without nausea or vomiting • demonstrate cooperation with mobility restrictions and safety measures • verbalize control of incisional pain • participate in progressive gait training program and begin stair climbing • exhibit effective coping • remain free of infection and injury	Client is afebrile, with stable vital signs and aequate CSMs Client has a clean, dry wound with edges well-approximated, healing by first intention Client has clear breath sounds Client manages pain with non–pharmacologic measures and/or with oral medications Client is independent in self-care Client independently and safely transfers and ambulates 50–70 feet qid with ordered assistive devices Client has resumed preadmission urine and bowel elimination pattern Client verbalizes/demonstrates home care instructions Client tolerates usual diet Client exhibits effective coping Client remains free of injury and infection
Assessments, tests, and treatments	Hemoglobin and hematocrit Prothrombin time Vital signs BID CSMs q8hr and prn Change dressing Assess wound healing Transfuse if ordered	Prothrombin time Vital signs CSMs q8hr and prn Remove dressing Assess wound healing
Knowledge deficit	Review plan of care Continue discharge teaching regarding wound care, activity, and diet Review safety measures for transfers and ambulation for home care Evaluate understanding of teaching	Patient and/or family verbalizes understanding of discharge teaching including wound care, activity, safety measures, diet, signs and symptoms to report, follow-up care, and home care arrangements Evaluate understanding of teaching

Fractured Hip with Prosthesis or Internal Fixation *(continued)*

	Date _____ **5th Postoperative Day**	Date _____ **6th Postoperative Day**

Diet	Regular diet as tolerated
	Encourage oral fluids to 2000 mL/
	    day
	Encourage high-fiber diet, rich in
	    vitamin C and iron and high in
	    protein
		Regular diet as tolerated
		Encourage oral fluids to 2000 mL/
		    day
		Encourage high-fiber diet, rich in
		    vitamin C and iron and high in
		    protein

Activity	Continue Day 1 activities
	  Ambulate 30–50 feet qid
	  (Weightbearing and assistive
	    devices per physical therapy)
		Continue Day 1 activities
		  Ambulate 50–70 feet qid
		  (Weightbearing and assistive
		    devices per physical therapy)

Psychosocial	Assess level of anxiety
	Encourage verbalization of
	    ongoing concerns
	Provide information and ongoing
	    support and encouragement to
	    client and family
		Assess level of anxiety
		Encourage verbalization of
		    ongoing concerns
		Provide information and ongoing
		    support and encouragement to
		    client and family

Medications	Oral analgesics
	Stool softener
	Laxative if no BM in 3 days
	Coumadin or aspirin therapy as
	    ordered
		Oral analgesics
		Stool softener
		Coumadin or aspirin therapy as
		    ordered

*Transfer/
discharge plans*
	Review with client and family dis-
	    charge objectives regarding
	    activity and home care
	Collaborate with physical therapy
	Complete referrals for home
	    health care; including home
	    health aides, visiting nurse, and
	    physical and occupational
	    therapy if indicated
		Discharge with referrals for home
		    health care or skilled care or
		    rehab facility

Potential Client Variances
Fractured Hip with Prosthesis or Internal Fixation

Possible Complications

- Hemorrhage
- Infection
- Thromboembolism
- Prosthesis dislocation

Health Conditions

- Neurologic disorders
- Mobility problems

- Pre-existing cardiac or respiratory disorders
- Peripheral vascular disease

Nursing Diagnoses

- Acute pain
- Risk for injury
- Risk for infection
- Activity intolerance

Discharge Teaching for Client Following
Fractured Hip with Prosthesis or Internal Fixation

Activity

- Gradually return to usual level of activity by increasing activity each day. Alternate activity with rest periods. Avoid fatigue.
- Continue exercise program as instructed by physical therapist.
- Avoid crossing legs and externally rotating hip as instructed.
- When sitting, use a solid armchair with a pillow behind your back and one under your buttocks. If you sit as long as an hour, then stand up and walk around for a few minutes.
- Use elevated commode chair or toilet seat.
- No strenuous activity until okayed by physician.
- Avoid driving for the period designated by physician.
- Continue range of motion exercises four times a day or as recommended by your physician.
- Wear well-fitting, sturdy shoes at all times.
- Increase distance walked each day using crutches or walker as instructed.
- Avoid bending your hip more than 90 degrees, kneeling or bending to pick up things, twisting motions, crossing legs, and sitting in low chairs of any type.

Diet

- Eat a well balanced diet, including foods from all food groups: fruits, vegetables, meats, milk products, and starches and bread.
- Drink 6–8 glasses of fluid each day.

Signs and Symptoms to Report

Notify physician if any of these symptoms occur:
- Increase in pain, redness, or swelling in wound
- Sudden increase in wound drainage, especially if drainage has pus or a foul odor
- Chills, or fever greater than 100F or 38C

Follow-Up Care and General Health Care

- Schedule follow-up appointment with physician as directed.
- Use elevated toilet seat, handrails, and assistive devices as instructed.
- Remove obstacles in your home, including throw rugs.

Medications

- Review written list of medications including dose, frequency, food interactions, and side effects.
- Avoid over-the-counter medications unless recommended by physician.
- Discuss alcohol use with physician.

Wound and Dressing Care

- Cleanse skin around incision daily with mild soap and water.
- If dressing present, change it daily and as often as necessary to keep dressing dry and clean.
- Drainage, if present, should gradually decrease.
- If there is marked increase in drainage, swelling, tenderness, or fever, or if drainage is foul-smelling, notify physician.

Critical Pathway for Client Following
Total Hip Replacement

Expected length of stay: 6–7 days

	Date _____ **1st 24 Hours Postoperative**	Date _____ **2nd Day Postoperative**	Date _____ **3rd Day Postoperative**
Daily outcomes	Client will: • have stable vital signs • have a clean wound with edges well-approximated, healing by first intention • recover from anesthesia, as evidenced by VS return to baseline and being awake, alert, and oriented • verbalize understanding of and demonstrate cooperation with turning, coughing, deep breathing, and splinting • tolerate ordered diet without nausea or vomiting • verbalize understanding of and demonstrate cooperation with hip precautions • verbalize control of incisional pain • pivot to chair with 2 assists morning after surgery • exhibit effective coping	Client will: • have stable vital signs and be awake, alert, and oriented • have a clean wound with edges well-approximated, healing by first intention • demonstrate cooperation with turning, coughing, deep breathing, and splinting • tolerate ordered diet without nausea or vomiting • demonstrate cooperation with hip precautions • verbalize control of incisional pain • pivot to chair with 2 assists 3 times with steps as tolerated • exhibit effective coping	Client will: • have stable vital signs and be afebrile • demonstrate cooperation with turning, coughing, deep breathing, and splinting • have a clean wound with edges well-approximated, healing by first intention • tolerate ordered diet without nausea or vomiting • demonstrate cooperation with hip precautions • verbalize control of incisional pain • ambulate 10 ft with walker 3 or 4 times • exhibit effective coping
Assessments, tests, and treatments	Hemoglobin and hematocrit Prothrombin time A and P of hip in PACU Vital signs and O_2 saturation, neurovascular assessment, and dressing and hemovac assessment q15min × 4; q30min × 4; q1hr × 4; q4hr × 24 hours and prn Incentive spirometer q2hr O_2 as indicated Assess calves for redness, tenderness, swelling, heat, and edema q4hr TED stockings—remove and replace every shift Intake and output every shift Empty hemovac q8hr and prn	Hemoglobin and hematocrit Prothrombin time Vital signs and O_2 saturation, neurovascular assessment, and dressing and hemovac assessment q4hr and prn Intake and output every shift Empty hemovac q8hr and prn Assess Foley catheter or voiding—catheterize q8hr or prn if unable to void Incentive spirometer q2hr O_2 as indicated Assess calves for redness, tenderness, swelling, heat, edema every shift TED stockings—remove and replace every shift	Prothrombin time Vital signs and O_2 saturation, neurovascular assessment, and dressing assessment q4hr and prn Intake and output every shift Hemovac removed if drainage less than 30 mL/shift Change dressing and assess wound healing Incentive spirometer q2hr O_2 as indicated Assess calves for redness, tenderness, swelling, heat, edema every shift TED stockings—remove and replace every shift

➤

Total Hip Replacement *(continued)*

	Date _____ **1st 24 Hours Postoperative**	Date _____ **2nd Day Postoperative**	Date _____ **3rd Day Postoperative**
Assessments, tests, and treatments (continued)	Assess Foley catheter or voiding—use suggestive voiding techniques and/or catheterize q8hr or prn if unable to void Reinfuse drainage via blood retrieval system as ordered Transfuse as ordered Maintain dry, sterile dressing	Maintain dry, sterile dressing; assess wound and change dressing per MD order	Assess wound and change dressing every day and prn
Knowledge deficit	Orient to room and postoperative routine, including hip precautions Include family in teaching Review plan of care and importance of early mobilization Review importance of coughing, deep breathing, splinting incision, incentive spirometer, mobilization, any drainage of intraveneous tubes, and pain management Evaluate understanding of teaching	Review importance of early progressive exercise Review plan of care with client and family Reinforce hip precautions and safety measures for transfers and ambulation Evaluate understanding of teaching	Review plan of care Include family in teaching Initiate discharge teaching regarding wound care, activity, and diet Evaluate understanding of teaching
Diet	NPO to clear liquids as tolerated	If clear liquids are tolerated, advance to full to regular diet as tolerated; 2000 mL fluid/day	Regular diet as tolerated; 2000 mL fluid/day Encourage high-fiber diet, rich in vitamin C and iron and high in protein
Activity	Use abductor pillow when supine and with turning; check MD order regarding turning The morning after surgery, pivot to chair with 2 assists on affected side Turn, cough, and deep breathe q2hr Encourage muscle strengthening exercises: quadriceps, gluteal sets, plantar flexion, and leg lifts q2hr Assess safety needs and maintain appropriate precautions	Continue Day 1 activities From affected side, pivot to chair with 2 assists 1–3 times; steps as tolerated Weightbearing per physical therapy Maintain safety precautions	Continue Day 1 activities Ambulate 10 ft with walker 3–4 times Weightbearing per physical therapy Maintain safety precautions
Medications	Analgesics as ordered IV antibiotics Stool softener Antipyretics prn Evening of surgery: initiate aspirin or coumadin therapy if ordered IV fluids	Analgesics as ordered IV antibiotics Stool softener Antipyretics prn Laxative if no BM in 3 days Coumadin or aspirin therapy if ordered IV fluids or IV—KVO	D/C antibiotics D/C PCA or epidural and/or wean to oral analgesics Stool softener Coumadin or aspirin therapy if ordered Intermittent IV device, if needed

Total Hip Replacement *(continued)*

	Date _____ **1st 24 Hours Postoperative**	Date _____ **2nd Day Postoperative**	Date _____ **3rd Day Postoperative**
Transfer/ discharge plans	Home assessment if not previously completed Consult with social service regarding projected needs for home health care; including home health aides, visiting nurse, and physical and occupational therapy Establish discharge objectives with client and family	Review with client and family discharge objectives regarding activity and home care Consult and collaborate with physical therapy	Review with client and family progress toward discharge objectives Collaborate with physical therapy

	Date _____ **4th Day Postoperative**	Date _____ **5th Day Postoperative**	Date _____ **6th–7th Days Postoperative**
Daily outcomes	Client will: • have stable vital signs and be afebrile • demonstrate cooperation with turning, coughing, deep breathing, and splinting • have a clean wound with edges well-approximated, healing by first intention • tolerate ordered diet without nausea or vomiting • demonstrates cooperation with hip precautions • demonstrate ability to use PCA • verbalize control of incisional pain • ambulate 20–30 ft with walker 4 times • exhibit effective coping	Client will: • have stable vital signs and be afebrile • demonstrate cooperation with turning, coughing, deep breathing, and splinting • have a clean wound with edges well-approximated, healing by first intention • tolerate ordered diet without nausea or vomiting • demonstrate cooperation with hip precautions • demonstrate ability to use PCA • verbalize control of incisional pain • ambulate 30–50 ft with walker 4 times • exhibit effective coping	Client is afebrile and has stable vital signs Client has a clean, dry wound with edges well-approximated, healing by first intention Client manages pain with non-pharmacologic measures Client is independent in self-care Client is independent in transfers and ambulates 50–70 ft qid with ordered assistive devices Client has resumed preadmission urine and bowel elimination pattern Client verbalizes/demonstrates home care instructions Client tolerates usual diet Client exhibits effective coping with ongoing stressors
Assessments, tests, and treatments	Prothrombin time Vital signs BID Change dressing every day and prn Assess wound healing TED stockings—remove and replace every shift Assess calves for redness, tenderness, swelling, heat, edema every shift Intake and output every shift—assess urine output	Hemoglobin and hematocrit Prothrombin time Vital signs BID Change dressing every day and prn Assess wound healing TED stockings—remove and replace every shift Transfuse if ordered	Prothrombin time Vital signs Remove dressing Assess wound

➤

Total Hip Replacement *(continued)*

	Date _____ **4th Day Postoperative**	Date _____ **5th Day Postoperative**	Date _____ **6th–7th Days Postoperative**
Knowledge deficit	Review plan of care Include family in teaching Continue discharge teaching regarding wound care, activity, and diet Evaluate understanding of teaching	Review plan of care with client and family Continue discharge teaching regarding wound care, activity, and diet Review safety measures for transfers and ambulation for home care Evaluate understanding of teaching	Client and/or family verbalizes understanding of discharge teaching, including wound care, activity, safety measures, diet, signs and symptoms to report, follow-up care and MD appointment, home care arrangements, and medications: name, purpose, dose, frequency, route, dietary interactions and side effects Evaluate understanding of teaching
Diet	Regular diet as tolerated; 2000 mL fluids/day Encourage high-fiber diet, rich in vitamin C and high in protein	Regular diet as tolerated; 2000 mL fluids/day Encourage high-fiber diet, rich in vitamin C and high in protein	Regular diet as tolerated; 2000 mL fluids/day Encourage high-fiber diet, rich in vitamin C and high in protein
Activity	Continue Day 1 activities Ambulate 20–30 ft qid Weightbearing and assistive devices per physical therapy	Continue Day 1 activities Ambulate 30–50 ft qid Weightbearing and assistive devices per physical therapy	Continue Day 1 activities Ambulate 50–70 ft qid Weightbearing and assistive devices per physical therapy
Medications	Analgesics as ordered Stool softener Aspirin or coumadin therapy if ordered D/C intermittent IV device	Analgesics as ordered Stool softener Laxative if no BM in 3 days Coumadin or aspirin therapy if ordered	Analgesics as ordered Stool softener Coumadin or aspirin therapy if ordered
Transfer/ discharge plans	Review with client and family discharge objectives regarding activity and home care Collaborate with physical therapy	Review with client and family discharge objectives regarding activity and home care Collaborate with physical therapy Complete referrals for home health care; including home health aides, visiting nurse, and physical and occupational therapy	Discharge with referrals for home health care

Potential Client Variances
Total Hip Replacement

Possible Complications

- Hemorrhage
- Infection
- Thromboembolism
- Prosthesis dislocation

Health Conditions

- Neurologic disorders

- Mobility problems
- Pre-existing cardiac or respiratory disorders
- Peripheral vascular disease

Nursing Diagnoses

- Acute pain
- Risk for injury
- Risk for infection

Discharge Teaching for Client Following
Total Hip Replacement

Activity

- Gradually return to usual level of activity by increasing activity each day. Alternate activity with rest periods. Avoid fatigue.
- Avoid flexing hip more than instructed.
- Avoid crossing legs and externally rotating hip as instructed.
- When sitting, use a solid armchair with one pillow behind your back and another under your buttocks. If you sit longer than an hour, stand up and walk around for a few minutes each hour.
- Use elevated commode chair or toilet seat.
- No strenuous activity until okayed by physician.
- Avoid driving for the period designated by physician.
- Continue range of motion exercises four times a day or as recommended by physician.
- Wear well-fitting, sturdy shoes at all times.
- Increase distance walked each day using crutches or walker as instructed.

Diet

- Eat a well-balanced diet, including all food groups.
- Drink 6–8 glasses of fluid every day.

Signs and Symptoms to Report

Notify physician if any of these symptoms occur:
- Increase in pain, redness, or swelling
- Sudden increase in wound drainage, especially if drainage has pus or a foul odor.

- Chills, or fever greater than 100F or 38C
- Unusual pain in legs or hip area

Follow-Up Care and General Health Care

- Schedule follow-up appointment with physician as directed.
- Wear well-fitting shoes and use elevated chairs, an elevated toilet seat, handrails, and a walker or crutches.
- Remove any obstacles in your home, including throw rugs.
- Use a pillow between your legs for 6 weeks or as directed by physician.
- Alert all other physicians and dentists that you have a total joint replacement prior to undergoing any procedure so that antibiotic prophylaxis can be ordered.

Medications

- Review written list of medications, including dose, frequency, food interactions, and side effects.
- Avoid over-the-counter medications unless recommended by physician.

Wound and Dressing Care

- Cleanse skin around incision daily with mild soap and water.
- If dressing present, change it daily and as often as necessary to keep dressing dry and clean.
- Remove dressing prior to showering and replace with a clean dressing afterward.
- Drainage, if present, should gradually decrease.
- If there is a marked increase in drainage, swelling, tenderness, or fever, or if drainage is foul-smelling, notify physician.

Critical Pathway for Client Following

Abdominal Hysterectomy

Expected length of stay: 3 days

	Date _____ **Preoperative**	Date _____ **1st Day Postoperative**
Daily outcomes	Client verbalizes understanding of preoperative teaching, including: turning, coughing, deep breathing, incentive spirometer, mobilization, possible tubes, and pain management (PCA or prn medications) Client exhibits effective coping with preoperative preparation Client verbalizes understanding of procedure, indications for procedure, comparative risks, benefits, and implications	Client will: • have stable vital signs • have clean, dry wound with edges well-approximated, healing by first intention • recover from anesthesia, as evidenced by VS return to baseline and being awake, alert, and oriented • verbalize understanding of and demonstrates cooperation with turning, coughing, deep breathing, and splinting • tolerate ordered diet without nausea or vomiting • verbalize control of incisional pain • exhibit effective coping
Assessments, tests, and treatments	CBC Urinalysis Baseline physical assessment with a focus on respiratory status and gastrointestinal function Betadine douche if ordered Fleet enema AM of admission	CBC Vital signs and O_2 saturation, neurovascular assessment, dressing and wound and vaginal drainage assessment q15min × 4; q30min × 4; q1hr × 4 and then q4hr and prn Assess respiratory status and urinary and gastrointestinal function q4hr and prn Incentive spirometer q2hr Intake and output every shift Assess voiding—if unable to void, try suggestive voiding techniques or, if still unable, catheterize q8hr or prn
Knowledge deficit	Orient to room and surroundings Provide simple, brief instructions Include family in teaching Review preoperative preparation including hospital and surgical routines Discuss surgery and specific postoperative care: turning, coughing, deep breathing, incentive spirometer, mobilization, possible drainage and intravenous tubes, and pain management Evaluate understanding of teaching	Reorient to room and postoperative routine Include family in teaching Review plan of care and importance of early mobilization Begin discharge teaching regarding wound care/ dressing change Evaluate understanding of teaching
Psychosocial	Assess anxiety related to diagnosis and pending surgery Assess fears of the unknown related to surgery Provide support to client and family Encourage verbalization of concerns regarding loss of reproductive capability Minimize external stimuli (eg, noise, movement)	Assess level of anxiety Encourage verbalization of concerns Provide ongoing support and encouragement to client and family

Abdominal Hysterectomy *(continued)*

	Date _____ **Preoperative**	Date _____ **1st 24 Hours Postoperative**
Diet	NPO after midnight Baseline nutritional assessment	Advance to clear liquids
Activity	Assess safety needs and implement appropriate precautions Bed rest or bathroom privileges with assistance	Maintain safety precautions Bathroom privileges with assistance Dangle evening of surgery and ambulate 4 times with assistance
Medications	Preoperative medications as ordered	Analgesics as ordered IV fluids
Transfer/ discharge plans	Assess discharge plans and support system Identify potential referral needs	Determine needs at time of discharge Make appropriate referrals Begin home care teaching

	Date _____ **2nd Day Postoperative**	Date _____ **3rd Day Postoperative**
Daily outcomes	Client will: • be afebrile and have stable vital signs • have clean, dry wound with edges well-approximated, healing by first intention • demonstrate cooperation with turning, coughing, deep breathing, and splinting • tolerate ordered diet without nausea or vomiting • ambulate 4 times per day • verbalize control of incisional pain • exhibit effective coping • verbalize beginning understanding of home care instructions	Client is afebrile and has stable vital signs Client has a clean, dry wound with edges well-approximated, healing by first intention Client manages pain with non-pharmacologic measures Client is independent in self-care Client is fully ambulatory Client has resumed preadmission urine and bowel elimination patterns Client verbalizes/demonstrates home care instructions Client tolerates usual diet Client verbalizes ability to cope with ongoing stressors
Assessments, tests, and treatments	Vital signs and dressing and wound and vaginal drainage assessment q4hr and prn Assess respiratory status and urinary and gastrointestinal function q4hr Incentive spirometer q2hr until fully ambulatory Intake and output every shift Assess voiding pattern every shift	Vital signs, dressing, wound, and vaginal drainage assessment q4hr Assess respiratory status and urinary and gastrointestinal function
Knowledge deficit	Initiate discharge teaching regarding wound care, diet, and activity Include family in teaching Review written discharge instructions Evaluate understanding of teaching	Complete discharge teaching to include wound care, diet, follow-up care, signs and symptoms to report, activity, and medications: name, purpose, dose, frequency, route, dietary interactions, and side effects Evaluate understanding of teaching Provide client with written discharge instructions Include family in discharge teaching

➤

	Date _____ **2nd Day Postoperative**	Date _____ **3rd Day Postoperative**
Psychosocial	Encourage verbalization of concerns Provide ongoing support and encouragement to client and family Continue to explore issues related to perceived body image changes	Encourage verbalization of concerns Provide ongoing support and encouragement
Diet	If tolerating clear liquids, advance diet to full liquids and then to regular diet as tolerated	Regular diet as tolerated
Activity	Maintain safety precautions Ambulate independently at least 4 times Shower/shampoo	Fully ambulatory
Medications	Analgesics as ordered Stool softener, laxative, or suppository as ordered	Analgesics as ordered Stool softener
Transfer/ discharge plans	Complete discharge plans Continue home care instructions	Complete discharge instructions

Potential Client Variances
Abdominal Hysterectomy

Possible Complications

- Hemorrhage
- Infection
- Deep vein thrombosis
- Urinary retention

Health Conditions

- Obesity
- History of clotting disorders
- History of bleeding tendencies

Nursing Diagnoses

- Body image disturbance
- Altered sexuality patterns

Discharge Teaching for Client Following
Abdominal Hysterectomy

Activity

- Gradually return to usual level of activity by increasing activity each day. Alternate activity with rest periods. Avoid fatigue.
- You may go up and down stairs.
- Avoid heavy housework, working, straining, heavy lifting, and driving for the period designated by your physician.

Diet

- Eat a well-balanced diet, including all food groups.
- Report nausea, vomiting, or change in bowel habits.
- Drink 6–8 glasses of fluid each day.

Signs and Symptoms to Report

Notify physician if any of these symptoms occur:
- Increase in pain or any redness or swelling in wound
- Sudden increase in wound and/or vaginal drainage, especially if drainage has pus or a foul odor
- Chills, or fever greater than 100F or 38C
- Vaginal bleeding or abdominal pain

Follow-Up Care and General Health Care

- Schedule follow-up appointment with physician as directed.
- Consult with physician regarding resumption of sexual activity.

Medications

- Review written list of medications, including dose, route, frequency, food interactions, and side effects.
- Discuss use of estrogen replacement therapy with physician.
- Avoid alcohol if taking medication.

Wound and Dressing Care

- Cleanse skin around incision daily with mild soap and water.
- If you still need a dressing, change it daily and as often as necessary to keep dressing dry and clean.
- Remove dressing prior to showering and replace with a clean dressing afterward.
- Drainage, if present, should gradually decrease.
- If there is a marked increase in drainage, swelling, tenderness, or fever, or if drainage is foul-smelling, notify physician.

Vaginal Hysterectomy

Expected length of stay: 2–3 days

	Date _____ **Preoperative**	Date _____ **1st Day Postoperative**
Daily outcomes	Client verbalizes understanding of preoperative teaching, including: turning, coughing, deep breathing, incentive spirometer, mobilization, possible tubes, and pain management Client verbalizes feelings regarding surgery Client exhibits effective coping with pending surgery Client verbalizes understanding of procedure, indications for procedure, comparative risks, benefits, and implications of options	Client will: • be afebrile, with stable vital signs • recover from anesthesia as evidenced by VS return to baseline and being awake, alert, and oriented • remain free of hemorrhage and urinary tract or wound infection • verbalize understanding of and demonstrate cooperation with turning, coughing, deep breathing, and splinting • maintain urine output >30 mL/hr • tolerate ordered diet without nausea or vomiting • verbalize control of discomfort • verbalize feelings regarding surgical procedure • exhibit effective coping
Assessments, tests, and treatments	CBC Urinalysis Baseline physical assessment with a focus on respiratory status and gastrointestinal function Betadine douche if ordered Fleet enema AM of admission Measure for TED stockings	CBC Vital signs and O_2 saturation, neurovascular assessment, and vaginal drainage assessment q15min × 4; q30min × 4; q1hr × 4 and then q4hr and prn Assess respiratory status and urinary and gastrointestinal function q4hr and prn Incentive spirometer q2hr Intake and output every shift Foley catheter Assess urine output q4hr and prn Remove and replace TED stockings every shift
Knowledge deficit	Orient to room and surroundings Provide simple, brief instructions Include family in teaching Review preoperative preparation, including hospital and surgical routines Discuss surgery and specific postoperative care: turning, coughing, deep breathing, incentive spirometer, mobilization, any drainage tubes or intravenous tubes, and pain management Evaluate understanding of teaching	Reorient to room and postoperative routine Include family in teaching Review plan of care and importance of early mobilization Initiate discharge teaching regarding postoperative care including diet, activity, and follow–up care Evaluate understanding of teaching
Psychosocial	Assess anxiety related to diagnosis and pending surgery Assess fears of the unknown related to surgery Provide support to client and family Encourage verbalization of concerns regarding loss of reproductive capability Minimize external stimuli (eg, noise, movement)	Assess level of anxiety Encourage verbalization of concerns Provide ongoing support and encouragement to client and family

Vaginal Hysterectomy *(continued)*

	Date _____ **Preoperative**	Date _____ **1st Day Postoperative**
Diet	NPO after midnight Baseline nutritional assessment	Advance to clear liquids
Activity	Assess safety needs and implement appropriate precautions Bed rest or bathroom privileges with assistance	Maintain safety precautions Bathroom privileges with assistance Dangle evening of surgery and ambulate 4 times with assistance the following day
Medications	Preoperative medications as ordered	Analgesics as ordered IV fluids
Transfer/ discharge plans	Assess discharge plans and support system Identify potential referral needs	Determine needs at time of discharge Make appropriate referrals Begin home care teaching

	Date _____ **2nd Day Postoperative**	Date _____ **3rd Day Postoperative**
Daily outcomes	Client will: • be afebrile with stable vital signs • demonstrate cooperation with turning, coughing, deep breathing, and splinting • remain free of hemorrhage, and urinary tract or wound infection • maintain urine output >30 mL/hr • tolerate ordered diet without nausea or vomiting • ambulate 4 times per day • verbalize control of incisional pain • exhibit effective coping • begin to verbalize feelings regarding change in body function • verbalize beginning understanding of home care instructions	Client is afebrile with stable vital signs Client has a clean, dry wound with edges well-approximated, healing by first intention Client manages pain with non-pharmacologic measures Client is independent in self-care Client is fully ambulatory Client has resumed preadmission urine and bowel elimination patterns Client verbalizes/demonstrates home care instructions Client tolerates usual diet Client verbalizes feelings regarding change in body functions Client exhibits effective coping with ongoing stressors
Assessments, tests, and treatments	Vital signs and dressing, wound, and vaginal drainage assessment q4hr and prn Assess respiratory status and urinary and gastrointestinal function q4hr Incentive spirometer q2hr until fully ambulatory Intake and output every shift Foley catheter/bladder training if ordered Assess urinary output every shift Remove and replace TED stockings every shift	Vital signs, dressing, wound, and vaginal drainage assessment q4hr Assess respiratory status and urinary and gastrointestinal function Remove Foley catheter if ordered and assess voiding pattern. Catheterize for residual if ordered. Replace Foley catheter if urine residual over 100 mL

►

	Date _____ **2nd Day Postoperative**	Date _____ **3rd Day Postoperative**
Knowledge deficit	Review and reinforce discharge teaching regarding diet, activity, and follow-up care Initiate discharge teaching regarding medications Include family in teaching Review written discharge instructions Evaluate understanding of teaching	Complete discharge teaching to include wound care, diet, follow-up care, signs and symptoms to report, activity, and medications: name, purpose, dose, frequency, route, dietary interactions, and side effects Provide teaching regarding home Foley catheter care if discharged home with catheter. Have client demonstrate home care procedures Provide client with written discharge instructions Include family in discharge teaching Evaluate understanding of teaching
Psychosocial	Encourage verbalization of concerns Provide ongoing support and encouragement to client and family Continue to explore issues related to perceived body image changes	Encourage verbalization of concerns Provide ongoing support and encouragement
Diet	If tolerating clear liquids, advance diet to full liquids to regular diet to tolerance	Regular diet as tolerated
Activity	Maintain safety precautions Ambulate independently at least 4 times Shower/shampoo	Fully ambulatory
Medications	Analgesics as ordered Stool softener, laxative, or suppository as ordered	Analgesics as ordered Stool softener
Transfer/ discharge plans	Complete discharge plans Continue home care instructions	Complete discharge instructions

Potential Client Variances
Vaginal Hysterectomy

Possible Complications

- Hemorrhage
- Infection
- Deep vein thrombosis
- Urinary retention

Health Conditions

- Obesity
- History of clotting disorders
- History of bleeding tendencies

Nursing Diagnoses

- Body image disturbance
- Altered sexuality patterns

Discharge Teaching for Client Following
Vaginal Hysterectomy

Activity

- Gradually return to usual level of activity by increasing activity each day. Alternate activity with rest periods. Avoid fatigue.
- You may go up and down stairs.
- Avoid heavy housework, straining, heavy lifting, and driving for the period designated by your physician.

Diet

- Eat a well-balanced diet, including all food groups.
- Drink 6–8 glasses of fluid each day.

Signs and Symptoms to Support

Notify physician if any of these symptoms occur:
- Sudden increase in vaginal drainage, especially if discharge has pus or has a foul odor
- Chills or fever greater than 100F or 38C
- Vaginal bleeding or abdominal pain
- Nausea, vomiting, or change in bowel habits

Follow-Up Care and General Health Care

- Schedule follow-up appointment with physician as directed.
- Consult with physician regarding resumption of sexual activity.
- Do not douche or use tampons until okayed by physician.

Medications

- Review written list of medications, including dose, route, frequency, food interactions, and side effects.
- Avoid alcohol if taking medication.

Total Knee Replacement

Expected length of stay: 6–7 days

	Date _____ **1st 24 Hours Postoperative**	Date _____ **2nd Day Postoperative**	Date _____ **3rd Day Postoperative**
Daily outcomes	Client will: • have adequate CSMs • have a clean wound with edges well-approximated, healing by first intention • recover from anesthesia, as evidenced by VS return to baseline, and being awake, alert, and oriented • verbalize understanding of and demonstrate cooperation with turning, coughing, deep breathing, and splinting • have clear breath sounds and use incentive spirometer q1hr while awake • maintain urine output >30 mL/hr • have active bowel sounds • tolerate ordered diet without nausea or vomiting • verbalize understanding and demonstrate cooperation with mobility restrictions and safety measures • demonstrate ability to use PCA/epidural • verbalize control of incisional pain • pivot to chair with 2 assists morning after surgery • exhibit effective coping	Client will: • have stable vital signs and adequate CSMs • have a clean wound with edges well-approximated, healing by first intention • have stable vital signs and be awake, alert, and oriented • demonstrate cooperation with turning, coughing, deep breathing, and splinting • have clear breath sounds and use incentive spirometer q1hr while awake • maintain urine output >30 mL/hr • have active bowel sounds • tolerate ordered diet without nausea or vomiting • demonstrate cooperation with mobility restrictions and safety measures • demonstrate ability to use PCA/epidural • verbalize control of incisional pain • pivot to chair with 2 assists 3 times • exhibit effective coping • remain free of infection and injury	Client will: • be afebrile, with stable vital signs, and adequate CSMs • have a clean wound with edges well-approximated, healing by first intention • demonstrate cooperation with turning, coughing, deep breathing, and splinting • have clear breath sounds and use incentive spirometer q1hr while awake • maintain urine output >30 mL/hr • have active bowel sounds • tolerate ordered diet without nausea or vomiting • demonstrate cooperation with mobility restrictions and safety measures • demonstrate ability to use PCA/epidural • verbalize control of incisional pain • begin gait training in room with assistive device per physical therapy • exhibit effective coping • remain free of infection and injury

Total Knee Replacement *(continued)*

	Date _____ **1st 24 Hours Postoperative**	Date _____ **2nd Day Postoperative**	Date _____ **3rd Day Postoperative**
Assessments, tests, and treatments	Hemoglobin and hematocrit Prothrombin time A & P of knee in PACU Vital signs and O_2 saturation, and neurovascular, dressing, and hemovac assessment q15min × 4; q30min × 4; q1hr × 4; q4hr and prn Incentive spirometer q1hr while awake O_2 as indicated Assess calves for redness, tenderness, swelling, heat, and edema q4hr TED stockings—remove and replace every shift Intake and output every shift Drain care q4hr and prn Foley catheter care Reinfuse drainage via blood retrieval system as ordered Transfuse as ordered Maintain dry, sterile dressing	Hemoglobin and hematocrit Prothrombin time Vital signs, O_2 saturation, and neurovascular, dressing, and hemovac assessment q4hr and prn Intake and output every shift Drain care q8hr and prn Foley catheter care q8hr Incentive spirometer q1–2hr while awake O_2 as indicated Assess calves for redness, tenderness, swelling, heat, and edema every shift TED stockings—remove and replace every shift Maintain dry, sterile dressing. Assess wound and change dressing per MD order	Prothrombin time Vital signs, O_2 saturation, and neurovascular, dressing, and hemovac assessment q4hr Intake and output every shift Remove drain per order Change dressing and assess wound healing Incentive spirometer q2hr while awake O_2 as indicated Assess calves for redness, tenderness, swelling, heat, and edema every shift TED stockings—remove and replace every shift Assess wound and change dressing every day and prn
Knowledge deficit	Orient to room and postoperative routine, including hip precautions Include family in teaching Review plan of care and importance of early mobilization Review importance of coughing, deep breathing, splinting incision, incentive spirometer, mobilization, any drainage or intravenous tubes, and pain management Evaluate understanding of teaching	Review importance of early progressive exercise Review plan of care with client and family Reinforce safety measures for transfers and ambulation Evaluate understanding of teaching	Review plan of care Include family in teaching Initiate discharge teaching regarding wound care, activity, and diet Coumadin teaching Evaluate understanding of teaching
Diet	NPO to clear liquids to tolerance	If clear liquids are tolerated, advance to full to regular diet as tolerated; 2000 mL fluid/day	Regular diet as tolerated; 2000 mL fluid/day Encourage high-fiber diet, rich in vitamin C and iron and high in protein

Total Knee Replacement *(continued)*

	Date _____ **1st 24 Hours Postoperative**	Date _____ **2nd Day Postoperative**	Date _____ **3rd Day Postoperative**
Activity	Bed rest for 12 hr Trapeze to bed Encourage frequent ankle and toe exercises CPM as ordered The morning after surgery, pivot to chair with 2 assist, legs elevated Partial weight bearing to tolerance Turn, cough, and deep breathe q1–2hr while awake Encourage muscle strengthening exercises: quadriceps, gluteal sets, plantar flexion, and leg lifts every shift Assess safety needs and maintain appropriate precautions	CPM as ordered Pivot to chair with 2 assists 2–3 times Partial weight bearing in room Encourage muscle strengthening exercises: quadriceps, gluteal sets, plantar flexion and leg lifts q4hr while awake Maintain safety precautions	CPM as ordered Begin gait training with assistive device per physical therapy Encourage muscle strengthening exercises: quadriceps, gluteal sets, plantar flexion and leg lifts q2–4hr while awake Maintain safety precautions
Medications	Analgesics as ordered Stool softener Antipyretics prn Coumadin if ordered IV fluids	Analgesics as ordered Stool softener Antipyretics prn Laxative if no BM in 3 days Coumadin if ordered IV fluids or IV—KVO	D/C PCA or epidural and/or wean to oral analgesics Stool softener Coumadin if ordered Intermittent IV device
Transfer/ discharge plans	Home assessment if not previously completed Consult with social service regarding projected needs for home health care, including home health aides, visiting nurse, and physical and occupational therapy Establish discharge objectives with client and family	Review with client and family discharge objectives regarding activity and home care Consult and collaborate with physical therapy	Review with client and family progress toward discharge objectives Collaborate with physical therapy

Total Knee Replacement (*continued*)

	Date _____ **4th Day Postoperative**	Date _____ **5th Day Postoperative**	Date _____ **6th–7th Days Postoperative**
Daily outcomes	Client will: • be afebrile, with stable vital signs, and adequate CSMs • have a clean wound with edges well-approximated, healing by first intention • demonstrate cooperation with turning, coughing, deep breathing, and splinting • have clear breath sounds and use incentive spirometer q4hr while awake • maintain urine output >30 mL/hr and void following removal of catheter • have active bowel sounds and have a bowel movement • tolerate ordered diet without nausea or vomiting • demonstrate cooperation with hip precautions • verbalize control of incisional pain • participate in progressive gait training program • exhibit effective coping • remain free of infection and injury	Client will: • be afebrile, with stable vital signs, and adequate CSMs • have a clean wound with edges well-approximated, healing by first intention • demonstrate cooperation with turning, coughing, deep breathing, and splinting • have clear breath sounds and use incentive spirometer q4hr while awake • maintain urine output >30 mL/hr • have active bowel sounds • tolerate ordered diet without nausea or vomiting • demonstrate cooperation with hip precautions • verbalize control of incisional pain • participate in progressive gait training program and begin stair training • exhibit effective coping • remain free of infection and injury	Client is afebrile, with stable vital signs and adequate CSMs Client has a clean, dry wound with edges well-approximated, healing by first intention Client has clear breath sounds Client manages pain with non-pharmacologic measures and/or oral medications Client is independent in self-care Client independently and safely transfers and ambulates 50–70 feet qid with ordered assistive devices Client has resumed preadmission urine and bowel elimination pattern Client verbalizes/demonstrates home care instructions Client tolerates usual diet Client exhibits effective coping with ongoing stressors Client remains free of infection and injury
Assessments, tests, and treatments	Prothrombin time Vital signs q8hr CSMs q4hr and prn Change dressing every day and prn Assess wound healing Incentive spirometer q4hr while awake Remove Foley catheter and assess voiding Intake and output every shift TED stockings—remove and replace every shift Assess calves for redness, tenderness, swelling, heat, and edema every shift Intake and output every shift—assess urine output	Hemoglobin and hematocrit Prothrombin time Vital signs BID CSMs q8hr and prn Change dressing every day and prn Assess wound healing Incentive spirometer q2–4hr while awake Transfuse if ordered TED stockings—remove and replace every shift	Prothrombin time Vital signs CSMs q8hr and prn Remove dressing Assess wound Incentive spirometer q4hr while awake

Total Knee Replacement *(continued)*

	Date _____ **4th Day Postoperative**	Date _____ **5th Day Postoperative**	Date _____ **6th–7th Days Postoperative**
Knowledge deficit	Review plan of care Include family in teaching Continue discharge teaching regarding wound care, activity, and diet Evaluate understanding of teaching	Review plan of care with client and family Continue discharge teaching regarding wound care, activity, and diet Review safety measures for transfers and ambulation for home care Evaluate understanding of teaching	Client and/or family verbalizes understanding of discharge teaching including wound care, activity, safety measures, diet, signs and symptoms to report, follow-up care and MD appointment, home care arrangements, and medications: name, purpose, dose, frequency, route, dietary interactions, and side effects Evaluate understanding of teaching
Diet	Regular diet as tolerated; 2000 mL fluids/day Encourage high-fiber diet, rich in vitamin C and high in protein	Regular diet as tolerated; 2000 mL fluids/day Encourage high-fiber diet, rich in vitamin C and high in protein	Regular diet as tolerated; 2000 mL fluids/day Encourage high-fiber diet, rich in vitamin C and high in protein
Activity	Progressive gait training Ambulate 20–30 feet qid Weightbearing and assistive devices per physical therapy CPM as ordered Shower	Progressive gait training Ambulate 30–50 feet qid Begin stair training Weightbearing and assistive devices per physical therapy CPM as ordered	Progressive gait training Continue Day 1 activities Ambulate 50–70 feet qid Weightbearing and assistive devices per physical therapy CPM as ordered
Medications	Analgesics as ordered Stool softener Laxative if no BM in 3 days Coumadin if ordered D/C intermittent IV device	Analgesics as ordered Stool softener Coumadin if ordered	Analgesics as ordered Stool softener Coumadin if ordered
Transfer/ discharge plans	Review with client and family discharge objectives regarding activity and home care Collaborate with physical therapy Assess needs for equipment at home and make appropriate referrals	Review with client and family discharge objectives regarding activity and home care Collaborate with physical therapy Complete referrals for home health care; including home health aides, visiting nurse, and physical and occupational therapy	Discharge with referrals for home health care

Potential Client Variances
Total Knee Replacement

Possible Complications
- Hemorrhage
- Infection
- Thrombophlebitis
- Prosthesis dislocation
- Neurovascular compromise

Health Conditions
- Neurologic conditions
- Mobility problems
- Pre-existing cardiac or respiratory problems
- Peripheral vascular disease

Nursing Diagnoses
- Impaired physical mobility
- Risk for infection
- Risk for injury
- Acute pain

Discharge Teaching for Client Following
Total Knee Replacement

Activity
- Gradually return to usual level of activity by increasing activity each day. Alternate activity with rest periods. Avoid fatigue.
- Continue exercise program as instructed by physical therapist.
- Avoid heavy housework, working, straining, and driving for the period designated by your physician.
- Avoid excessive bending, lifting, crossing legs, kneeling, or exercise that includes jumping or kneeling.
- Use assistive devices as directed.
- Continue leg and knee exercises as directed.
- Wear antiembolic hose—remove and replace for 30 minutes twice each day.
- Review instructions for continuous passive motion at home.
- Wear well-fitting shoes and use elevated chairs, an elevated toilet seat, and handrails.

Diet
- Eat a well-balanced diet including all food groups.
- Drink 6–8 glasses of fluid every day.

Signs and Symptoms to Report
Notify physician if any of these symptoms occur:
- Increase in pain, redness, or swelling
- Sudden increase in wound drainage, especially if drainage has pus or a foul odor
- Chills or fever greater than 100F or 38C
- Unusual pain in legs or the knee area
- Change in temperature of affected extremity

Follow-Up Care and General Health Care
- Schedule follow-up appointment with physician as directed
- Continue physical therapy routine until directed otherwise

Medications
- Review written list of medications, including dose, frequency, food interactions, and side effects.
- Provide teaching sheets related to medications and any antico- agulant therapy.

Wound and Dressing Care
- Cleanse skin around incision daily with mild soap and water.
- If dressing present, change it daily and as often as necessary to keep dressing dry and clean.
- Remove dressing prior to showering and replace with a clean dressing afterward.

Critical Pathway for Client Following
Lumbar Laminectomy

Expected length of stay: 3–4 days following surgery

	Date _____ **Operative Day**	Date _____ **1st Day Postoperative**
Daily outcomes	Client will: • have stable vital signs • have a dry, sterile dressing • recover from anesthesia, as evidenced by VS return to baseline and being awake, alert, and oriented, with clear lungs • verbalize understanding of and demonstrate cooperation with turning, coughing, deep breathing, and prescribed activity level • maintain full and equal circulation, sensation, and motion to lower extremities • maintain urine output >30 mL/hr • have active bowel sounds and a soft, non-distended abdomen • state pain controlled with ordered medication • tolerate ordered diet without nausea or vomiting • exhibit effective coping	Client will: • be afebrile • have stable vital signs and clear lungs • be alert and oriented • verbalize understanding of and demonstrate cooperation with turning, coughing, deep breathing, and prescribed activity level • maintain full and equal circulation, sensation, and motion to lower extremities • maintain urine output >30 mL/hr • have active bowel sounds and a soft, non-distended abdomen • state pain controlled with ordered medication • tolerate ordered diet without nausea or vomiting • exhibit effective coping
Assessments, tests, and treatments	Hct/Hgb Vital signs and O_2 saturation, neurovascular assessment and wound assessment q15min × 4; q30min × 4; q1hr × 4 and then q4hr and prn Physical assessment q4–8hr with focus on neurologic, respiratory, musculoskeletal, gastrointestinal, and urinary status Incentive spirometer q2hr Intake and output q4hr and prn—straight cath q8hr and prn Measure for TED stockings and remove and replace every shift Assess wound drainage q2–4hr and prn	Vital signs and O_2 saturation, neurovascular assessment and wound assessment q4hr and prne Physical assessment q4–8hr with focus on neurologic, respiratory, musculoskeletal, gastrointestinal, and urinary status Incentive spirometer q2hr Intake and output every shift and prn-straight cath q8hr and prn Remove and replace TED stockings every shift Assess wound drainage q2–4hr and prn Assess wound and remove and replace dressing BID and prn Maintain sterile technique
Knowledge deficit	Orient to room and surroundings Provide simple, brief instructions Review plan of care and importance of specific postoperative care, including turning, coughing, deep breathing, incentive spirometer, mobilization, possible intravenous tubes, and pain management Include family in teaching Evaluate understanding of teaching	Review plan of care and importance of early mobilization Initiate discharge teaching regarding diet, activity, and strategies to prevent re-injury Include family in teaching Evaluate understanding of teaching
Psychosocial	Assess anxiety related to diagnosis and surgery Assess fears of the unknown related to surgery Encourage verbalization of concerns Minimize external stimuli (eg, noise, movement)	Assess level of anxiety Encourage verbalization of concerns Provide ongoing support and encouragement

	Date ____ **Operative Day**	Date ____ **1st Day Postoperative**
Diet	Advance from clear liquids to full liquids as tolerated Baseline nutritional assessment	Advance from full liquids to regular diet as tolerated Encourage fluids to 2000 mL/day
Activity	Assess safety needs and provide appropriate precautions Reposition q2hr and prn (log roll) Bed rest; stand to void Assist client with full range of motion to all extremities 3–4 × daily Encourage client to participate in activities of daily living as much as possible	Maintain safety precautions Encourage client to participate in activities of daily living as much as possible Review principles of good body mechanics Ambulate with assistance in room qid When in bed, continue log rolling
Medications	Analgesics as ordered IV antibiotics IV fluids Antipyretics Stool softener	Analgesics as ordered IV antibiotics IV fluids or intermittent IV device Antipyretics Stool softener
Transfer/ discharge plans	Assess potential discharge needs and support system	Determine needs for referrals at time of discharge Begin home care teaching

	Date ____ **2nd Day Postoperative**	Date ____ **3rd Day Postoperative**
Daily outcomes	Client will: • have stable vital signs and clear lungs • be alert and oriented • have a clean, dry wound with edges well approximated, healing by first intention • demonstrate cooperation with turning, coughing, deep breathing, and prescribed activity level • maintain full and equal circulation, sensation, and motion to lower extremities • state pain controlled with ordered medication • maintain urine output >30 mL/hr • have active bowel sounds and a soft, non-distended abdomen • tolerate ordered diet without nausea or vomiting • exhibit effective coping • verbalize beginning understanding of home care instructions	Client is afebrile, with stable vital signs and clear lungs Client has intact neurovascular status to lower extremities Client has a clean, dry wound with edges well-approximated, healing by first intention Client manages pain with oral medications Client is independent in self-care Client is fully ambulatory Client has resumed preadmission urine and bowel elimination pattern Client verbalizes/demonstrates understanding of home care instructions Client tolerates usual diet Client exhibits effective coping with ongoing stressors

	Date _____ **2nd Day Postoperative**	Date _____ **3rd Day Postoperative**
Assessments, tests, and treatments	Vital signs q4hr and prn Physical assessment q4–8hr with focus on neurologic, respiratory, musculoskeletal, gastrointestinal, and urinary status Incentive spirometer q2hr until fully ambulatory Intake and output every shift Remove and replace TED stockings every shift Assess wound drainage q2–4hr and prn Assess wound and remove and replace dressing BID and prn Maintain sterile technique	Vital signs assessment q4hr Neurologic, respiratory, musculoskeletal, gastrointestinal, and urinary assessment every shift Incentive spirometer q2hr until fully ambulatory D/C intake and output if taking adequate fluids and balanced with output Remove and replace TED stockings every shift Remove dressing and assess wound
Knowledge deficit	Review and reinforce discharge teaching regarding diet, signs and symptoms to report, and activity level Initiate medication teaching Review written discharge instructions Include family in teaching Evaluate understanding of teaching	Provide client with written discharge instructions that discuss: 1) signs and symptoms of infection , 2) importance of regular follow-up care, 3) care of wound, and 4) monitoring neurovascular status Complete discharge teaching to include diet, follow-up care, signs and symptoms to report, activity, and medications: name, purpose, dose, frequency, route, food interactions, and side effects Include family in teaching Evaluate understanding of teaching
Psychosocial	Encourage verbalization of concerns Provide ongoing support and encouragement	Encourage verbalization of concerns Provide ongoing support and encouragement to client and family
Diet	Regular diet as tolerated Encourage fluid intake of 2000 mL/day	Regular diet as tolerated Encourage fluids to 2000mL/day
Activity	Maintain safety precautions Encourage client to participate in activities of daily living as much as possible Ambulate daily 4 times with assistance, increasing distance each time as tolerated When in bed, continue log rolling	Provide safety precautions Encourage ambulation ad lib Encourage client to participate in activities of daily living as much as possible Reinforce teaching regarding turning, positioning, and body mechanics
Medications	Analgesics as ordered IV antibiotics Intermittent IV device Stool softener Laxative if no BM in 3 days	Analgesics as ordered D/C intermittent IV device Stool softener Laxative if no BM in 3 days
Transfer/ discharge plans	Complete discharge plans Make appropriate referrals Continue home care instructions	Complete discharge instructions Refer to outpatient physical therapy if indicated

Lumbar Laminectomy

Possible Complications

- Respiratory distress
- Hemorrhage
- Infection
- Altered bowel and urine elimination

Health Conditions

- Obesity
- Peripheral vascular disease
- Neurologic disorders

Nursing Diagnoses

- Impaired physical mobility
- Activity intolerance
- Risk for injury
- Self-care deficits
- Acute pain

Discharge Teaching for Client Following
Lumbar Laminectomy

Activity

- Gradually return to usual level of activity by increasing activity each day. Alternate activity with rest periods. Avoid fatigue.
- You may sit on a bar stool to comfort.
- You may go up and down stairs.
- Avoid heavy housework, working, straining, lifting, riding, and driving for the period designated by physician.
- You may do light chores (washing dishes, preparing vegetables, or hobbies) for periods of 10–15 minutes if tolerated.
- When picking things up off the floor, hold onto a sturdy chair or table and kneel or do deep knee bend.

Diet

- Eat a well-balanced diet, including all food groups.
- Drink 6–8 glasses of fluid each day.

Signs and Symptoms to Support

Notify physician if any of these symptoms occur:
- Increase in pain, redness, or swelling
- Sudden increase in wound drainage, especially if drainage has pus or a foul odor
- Chills, or fever greater than 100F or 38C
- Nausea or vomiting
- Change in bladder or bowel habits

Follow-Up Care and General Health Care

- Schedule follow-up appointment with physician as directed.

Medications

- Review written list of medications including dose, route, frequency, food interactions, and side effects.

Wound and Dressing Care

- Cleanse skin around incision daily with mild soap and water
- If dressing present, change it daily and as often as necessary to keep dressing dry and clean.
- Remove dressing prior to showering and replace with a clean dressing afterward.
- Drainage, if present, should gradually decrease.
- If there is a marked increase in drainage, swelling, tenderness, or fever, or if drainage is foul-smelling, notify physician.

Laryngectomy

Expected length of stay: 7 days

	Date _____ **Preoperative**	Date _____ **1st 24 Hours Postoperative**	Date _____ **2nd Day Postoperative**
Daily outcomes	Client verbalizes understanding of preoperative teaching including: turning, deep breathing, coughing, moblization, oxygen therapy, suctioning and stoma care, possible tubes (nasogastric or gastrostomy tube, IV, Foley catheter, drains), pain management, and possible transfer to ICU following surgery Client communicates using an alternate mode of communication Client exhibits effective coping Client verbalizes understanding of procedure, indications for procedure, comparative risks, benefits, and implications of all options	Client will: • maintain a patent airway, with an effective breathing pattern and cough • recover from anesthesia, as evidenced by VS return to baseline and being responsive to stimuli • have a stable cardiac rhythm • have a clean wound with edges well-approximated, healing by first intention • communicate needs to staff with minimal frustration • communicate understanding of and demonstrate cooperation with turning, deep breathing, and splinting • communicate control of incisional pain with ordered medications • exhibit effective coping	Client will: • have stable vital signs and a stable cardiac rhythm, and be awake, alert, and oriented • maintain a patent airway and an effective breathing pattern and cough • maintain urine output >30 mL/hr • remain free of fluid overload or deficit • have a clean wound with edges well-approximated, healing by first intention • communicate needs to staff with minimal frustration • demonstrate cooperation with turning, deep breathing, and splinting • verbalize control of incisional pain • ambulate 2–3 times/day as tolerated • exhibit effective coping
Assessments, tests, and treatments	CBC Serum chemistries Urinalysis Chest x-ray Coagulation studies Type and cross match for designated number of units Baseline physical assessment Weight	Vital signs and O_2 saturation, neurovascular assessment, and dressing and wound drainage assessment q15min × 4, q30min × 4, then q1hr and prn Respiratory assessment: breath sounds, respiratory rate and quality, effectiveness of cough, and color and consistency of secretions q1hr and prn ABGs prn Respiratory therapy consult Cardiac monitoring Elevate head of bed at least 30 degrees Head to toe assessment q4hr Tracheostomy care per clinical protocol Suction as needed Turn, cough and deep breathe q1–2hr and prn	Vital signs and O_2 saturation, neurovascular assessment, and dressing and wound drainage assessement q2–4hr and prn Respiratory assessment q1–2hr Tracheostomy care per clinical protocol Suction as needed Intake and output q4–8hr D/C Foley catheter and assess voiding Elevate head of bed 30 degrees O_2 via humified mist collar Assess calves for redness, tenderness, swelling, heat, and edema every shift TED stockings—remove and replace every shift Head to toe assessment q4hr and prn

Laryngectomy (continued)

	Date _____ **Preoperative**	Date _____ **1st 24 Hours Postoperative**	Date _____ **2nd Day Postoperative**
Assessments, tests, and treatments (continued)		Hemoglobin and hematocrit Oxygen via humidified mist collar Small bore NG tube or gastrostomy tube to low continous suction Foley catheter to constant drainage Assess calves for redness, tenderness, swelling, heat, and edema q4hr TED stockings—remove and replace every shift Head to toe assessment q4hr and prn Intake and output q2–4hr Maintain sterile dressing—reinforce prn Mouth care q2hr and prn while awake	Maintain dry, sterile dressing—reinforce prn Assess wound and change dressing per MD order Intake and output every shift Mouth care q2hr and prn while awake
Communication	Listen carefully and provide adequate time for communication Explore use of word cards, magic slate, or portable computer to enhance communication Speech therapy consult	Listen carefully and provide adequate time for communication Observe nonverbal communication Use alternate methods for communication as determined preoperatively Answer call bell immediately and in person Anticipate needs Speech therapy consult	Listen carefully and provide adequate time for communication Observe nonverbal communication Use alternate methods for communication as determined preoperatively Answer call bell immediately and in person Encourage client and family to express feelings regarding changes in body image and function Anticipate needs Collaborate with speech therapy
Knowledge deficit	Orient to room and surroundings Provide simple, brief instructions Review preoperative preparation including hospital and surgical routines Include family in teaching Discuss surgery and specific postoperative care Instruct in relaxation techniques Evaluate understanding of teaching	Orient client and family to room and postoperative routine Include family in teaching Review plan of care Review importance of deep breathing, coughing, incentive spirometer, mobilization, and any drainage or intravenous tubes, and pain management Evaluate understanding of teaching Assess level of anxiety and offer emotional support	Review importance of early progressive exercise Review plan of care with client and family Reinforce safety measures Evaluate understanding of teaching Assess level of anxiety and offer emotional support
Diet	NPO Baseline nutritional and hydration assessment	NPO Dietary consult	NPO Dietary consult

➤

Laryngectomy *(continued)*

	Date _____ **Preoperative**	Date _____ **1st 24 Hours Postoperative**	Date _____ **2nd Day Postoperative**
Activity	Assess safety needs and provide appropriate measures Activity as ordered	Bed rest Turn, cough, and deep breathe q1–2hr ROM every shift Assess safety needs and maintain appropriate precautions	Maintain safety precautions turning, coughing, and deep breathing q2hr Assist out of bed 2–3 times Begin ambulation (25–50 ft)
Medications	Preoperative medications as ordered	Analgesics as ordered IV antibiotics IV fluids per order	Analgesics as ordered IV antibiotics Stool softener IV fluids per order
Transfer/ discharge plans	Assess potential discharge needs and support system Establish discharge goals with client and family	Home assessment if not previously completed Consult with social service regarding projected needs for home health care; including home health aides, visiting nurse, and speech therapy Establish discharge objectives with client and family	Review with client and family discharge objectives regarding activity and home care Consult and collaborate with speech therapy Complete discharge planning

	Date _____ **3rd Day Postoperative**	Date _____ **4th Day Postoperative**
Daily outcomes	Client will: • be afebrile, with stable vital signs • have a patent airway, with an effective breathing pattern and cough • have lungs clear to auscultation • have a clean wound with edges well-approximated, healing by first intention • have stable vital signs • communicate needs to staff with minimal frustration • demonstrate cooperation with turning, deep breathing, and splinting • verbalize control of incisional pain • ambulate 50–100 ft 2 times • exhibit effective coping	Client will: • be afebrile, have stable vital signs, and be awake, alert and oriented • have a patent airway, lungs clear to auscultation, and an effective cough • have a clean wound with edges well-approximated, healing by first intention • communicate needs with minimal frustration • communicate satisfaction with alternate means of communication • demonstrate cooperation with turning, deep breathing, and splinting • tolerate ordered feedings without nausea or vomiting • verbalize control of incisional pain • ambulate 150–200 ft 4 times • exhibit effective coping

Laryngectomy *(continued)*

	Date _____ **3rd Day Postoperative**	Date _____ **4th Day Postoperative**
Daily outcomes (continued)		• tolerate activity level without dyspnea, shortness of breath, or chest pain
Assessments, tests, and treatments	Vital signs and O_2 saturation, neurovascular assessment, and dressing assessment q4hr Respiratory assessment q1–2hr Tracheostomy care per clinical protocol Suction as needed Air or O_2 via mist collar Intake and output every shift Change dressing and assess wound healing BID Assess calves for redness, tenderness, swelling, heat, and edema every shift TED stockings—remove and replace every shift day and prn Head to toe assessment q4hr and prn Weight D/C oxygen when O_2 saturation >92% Mouth care q2hr and prn while awake	Vital signs and O_2 saturation q4hr and prn Respiratory assessment q2 4hr and prn Tracheostomy care per clinical protocol Head to toe assessment every shift Change dressings every day and prn Assess wound healing BID TED stockings—remove and replace every shift Assess calves for redness, tenderness, swelling, heat, and edema every shift Intake and output every shift Weight D/C oxygen if O_2 saturation >92% Mouth care q2hr and prn while awake
Communication	Listen carefully and provide adequate time for communication Observe nonverbal communication Use alternate methods for communication as determined preoperatively Answer call bell immediately and in person Encourage client and family to express feelings regarding changes in body image and function Anticipate needs Collaborate with speech therapy	Listen carefully and provide adequate time for communication Observe nonverbal communication Use alternate methods for communication as determined preoperatively Answer call bell immediately and in person Anticipate needs
Knowledge deficit	Review plan of care Include family in teaching Initiate discharge teaching regarding wound care and tracheostomy care Evaluate understanding of teaching Assess level of anxiety and offer emotional support	Review plan of care Include family in teaching Continue discharge teaching regarding wound care, tracheostomy care, activity, and diet Evaluate understanding of teaching Offer emotional support

➤

Laryngectomy *(continued)*

	Date _____ **3rd Day Postoperative**	Date _____ **4th Day Postoperative**
Diet	NPO Initiate NG/GT feedings if ordered	NG/GT feedings as ordered
Activity	Maintain safety precautions turning, coughing, and deep breathing q2hr Assist out of bed 2–3 times Begin ambulation (50–100Ft) BID	Encourage self-care Ambulate 150–200 ft qid
Medications	Analgesics as ordered IV antibiotics Stool softener IV fluids as ordered	Analgesics as ordered Stool softener Intermittent IV device

*Transfer/
discharge plans*
	Review with client and family
	   progress toward discharge
	   objectives
	Collaborate with speech therapy
	Make appropriate referrals for
	   discharge care
		Review with client and family
		   discharge objectives regarding
		   activity and home care
		Arrange visit from laryngectomy
		   support group

	Date _____ **5th–6th Days Postoperative**	Date _____ **7th Day—Discharge Day**
Daily outcomes	Client will: • be afebrile, have stable vital signs, and be awake, alert, and oriented • have a patent airway, lungs clear to auscultation, and an effective cough • have a clean wound with edges well-approximated, healing by first intention • communicate needs with minimal frustration • communicate satisfaction with alternate means of communication • demonstrate cooperation with turning, coughing, deep breathing, and splinting • tolerate ordered feedings without nausea or vomiting • verbalize control of incisional pain • ambulate 150–300 ft 4 times • exhibits effective coping	Client is afebrile Client is alert and oriented Client has a patent airway, lungs clear to auscultation, and an effective cough Client has a dry, clean wound with edges well-approximated, healing by first intention Client has stable vital signs Client manages pain with non-pharmacologic measures and ordered medications Client communicates needs with minimal frustration Client and family communicate satisfaction with alternate means of communication Client is independent in self-care Client ambulates 300–500 ft qid Client has resumed preadmission urine and bowel elimination pattern Client verbalizes/demonstrates home care instructions

Laryngectomy *(continued)*

	Date _____ **5th–6th Days Postoperative**	Date _____ **7th Day—Discharge Day**
Daily outcomes (continued)		Client and/or family demonstrates tracheostomy care safely and correctly Client tolerates ordered feedings Client and family demonstrate ability to safely and correctly administer tube feedings Client exhibits effective coping with ongoing stressors
Assessments, tests, *and treatments*	CBC, electrolytes, glucose, serum protein and albumin Vital signs q4hr and prn Respiratory assessment q4hr and prn Tracheostomy care per clinical protocol Head to toe assessment every shift Remove dressings Assess wound healing BID Intake and output Weight Mouth care q2hr and prn while awake	Vital signs every shift Respiratory assessment q4hr and prn Tracheostomy care per clinical protocol Head to toe assessment Assess wounds Weight Mouth care q2hr and prn while awake
Communication	Listen carefully and provide adequate time for communication Observe nonverbal communication Use alternate methods for communication as determined preoperatively Answer call bell immediately and in person Anticipate needs	Listen carefully and provide adequate time for communication Observe nonverbal communication Use alternate methods for communication Answer call bell immediately and in person Anticipate needs
Knowledge deficit	Review plan of care with client and family Continue discharge teaching regarding wound care, tracheostomy care, activity, and diet Instruct client and family regarding home tube feedings if indicated Evaluate understanding of teaching Offer emotional support	Client and/or family verbalizes understanding of discharge teaching including wound care, tracheostomy care, activity, safety measures, diet, signs and symptoms to report, follow-up care and MD appointment, postoperative treatment, home care arrangements, and medications: name, purpose, dose, frequency, route, dietary interactions, and side effects Evaluate understanding of teaching Refer learning needs to community resources

➤

Laryngectomy *(continued)*

	Date _____ **5th–6th Days Postoperative**	Date _____ **7th Day—Discharge Day**
Diet	NG/GT feedings or diet as ordered	NG/GT feedings or diet as ordered
Activity	Ambulate 150–300 ft qid Shower	Ambulate 300–500 ft qid Shower
Medications	Analgesics as ordered Stool softener D/C intermittent IV device	Analgesics as ordered Stool softener
Transfer/ discharge plans	Review with client and family discharge objectives regarding activity and home care Complete referrals for home health care; including home health aides, visiting nurse, and speech therapy Refer to any appropriate support services, such as American Cancer Society	Discharge with referrals for home health care and speech therapy

Potential Client Variances
Laryngectomy

Possible Complications
- Hemorrhage
- Fistula formation
- Airway obstruction

Health Conditions
- Pre-existing respiratory problems
- Smoker
- History of alcohol abuse

Nursing Diagnoses
- Self-concept disturbance
- Constipation
- Altered oral mucous membranes
- Risk for infection

Discharge Teaching for Client Following
Laryngectomy

Activity

- Gradually return to usual level of activity by increasing activity each day. Alternate activity with rest periods. Avoid fatigue.
- No swimming.
- You may shower—but wear a shield over your stoma, direct spray below stoma, and avoid getting soap in stoma.
- Return to work following physician approval.

Diet

- Follow diet as prescribed by physician. If allowed, eat a well-balanced diet, including fruits, vegetables, meat, breads and starch, and milk products.
- Food may taste dull because of the loss of the sense of smell.
- If you have any difficulty swallowing or you notice anything unusual about eating, report it immediately to your physician.

Signs and Symptoms to Report

Notify physician if any of these symptoms occur:
- Difficulty breathing or shortness of breath
- Difficulty swallowing or eating
- Swelling in the neck area
- Shrinking around the stoma
- Sudden increase in wound drainage, especially if drainage has pus or a foul odor
- Chills, or fever greater than 100F or 38C

Follow-Up Care and General Health Care

- Schedule follow-up appointment with physician as directed.
- Cover your stoma when coughing.
- Keep your stoma covered at all times with a trach bib.
- Keep air humidified at home.
- No smoking; avoid secondhand smoke.
- Avoid individuals with respiratory infections.
- If you notice signs or symptoms of a respiratory infection, notify your physician.
- Wear a MedicAlert bracelet at all times and carry an identification card that identifies you as a neck breather.

Medications

- Review written list of medications, including dose, route, frequency, food interactions, and side effects.
- Avoid over-the-counter drugs unless recommended by your physician.
- Ask your physician regarding flu and pneumonia vaccines.

Wound and Dressing Care

Dressing care:
- Cleanse skin around incision daily with mild soap and water and pat dry.
- If there is a marked increase in drainage, swelling, tenderness, or fever, or if drainage is foul-smelling, notify physician.

Stoma care:
- Sit in a well-lighted area.
- Using a mirror, cleanse stoma twice a day as directed and pat dry.
- Keep stoma clean and free of dried secretions.

Open Reduction and Internal Fixation of Lower Leg Fracture

Expected length of stay: 3–4 days following surgery

	Date _____ **Operative Day**	Date _____ **1st Postoperative Day**
Daily outcomes	Client will: • have stable vital signs • recover from anesthesia, as evidenced by VS return to baseline, clear lungs, and being awake, alert, and oriented • verbalize understanding and demonstrate cooperation with turning, coughing, deep breathing, and prescribed activity level • state pain controlled with ordered medication • tolerate ordered diet without nausea or vomiting • exhibit effective coping	Client will: • have stable vital signs • have clear lungs, and be awake, alert, and oriented • verbalize understanding and demonstrate cooperation with turning, coughing, deep breathing, and prescribed activity level • state pain control with ordered medication • tolerate ordered diet without nausea and vomiting • exhibit effective coping
Assessments, tests, and treatments	Hct/Hgb Vital signs and O_2 saturation, neurovascular assessment and wound/cast assessment q15min × 4; q30min × 4; q1hr × 4 and then q4hr and prn Physical assessment q4–8hr with a focus on respiratory, cardiovascular, neurologic, musculoskeletal, gastrointestinal, and urinary status Incentive spirometer q2hr Intake and output every shift	Vital signs and O_2 saturation, neurovascular assessment and wound/cast assessment q4hr and prn Head to toe assessment every shift and prn Incentive spirometer q2hr Intake and output every shift
Knowledge deficit	Orient to room and surroundings Provide simple, brief instructions Review plan of care and importance of specific postoperative care: turning, coughing, deep breathing, incentive spirometer, mobilization, possible intravenous tubes, and pain management Include family in teaching Evaluate understanding of teaching	Review plan of care and importance of early mobilization Begin discharge teaching regarding cast care and mobility Include family in teaching Evaluate understanding of teaching
Psychosocial	Assess anxiety related to diagnosis and surgery Assess fears of the unknown related to surgery Encourage verbalization of concerns Minimize external stimuli (eg, noise, movement)	Assess level of anxiety Encourage verbalization of concerns Provide ongoing support and encouragement
Diet	Advance from clear liquids to full liquids to tolerance Baseline nutritional assessment	Advance from full liquids to regular diet as tolerated Offer supplemental feedings high in protein and vitamins

	Date _____ **Operative Day**	Date _____ **1st Postoperative Day**
Activity	Assess safety needs and provide appropriate precautions Reposition q2hr and prn Assist client with full range of motion to all unaffected extremities 3–4 times daily Demonstrate isometric exercises for the lower limb Encourage client to participate in activities of daily living as much as possible Provide overhead trapeze Keep extremity elevated	Maintain safety precautions Reposition q2hr and prn Assist client with full range of motion to all unaffected extremities 3–4 times daily Encourage client to perform isometric exercises for the lower limb Encourage client to participate in activities of daily living as much as possible Encourage use of overhead trapeze Keep extremity elevated
Medications	Analgesics as ordered IV antibiotics IV fluids Antipyretics—prn	Analgesics as ordered IV antibiotics IV fluids or intermittent IV device Antipyretics—prn
Transfer/ discharge plans	Assess discharge needs and support system Establish discharge goals with client and family	Determine referral needs for time of discharge Begin home care teaching

	Date _____ **2nd Postoperative Day**	Date _____ **3rd–4th Days Postoperative**
Daily outcomes	Client will: • have stable vital signs and clear lungs • demonstrate cooperation with turning, coughing, deep breathing, and prescribed activity level • state pain controlled with ordered medication • tolerate ordered diet without nausea or vomiting • ambulate with crutches 2–3 times per day • exhibit effective coping • verbalize/demonstrate beginning understanding of home care instructions	Client is afebrile, with stable vital signs and clear lungs Client has intact neurovascular status to affected extremity Client manages pain with oral medications Client is independent in self-care Client is independent in transfers and ambulatory with crutches Client has resumed preadmission urine and bowel elimination pattern Client verbalizes/demonstrates home care instructions Client tolerates usual diet Client exhibits effective coping with ongoing stressors
Assessments, tests, and treatments	Vital signs and wound/cast assessment q4hr Head to toe assessment every shift and prn Neurovascular assessment q4hr Incentive spirometer q2hr until fully ambulatory Intake and output every shift	Vital signs and wound/cast assessment q4hr Head to toe assessment every shift Neurovascular assessment q4hr and prn Incentive spirometer q2hr until fully ambulatory D/C intake and output if taking adequate fluids and balanced with output

Open Reduction and Internal Fixation of Lower Leg Fracture (continued)

	Date _____ **2nd Postoperative Day**	Date _____ **3rd–4th Days Postoperative**
Knowledge deficit	Initiate discharge teaching regarding diet, signs and symptoms to report, and activity level Physical therapy consult for beginning instructions regarding crutch walking Review written discharge instructions Include family in teaching Evaluate understanding of teaching	Provide client with written discharge instructions that discuss: 1) weightbearing on affected extremity, 2) signs and symptoms of infection related to internal fixation device, 3) importance of regular follow-up care, 4) care of wound/cast, 5) monitoring neurovascular status, and 6) use of assistive devices Include family in teaching Complete discharge teaching to include diet, follow-up care, signs and symptoms to report, activity, and medications: name, purpose, dose, frequency, route, food interactions, and side effects Evaluate understanding of teaching
Psychosocial	Encourage verbalization of concerns Provide ongoing support and encouragement	Encourage verbalization of concerns Provide ongoing support and encouragement
Diet	Regular diet as tolerated Encourage fluid intake of 2000 mL per day Offer supplemental feedings high in protein and vitamins	Regular diet as tolerated Encourage fluids to 2000 mL/day Offer supplemental feedings high in protein and vitamins
Activity	Maintain safety precautions Assist client with full range of motion to all unaffected extremities 3–4 times daily Encourage client to perform isometric exercises for the lower limb Encourage client to participate in activities of daily living as much as possible Encourage client to use overhead trapeze Refer to physical therapy to begin non-weight bearing crutch walking Assist out of bed 2–3 times daily as tolerated Keep extremity elevated	Provide safety precautions Assist client with full range of motion to all unaffected extremities 3 or 4 times daily Encourage client to perform isometric exercises for the lower limb Encourage client to participate in activities of daily living as much as possible Encourage client to use overhead trapeze q3hr Continue to work with physical therapy to promote non-weight bearing crutch walking 4 times daily; begin stair training
Medications	Analgesics as ordered IV antibiotics Intermittent IV device	Analgesics as ordered D/C intermittent IV device
Transfer/ discharge plans	Complete discharge plans Make appropriate discharge referrals Continue home care instructions	Complete discharge instructions and referrals

Potential Client Variances

Open Reduction and Internal Fixation of Lower Leg Fracture

Possible Complications

- Hemorrhage
- Compartment syndrome
- Infection
- Altered peripheral tissue perfusion
- Deep vein thrombosis

Health Conditions

- Pre-existing respiratory problems
- Pre-existing mobility problems
- Bleeding tendencies
- Neurologic disorders

Nursing Diagnoses

- Impaired physical mobility
- Acute pain
- Risk for injury

Discharge Teaching for Client Following

Open Reduction and Internal Fixation of Lower Leg Fracture

Activity

- Gradually return to usual level of activity by increasing activity each day. Alternate activity with rest periods. Avoid fatigue.
- To prevent swelling, keep leg elevated except when walking. When in bed or on couch, elevate leg on pillow.
- If leg and/or foot is swollen and causes you pain, you are walking too much; cut back on activity and keep your leg elevated for longer periods.
- No strenuous activity until okayed by physician.
- Avoid driving for the period designated by physician.
- Continue exercises as recommended by physician.
- Return to work as directed by physician.
- Use crutches as instructed.
- Do not shower or tub bathe until okayed by physician.

Diet

- Eat a well-balanced diet, including all food groups.
- Drink 6–8 glasses of fluid each day.

Signs and Symptoms to Report

Notify physician if any of these symptoms occur:
- Increase in pain, redness, or swelling
- Sudden increase in wound drainage, especially if drainage has pus or a foul odor
- Chills, or fever greater than 100F or 38C

Follow-Up Care and General Health Care

- Schedule follow-up appointment with physician as directed.
- Have someone remove scatter rugs from floors at home.
- Have someone remove any potential safety hazards from home.
- Wear an apron or shoulder bag to carry small objects from room to room.

Medications

- Review written list of medications, including dose, frequency, food interactions, and side effects.

Wound and Dressing Care

If dressing is present:
- Cleanse skin around incision daily with mild soap and water.
- Change dressing daily and as often as necessary to keep dressing dry and clean.
- Drainage, if present, should gradually decrease.
- If there is a marked increase in drainage, swelling, tenderness, or fever, or if drainage is foul-smelling, notify physician.

If cast is present:
- Keep cast dry.
- Do not put any objects or material under cast.
- When cast is removed, minimize exposure to sun.

Mastectomy

Expected length of stay: 3–4 days

	Date _____ **1st 24 Hours Postoperative**	Date _____ **48 Hours Postoperative**	Date _____ **3–4 Days Postoperative**
Daily outcomes	Client will: • be afebrile and have stable vital signs • have a clean, dry dressing • recover from anesthesia, as evidenced by VS return to baseline and being awake, alert and oriented • verbalize understanding of and demonstrate cooperation with turning, coughing, deep breathing, and splinting • tolerate ordered diet without nausea or vomiting • verbalize control of incisional pain • exhibit effective coping	Client will: • be afebrile and have stable vital signs • have a clean, dry wound with edges well-approximated, healing by first intention • demonstrate cooperation with turning, coughing, deep breathing, and splinting • tolerate ordered diet without nausea or vomiting • ambulate 4 × daily in hallway • verbalize control of incisional pain • exhibit beginning ability to cope with changes in body image • verbalize beginning understanding of home care instructions	Cllient is afebrile and has stable vital signs Client has a clean, dry wound with edges well-approximated, healing by first intention Client manages pain with oral medications and/or non-pharmacologic measures Client is independent in self-care Client is fully ambulatory Client has resumed preadmission urine and bowel elimination pattern Client verbalizes home care instructions Client tolerates usual diet Client exhibits increasing ability to cope with changes in body image and ongoing stressors Client verbalizes knowledge of and demonstrates progessive upper extremity exercises that include external rotation and abduction of the affected shoulder when the stitches are removed 7–10 days after surgery
Assessments, tests, and treatments	Vital signs and O_2 saturation, neurovascular assessment, dressing and wound drainage assessment q15min × 4; q30min × 4; q1hr × 4 and then q4hr and prn NO BLOOD PRESSURES OR VENIPUNCTURES ON AFFECTED ARM Assess respiratory status q4hr and prn Incentive spirometer q2hr Intake and output every shift Assess voiding—if unable to void, try suggestive voiding techniqes or if still unable, catheterize q8hr or prn	Vital signs and dressing and wound drainage assessment q4hr and prn NO BLOOD PRESSURES OR VENIPUNCTURES ON AFFECTED ARM Assess respiratory status q4hr Incentive spirometer q2hr until fully ambulatory Intake and output every shift Assess voiding pattern every shift Dressing change by surgeon	Vital signs and dressing and wound drainage assessment q4–8hr NO BLOOD PRESSURES OR VENIPUNCTURES ON AFFECTED ARM Assess respiratory status q4–8hr Assess wound and apply dry sterile dressing every day and prn

	Date _____ **1st 24 Hours Postoperative**	Date _____ **48 Hours Postoperative**	Date _____ **3–4 Days Postoperative**
Knowledge deficit	Orient to room and surroundings Provide simple, brief instructions Review preoperative preparation, including hospital and specific postoperative care: turning, coughing, deep breathing, incentive spirometer, mobilization, intravenous and pain management (PCA or prn medications) Evaluate understanding of teaching	Review plan of care and importance of early mobilization Begin discharge teaching regarding wound care/dressing change, diet, and activity Review written discharge instructions with client and family Evaluate understanding of teaching	Complete discharge teaching to include wound care, diet, follow-up care, signs and symptoms to report, activity, and medication: dose, frequency, route, and side effects Provide client with written discharge instructions including upper arm and shoulder exercises for affected arm Evaluate understanding of teaching
Diet	Clear to full liquids as tolerated	Full liquids to usual diet as tolerated	Usual diet as tolerated
Activity	Provide safety precautions Ambulate 4 times in room Encourage finger, wrist, and elbow movement, and use of affected arm for ADLs and personal hygiene	Fully ambulatory in room Walk in hall 4–6 times per day Encourage finger, wrist, and elbow movement, and use of affected arm for ADLs and personal hygiene Instruct client in progressive upper arm exercises	Fully ambulatory Encourage finger, wrist, and elbow movement, and use of affected arm for ADLs and personal hygiene Instruct client in progressive upper arm exercises
Medications	Analgesics as ordered IV antibiotics if ordered IV fluids	Analgesics as ordered IV antibiotics if ordered Intermittent IV device	Analgesics as ordered D/C IV device
Psychosocial	Assess coping status Use active listening Provide a nonthreatening environment Determine support persons and resources available to client Assess responses of support persons Allow for client's input regarding sequence of care Be supportive of client's effective coping behaviors Establish a trusting relationship with client Encourage client and significant other to verbalize their feelings about the mastectomy Listen to client and significant other and show interest and concern rather than giving advice	Assess coping status Use active listening Provide a nonthreatening environment Assist client to identify and develop support systems and resources Assess responses of support persons Allow for client's input regarding sequence of care Be supportive of client's effective coping behaviors Maintain trusting relationship with client Encourage client and significant other to verbalize their feelings about the mastectomy Listen to client and significant other and show interest and concern rather than giving advice	Assess coping status Use active listening Provide a nonthreatening environment Determine support persons and resources available to the client Assess responses of support persons Allow for client's input regarding sequence of care Be supportive of client's effective coping behaviors Provide opportunities to verbalize ongoing concerns regarding changes in body image and self-concept Encourage and provide opportunities for self-care of wound and dressing Provide opportunity for client to meet with volunteer from Reach to Recovery

	Date _____ **1st 24 Hours Postoperative**	Date _____ **48 Hours Postoperative**	Date _____ **3–4 Days Postoperative**
Psychosocial *(continued)*	Allow the patient to respond to loss of body part and changed body image with denial, shock, anger, depression, and other grieving behaviors Support client's strengths and assist her to look at herself in totality	Allow the patient to respond to loss of body part and changed body image with denial, shock, anger, depression, and other grieving behaviors Support client's strengths and assist her to look at herself in totality	Assist client to obtain temporary breast prosthesis Answer questions and provide information regarding breast reconstruction
Transfer/ *discharge plans*	Determine discharge needs with client and significant other Begin home care instructions	Review progess toward discharge goals Finalize discharge plans Refer to Reach to Recovery	Complete discharge instructions

Potential Client Variances
Mastectomy

Potential Complications

- Lymphedema
- Impaired wound healing
- Hematoma formation

Health Conditions

- Pre-existing respiratory problems
- Pre-existing mobility problems

Nursing Diagnoses

- Body image disturbance
- Grieving
- Self-care deficits
- Ineffective individual coping

Discharge Teaching for Client Following
Mastectomy

Activity

- Gradually return to usual level of activity by increasing activity each day. Alternate activity with rest periods.
- Exercise affected arm as instructed to tolerance. Stop at the point of pain.
- Elevate affected arm several times a day, by combing hair, doing wall climbing exercises or eating with affected arm.
- Avoid heavy housework, working, straining, and driving for the period designated by your physician.

Diet

- Eat a well-balanced diet, including all food groups.
- Drink 6–8 glasses of fluid each day.

Signs and Symptoms to Report

Notify physician if any of these symptoms occur:
- Increase in pain, redness, or swelling
- Sudden increase in wound drainage, especially if drainage has pus or a foul odor.
- Chills, or fever greater than 100F or 38C

Follow-Up Care and General Health Care

- Schedule follow-up appointment with physician as directed.
- Examine remaining breast once per month.
- Refer to Reach to Recovery
- Reinforce safety precautions:
  - Avoid activities that could injure arm or hand; for example gardening, use of sharp objects
  - Avoid injections or blood drawing in affected arm
  - No B/P on affected arm
  - Treat burns, cuts, scratches on affected arm immediately
  - Wear gloves when working with sharp objects
  - Wear loose-fitting clothing until incision heals
  - Avoid sunburn
  - Use a thimble when sewing
  - Use an electric razor on affected underarm

Medications

- Review written list of medications, including dose, route, frequency, food interactions, and side effects.

Wound and Dressing Care

- Cleanse skin around incision daily with mild soap and water.
- If dressing present, change it daily and as often as necessary to keep dressing dry and clean.
- Remove dressing prior to showering and replace with a clean dressing afterward.
- Drainage, if present, should gradually decrease.
- If there is a marked increase in drainage or swelling, tenderness, or fever, or if drainage is foul-smelling, notify physician.

Microdiskectomy

Expected length of stay: less than 24 hours

	Date _____ **Preoperative**	Date _____ **1st 24 Hours Following Surgery**
Daily outcomes	Client verbalizes understanding of preoperative teaching, including: turning, deep breathing, incentive spirometer, mobilization, and pain management Client exhibits effective coping with preparations for surgery Client verbalizes understanding of procedure, indications for procedure, comparative risks, benefits, and implications Obtain informed consent	Client has stable vital signs and is alert and oriented Client has a clean, dry wound with edges well-approximated, healing by first intention Client has intact neurovascular assessments Client manages pain with non-pharmacologic measures and oral medications Client is independent in self-care with minimal assistance Client is fully ambulatory Client has resumed preadmission urine and bowel elimination pattern Client verbalizes/demonstrates home care instructions Client verbalizes strategies to prevent re-herniation Client tolerates usual diet Client demonstrates ability to cope with ongoing stressors
Assessments, tests, and treatments	CBC Urinalysis Baseline physical assessment with a focus on respiratory status and gastrointestinal and urinary function Measure for anti-emboli stockings and apply Anesthesia consult	Vital signs and O_2 saturation, mental status exam, dressing and wound drainage assessment q15min × 4; q30min × 4; q1hr × 4 and then q4hr and prn Neurovascular assessments to include distal pulse checks, capillary refill, skin color and temperature, muscle strength, movement, and sensation. Monitor for any numbness, tingling, or neurological impairment If there is serous drainage on the dressing, assess for presence or absence of glucose Maintain dry, sterile dressing and reinforce prn Monitor very carefully for changes in bladder/bowel function and check for distention Assess lung sounds q4–8hr and prn Assess gastrointestinal and urinary funtion q2–4hr and prn Intake and output every shift Assess voiding—if unable to void, try suggestive voiding techniques or, if still unable, catheterize q8hr or prn Remove and replace anti-emboli stockings for 30 minutes q8hr

	Date _____ **Preoperative**	Date _____ **1st 24 Hours Following Surgery**
Knowledge deficit	Orient to room and surroundings Include family in teaching Provide simple, brief instructions Review preoperative preparation, including hospital and surgical routines Reinforce preoperative teaching regarding specific postoperative care: turning, deep breathing, incentive spirometer, mobilization, and pain management Evaluate understanding of teaching	Reorient to room and postoperative routine Include family in teaching Review plan of care and importance of early mobilization, as well as any activity restrictions Complete discharge teaching regarding wound care/dressing change, follow-up care and appointment, signs and symptoms to report, diet, and medications: name, purpose, dose, route, frequency, food interactions, and side effects Instruct regarding the importance of a progressive exercise program with frequent rest periods and to avoid heavy lifting or driving until okayed by health care provider Evaluate understanding of teaching
Psychosocial	Assess anxiety related to pending surgery Assess fears of the unknown related to surgery Encourage verbalization of concerns Provide emotional support to client and family Minimize external stimuli (eg, noise, movement)	Assess level of anxiety Encourage verbalization of concerns Provide emotional support to client and family Provide information and ongoing support and encouragement
Diet	NPO Baseline nutritional assessment	Advance to clear liquids; if tolerated, advance to full liquids/regular diet morning following surgery
Activity	OOB ad lib until premedicated for surgery Assess safety needs and implement appropriate precautions	Maintain safety precautions Instruct regarding log-rolling and the importance of avoiding flexion, extension, stretching, flexing, twisting, and jarring movements Bathroom privileges with assistance evening after surgery; begin progressive ambulation as tolerated the morning following surgery until fully ambulatory
Medications	NPO except preoperative medications	Analgesics as ordered Muscle relaxants Nonsteroidal anti-inflammatory drugs Antibiotics if ordered IV fluids until adequate oral intake, then intermittent IV device. Discontinue prior to discharge
Transfer/ discharge plans	Assess potential discharge needs and availability of support system Establish discharge goals with client and family	Probable discharge within 24 hours of surgery Complete discharge instructions when fully awake and oriented and before discharge Provide a written copy of discharge instructions Make referral to physical therapy for progressive exercise program on an outpatient basis

Potential Client Variances
Microdiskectomy

Possible Complications

- Respiratory distress
- Hemorrhage
- Infection
- Altered bowel and urine elimination

Health Conditions

- Obesity
- Pre-existing mobility problems
- Peripheral vascular disease
- Neurologic disorders

Nursing Diagnoses

- Impaired physical mobility
- Activity intolerance
- Risk for injury
- Self-care deficits
- Acute pain

Discharge Teaching for Client Following
Microdiskectomy

Activity

- Gradually return to usual level of activity by increasing activity each day. Alternate activity with rest periods. Avoid fatigue.
- You may sit on a bar stool to comfort.
- You may go up and down stairs.
- Avoid heavy housework, working, straining, heavy lifting, riding, and driving for the period designated by your physician.
- You may do light chores (washing dishes, preparing vegtables, or hobbies) for periods of 10–15 minutes if tolerated.
- When picking things up off the floor, hold onto a sturdy chair or table and kneel or do a deep knee bend.

Diet

- Eat a well balanced diet including all food groups.
- Drink 6–8 glasses of fluid each day.

Signs and Symptoms to Report

Notify physician if any of these symptoms occur:
- Increase in pain, redness, or swelling
- Sudden increase in wound drainage, especially if drainage has pus or a foul odor
- Chills or fever greater than 100F or 38C
- Nausea or vomiting
- Change in bladder or bowel habits

Follow-Up Care and General Health Care

- Schedule follow-up appointment with physician as directed.

Medications

- Review written list of medications, including dose, route, frequency, food interactions, and side effects.

Wound and Dressing Care

- Cleanse skin around incision daily with mild soap and water.
- If dressing present, change it daily and as often as necessary to keep dressing dry and clean.
- Remove dressing prior to showering and replace with a clean dressing afterward.
- Drainage, if present, should gradually decrease.
- If there is a marked increase in drainage, swelling, tenderness, or fever, or if drainage is foul-smelling, notify physician.

Critical Pathway for Client Following
Nephrectomy

Expected length of stay: 6–7 days

	Date _____ **Preoperative**	Date _____ **1st 24 Hours Postoperative**	Date _____ **2nd–3rd Days Postoperative**
Daily outcomes	Client verbalizes understanding of preoperative teaching including: turning, coughing, deep breathing, incentive spirometer, mobilization, possible tubes (nasogastric tube, IV, Foley catheter, penrose or other drains), and pain management Client verbalizes understanding of procedure, indications for procedure, comparative risks, benefits, and implications of all options Obtain informed consent Client exhibits effective coping with preoperative preparations	Client will: • have stable vital signs • have a clean, dry wound with edges well-approximated, healing by first intention • recover from anesthesia, as evidenced by VS return to baseline, and being awake, alert, and oriented • verbalize understanding of and demonstrate cooperation with turning, coughing, deep breathing, and splinting • have lungs clear to auscultation • have urine output >30 mL/hr • remain free of nausea and vomiting • verbalize control of incisional pain with ordered medications and non-pharmacologic measures • transfer out of bed with assistance 2 times • exhibit effective coping	Client will: • have stable vital signs • have a clean, dry wound with edges well-approximated, healing by first intention • have a urine output >30 mL/hr • have active bowel sounds • tolerate ordered diet without nausea or vomiting • demonstrate cooperation with turning, coughing, deep breathing and splinting • have lungs clear to auscultation • ambulate 4 times each day • verbalize control of incisional pain with ordered medications and non-pharmacologic methods • exhibit effective coping • verbalize/demonstrate beginning understanding of home care instructions
Assessments, test, and treatments	CBC Electrolytes Chemistry profile Urinalysis Chest x-ray Baseline physical assessment with a focus on respiratory status and gastrointestinal and urinary function	CBC Electrolytes Vital signs and O_2 saturation, neurovascular assessment, dressing and wound drainage assessment q15min × 4; q30min × 4; q1hr × 4 and then q4hr and prn Assess respiratory status and gastrointestinal function q4hr and prn Assess patency of Foley catheter and urine output q1hr x 24 hr Report urine output <30 mL/hr Strict intake and output Incentive spirometer q2hr Intake and output every shift Assess patency of NG tube q2hr, noting volume, color, and character of drainage	Vital signs and dressing and wound drainage assessment q4hr and prn Assess respiratory status and gastrointestinal function q4hr Incentive spirometer q2hr until fully ambulatory Strict intake and output every 2–4 hr If still in place, assess patency and output of NG tube q4–8hr Assess Foley catheter and urine output q2–4hr and prn Report urine output <30 mL/hr Using sterile asepsis, change dressing; assess wound healing and wound drainage

Nephrectomy *(continued)*

	Date _____ **Preoperative**	Date _____ **1st 24 Hours Postoperative**	Date _____ **2nd–3rd Days Postoperative**
Assessments, tests, and treatments (continued)		Assess and record the description, location, duration, and characteristics of client's pain q2–4hr and prn Encourage verbalization of pain and discomfort Reduce or eliminate pain-producing factors and employ distraction or relaxation techniques Provide back rubs Encourage client to request analgesic or use PCA before pain becomes severe	Assess and record the description, location, duration, and characteristics of client's pain q4hr and prn Reduce or eliminate pain-producing factors, employ distraction or relaxation techniques, and offer back rubs
Knowledge deficit	Orient to room and surroundings Provide simple, brief instructions Review preoperative preparation including hospital and surgical routines Include family in teaching Discuss surgery and specific postoperative care: turning, coughing, deep breathing, splinting incision, incentive spirometer, mobilization, possible tubes (nasogastric [NG] and intravenous [IV]), and pain management Instruct regarding distraction techniques, such as slow rhythmic breathing and guided imagery, to produce pain relief Instruct in relaxation techniques, such as tensing and relaxing muscle groups and rhythmic breathing Evaluate understanding of teaching	Reorient to room and postoperative routine Include family in teaching Review plan of care and importance of early mobilization Review importance of turning, coughing, deep breathing, splinting incision, incentive spirometer, mobilization, possible tubes (drainage, Foley catheter, and intravenous), and pain management Evaluate understanding of teaching	Reinforce earlier teaching regarding ongoing care Include family in teaching Begin discharge teaching regarding activity level and wound care Evaluate understanding of teaching
Psychosocial	Assess anxiety related to diagnosis and pending surgery Assess fears of the unknown related to surgery Offer emotional support Encourage verbalization of concerns Minimize external stimuli (eg, noise, movement)	Assess client's and family's level of anxiety Encourage verbalization of concerns Provide information and ongoing support and encouragement to client and family	Encourage verbalization of concerns Provide ongoing support and encouragement to client and family
Diet	NPO Baseline nutritional and hydration assessment	NPO NG tube until return of bowel sounds	When NG tube removed, begin clear liquids as tolerated

	Date _____ **Preoperative**	Date _____ **1st 24 Hours Postoperative**	Date _____ **2nd–3rd Days Postoperative**
Activity	Assess safety needs and provide appropriate measures Activity as ordered	Maintain safety precautions Assist to chair 2 times	Maintain safety precautions Ambulate 4 times with assistance
Medications	Preoperative medications as ordered	IV fluids IV antibiotics if ordered Analgesics as ordered Evaluate effectiveness of analgesics	IV fluids IV antibiotics if ordered When ordered, convert IV to intermittent IV device Analgesics as ordered Evaluate effectiveness of analgesics
Transfer/ discharge plans	Assess potential discharge needs and support system Establish discharge goals with client and family	Review progress toward discharge goals with client and family Consult with social service regarding VNA and projected needs for home health care (if any)	Review progress toward discharge goals with client and family Make appropriate discharge referrals

	Date _____ **4th Day Postoperative**	Date _____ **5th Day Postoperative**	Date _____ **6th–7th Days Postoperative**
Daily outcomes	Client will: • be afebrile, with stable vital signs • be awake, alert, and oriented • have a clean, dry wound with edges well-approximated, healing by first intention • maintain urine output >30 mL/hr • have lungs clear to auscultation • tolerate ordered diet without nausea or vomiting • ambulate 4–6 times • verbalize control of incisional pain with ordered medications and non-pharmacologic measures • exhibit effective coping • verbalize/demonstrate beginning understanding of home care instructions	Client will: • be afebrile with stable vital signs • be awake, alert, and oriented • have a clean, dry wound with edges well-approximated, healing by first intention • maintain urine output >30 mL/hr • tolerate ordered diet without nausea or vomiting • ambulate 4–6 times • verbalize control of incisional pain with ordered medications and non-pharmacologic measures • exhibit effective coping • verbalize/demonstrate beginning understanding of home care instructions	Client is afebrile, with stable vital signs Client is awake, alert, and oriented Client has a clean, dry wound with edges well-approximated, healing by first intention Client has urine output >30 mL/hr Client manages pain with non-pharmacologic measures and any ordered medications Client is independent in self-care Client is fully ambulatory Client has resumed preadmission urine and bowel elimination patterns Client verbalizes home care instructions Client tolerates usual diet Client exhibits effective coping with ongoing stressors

➤

Nephrectomy *(continued)*

	Date _____ **4th Day Postoperative**	Date _____ **5th Day Postoperative**	Date _____ **6th–7th Days Postoperative**
Assessments, tests, and treatments	Vital signs, dressing, and wound drainage assessment q4hr and prn Incentive spirometer q2hr until fully ambulatory Intake and output every shift D/C Foley catheter and assess voiding pattern q2–4hr and prn Assess respiratory status and gastrointestinal function q4–8hr and prn Using sterile asepsis, change dressing: assess wound healing and wound drainage Assess and record description, location, duration, and characteristics of client's pain q4hr and prn Encourage client to employ distraction or relaxation techniques	Vital signs, dressing, and wound drainage assessment q4hr Assess respiratory status and gastrointestinal function q4–8hr Intake and output every shift and monitor urine output q4hr and prn Report urine output <30 mL/hr Remove dressing and assess wound healing and drainage Assess and record description, location, duration, and characteristics of client's pain q4hr and prn Encourage client to employ distraction or relaxation techniques	Vital signs and wound assessment q4–8hr Assess respiratory status and gastrointestinal function Intake and output Report urine output <30 mL/hr Assess wound healing Assess and record description, location, duration, and characteristics of client's pain q4hr and prn Encourage client to employ distraction or relaxation techniques
Knowledge deficit	Include family in teaching Initiate discharge teaching regarding wound care, diet, and activity Review written discharge instructions with client and family Evaluate understanding of teaching	Continue discharge teaching regarding wound care, diet, signs and symptoms to report, medications, and activity Include family in teachng Review written discharge instructions with client and family Evaluate understanding of teaching	Complete discharge teaching to include wound care, diet, follow-up care, signs and symptoms to report, activity, and medications: name, purpose, dose, frequency, route, dietary interactions, and side effects Provide client with written discharge instructions Evaluate understanding of teaching
Psychosocial	Encourage verbalization of concerns Provide ongoing support and encouragement	Encourage verbalization of concerns Provide ongoing support and encouragement	Encourage verbalization of concerns Provide ongoing support and encouragement
Diet	If tolerating clear liquids, advance to full liquids as tolerated	Advance diet to soft, regular diet as tolerated Encourage fluids	Regular diet as tolerated Encourage fluids
Activity	Ambulate independently at least 4 times Maintain safely precautions	Fully ambulatory Maintain safety precautions	Fully ambulatory

Nephrectomy *(continued)*

	Date _____ **4th Day Postoperative**	Date _____ **5th Day Postoperative**	Date _____ **6th–7th Days Postoperative**
Medications	Analgesics as ordered Evaluate effectiveness of analgesics Intermittent IV device for any IV medications—D/C when so ordered	Analgesics as ordered Evaluate effectiveness of analgesics	Analgesics as ordered Evaluate effectiveness of analgesics
Transfer/ discharge plans	Continue to review progress toward discharge goals Make appropriate discharge referrals	Finalize discharge plans Continue to review progress toward discharge goals Finalize plans for home care if needed	Complete discharge instructions

Potential Client Variances
Nephrectomy

Possible Complications
- Hemorrhage
- Pneumothorax
- Fluid and electrolyte disturbances

Health Conditions
- Pre-existing respiratory conditions
- Renal disease

Nursing Diagnoses
- Acute pain
- Ineffective breathing pattern
- Constipation

Discharge Teaching for Client Following
Nephrectomy

Activity

- Gradually return to usual level of activity by increasing activity each day. Alternate activity with planned rest periods. Avoid fatigue.
- You may go up and down stairs as long as you feel comfortable.
- Avoid heavy housework, working, straining, heavy lifting, and driving for the period designated by your physician.
- Avoid contact sports, horseback riding, motorcycle riding, skiing, and snowmobiling, until permitted by your physician.

Diet

- Follow the diet recommended by your physician. Eat a well-balanced diet, including all food groups.
- Drink 1-2 quarts of fluids each day.

Signs and Symptoms to Report

Notify physician if any of these symptoms occur:
- Increase in pain, redness, or swelling
- Sudden increase in wound drainage, especially if drainage has pus or a foul odor
- Nausea, vomiting, or change in bowel habits
- Chills, or fever greater than 100F or 38C

Follow-Up Care and General Health

- Schedule follow-up appointment with physician as directed.
- Avoid constipation and straining. Extra fiber and fluids may help prevent constipation. Do not use laxatives unless recommended by your physician.

Medications

- Review written list of medications, including dose, route, frequency, food interactions, and side effects.
- Avoid over-the-counter medications unless recommended by your physician.

Wound and Dressing Care

- Cleanse skin around incision daily with mild soap and water.
- If dressing present, change it daily and as often as necessary to keep dressing dry and clean.
- Remove dressing prior to showering and replace with a clean dressing afterward.
- Drainage, if present, should gradually decrease.
- If there is a marked increase in drainage, swelling, tenderness, or fever, or if drainage is foul-smelling, notify physician.

Permanent Pacemaker Insertion

Expected length of stay: 2–3 days post-procedure

	Date _____ **Pre-Procedure**	Date _____ **1st 24 Hours Post-Procedure**	Date _____ **Day 2 Until Discharge**
Daily outcomes	Client verbalizes understanding of pre-procedure teaching, including: activity restrictions, safety precautions, and pre-procedure sedation Client exhibits effective coping Client verbalizes understanding of procedure and reasons for permanent pacemaker insertion Client verbalizes understanding of comparative risks, benefits, and implications of treatment options Obtain informed consent	Client will: • maintain stable vital signs and be awake, alert, and oriented • maintain adequate cardiac output • remain free of signs of infection • have a clean, dry, wound with edges well-approximated, healing by first intention • maintain urine output >30 mL/hr • demonstrate understanding of any activity restrictions • have lungs clear to auscultation • have unlabored respirations • maintain oxygen saturation > 92% • demonstrate cooperation with activity restrictions • tolerate ordered diet without nausea or vomiting • exhibit effective coping • verbalize/demonstrate beginning understanding of home care instructions	Client is afebrile and remains free of signs and symptoms of infection Client has stable vital signs and B/P within specified range Client verbalizes understanding of pacemaker purpose, basic function, safety precautions, and monitoring procedures Client verbalizes understanding of diet, wound care, follow-up care, signs and symptoms to report, and medications: purpose, dose, frequency, route, food and drug interactions, and side effects Client has lungs clear to auscultation and unlabored respiration, with an oxygen saturation above >95% on room air Client manages pain with oral medications and/or non-pharmacologic measures Client is independent in self-care Client is fully ambulatory Client has resumed preadmission urine elimination pattern, maintaining urine output >30 mL/hr Client has a soft, non-distended abdomen, with active bowel sounds Client verbalizes ability to cope Client verbalizes/demonstrates home care instructions Client tolerates ordered diet without nausea or vomiting Client exhibits effective coping with ongoing stressors, including current illness

Permanent Pacemaker Insertion (continued)

	Date _____ Pre-Procedure	Date _____ 1st 24 Hours Post-Procedure	Date _____ Day 2 Until Discharge
Assessments, tests, and treatments	CBC Urinalysis PT/PTT Type and screen Chest x-ray EKG Continuous cardiac monitoring History and physical Vital signs and O_2 saturation, neurovascular and mental status assessment O_2 via nasal canula to maintain oxygen saturation >92% Assess coping status of client and family Provide ongoing emotional support to client and family Allow for client's input regarding care	Vital signs, CSM assessment, O_2 saturation and dressing assessment q15min × 4; q30min × 4; q1hr × 4 and prn Continuous cardiac monitoring Assess respiratory status q4hr and prn Turn, cough, and deep breathe q2hr until fully ambulatory O_2 via nasal canula to maintain oxygen saturation >92% Assess coping status of client and family Encourage client and family to verbalize feelings regarding any changes in appearance and functional abilities Provide ongoing emotional support to client and family	Vital signs, O_2 saturation, and dressing and wound drainage assessment q4–8hr and prn Continuous cardiac monitoring Assess respiratory status q4–8hr Turn, cough, and deep breathe q2hr until fully ambulatory Assess wound and apply dry sterile dressing every day and prn Encourage client to verbalize regarding any changes in appearance and functional ability Assist client and family to identify any resources or strategies to cope with changes in appearance and functional ability Assess coping status and provide appropriate emotional support
Knowledge deficit	Orient to room and surroundings Provide simple, brief instructions Include family in teaching Review specific post-procedure care Evaluate understanding of teaching	Review plan of care, including activity restrictions Begin discharge teaching regarding wound care, diet, and activity Review written discharge instructions with client and family Review medications: dose, purpose, frequency, and side effects Initiate and review discharge teaching regarding pacemaker—include activity restrictions, range of motion exercises to affected shoulder, safety precautions, and monitoring procedures Evaluate understanding of teaching	Complete discharge teaching to include wound care, diet, follow-up care and MD appointment, signs and symptoms to report, activity, and medication: name, purpose, dose, frequency, route, food interactions, and side effects Reinforce discharge teaching regarding pacemaker: include activity restrictions, range of motion exercises to affected shoulder, safety precautions and monitoring procedures Review written instructions regarding pacemaker for home care Evaluate understanding of teaching
Diet	NPO Consider referral to dietitian	Encourage fluids and advance to American Heart Association diet as tolerated	American Heart Association diet as tolerated
Activity	Assess safety needs and provide adequate precautions	Maintain safety precautions Activity restriction per order Passive ROM to affected shoulder Active ROM to all other extremities	Maintain safety precautions Begin progressive ambulation with assistance until fully ambulatory

	Date _____ **Pre-Procedure**	Date _____ **1st 24 Hours Post-Procedure**	Date _____ **Day 2 Until Discharge**
Medications	IV as ordered Routine meds as ordered Pre-procedure meds as ordered	IV fluids as ordered/intermittent IV device Analgesics as ordered Routine meds as ordered	Analgesics as ordered D/C IV device Routine meds as ordered
Transfer/ discharge plans	Establish discharge objectives with client and family Determine discharge needs and support system with client and family Consider consultation with cardiac rehab if indicated Begin home care instructions	Review progress toward discharge goals Make any referrals Finalize discharge plans	Finalize any home care arrangements Complete discharge instructions

Potential Client Variances
Permanent Pacemaker Insertion

Possible Complications
- Pacemaker malfunction
- Perforation of myocardium

Health Conditions
- Congestive heart failure
- Pre-existing respiratory disease
- Renal disease

Nursing Diagnoses
- Risk for injury
- Ineffective individual/family coping
- Self-care deficits

Discharge Teaching for Client Following
Permanent Pacemaker Insertion

Activity

- Gradually return to usual level of activity by increasing activity each day. Alternate activity with rest periods. Avoid fatigue. Plan rest periods each day.
- Gradually increase your walking and other activities. Monitor your response to activity and stop activity if shortness of breath, palpitations, or fatigue occur.
- No strenuous activity or return to work until okayed by physician.
- Check with physician about heavy housework or straining.

Diet

- Follow American Heart Association diet. Eat a well-balanced diet, including fruits, meat, vegetables, bread and starches, and milk products.
- Plan rest periods after meals.

Signs and Symptoms to Report

Notify physician if any of these symptoms occur:
- Shortness of breath, chest pain, lightheadedness, difficulty breathing, increasing fatigue, weakness, slow heart rate, or any symptoms you may have experienced before your pacemaker insertion.

Follow-Up Care and General Health Care

- Schedule follow-up appointment with physician as directed.
- Monitor pulse as instructed by taking your pulse for a full minute every day. Keep a record of your pulse to show to the doctor. Contact physician if your pulse is below the rate at which your pacemaker was set.
- Take your pulse if you feel dizzy, short of breath, or you have chest pain.

- Report signs and symptoms of pacemaker problems.
- Always carry a pacemaker identification card and a MedicAlert bracelet.
- Avoid contact sports.
- Avoid strenuous motion of the affected shoulder for at least one month.
- Alert other physicians and dentists regarding the presence of your pacemaker.
- If you travel by plane, alert airline personnel to the fact that you have a pacemaker.
- Avoid high-voltage electric equipment.

Medications

- Review written list of medications, including dose, frequency, food interactions, and side effects.
- Carry a list of medications, with doses listed on it.
- Avoid over-the-counter medications unless recommended by physician.
- Discuss alcohol use with physician.

Wound and Dressing Care

- Cleanse skin around incision daily with mild soap and water.
- If dressing present, change it daily and as often as necessary to keep dressing clean and dry.
- Remove dressing prior to shower and replace with a clean dressing afterward.
- Drainage, if present, should gradually decrease.
- If there is a marked increase in drainage, swelling, tenderness, or fever, or if drainage is foul-smelling, notify physician.
- Avoid using tight clothing or straps over the area of the pacemaker.

Total Proctocolectomy with Permanent Ileostomy

Expected length of stay: 6–7 days

	Date _____ **Preoperative**	Date _____ **1st 24 Hours Postoperative**	Date _____ **2nd–3rd Days Postoperative**
Daily outcomes	Client verbalizes understanding of preoperative teaching, including: turning, coughing, deep breathing, incentive spirometer, mobilization, possible tubes (nasogastric tube, IV, Foley catheter, penrose or other drains), ostomy, and pain management Client exhibits effective coping Client verbalizes understanding of procedure, indications for procedure, comparative risks, benefits, and implications of treatment options Obtain informed consent	Client will: • have stable vital signs • have a clean, dry dressing • recover from anesthesia as evidenced by VS return to baseline, and being awake, alert, and oriented • verbalize understanding and demonstrate cooperation with turning, coughing, deep breathing, and splinting, • have lungs clear to auscultation • have urine output >30 mL/hr and patent Foley catheter • have a patent NG tube and remain free of nausea and vomiting • have a patent ostomy and a soft, non-distended abdomen • verbalize control of incisional pain • transfer out of bed with assistance 2 times • begin to verbalize feelings regarding change in body image and functions • exhibit effective coping	Client will: • be afebrile • have a clean, dry wound with edges well-approximated, healing by first intention • have intact, non-reddened peristomal skin • tolerate ordered diet without nausea or vomiting • have urine output >30 mL/hr and patent Foley catheter • have a patent NG tube and remain free of nausea and vomiting • have a patent ostomy, a soft, non-distended abdomen, and active bowel sounds • demonstrate cooperation with turning, coughing, deep breathing, and splinting • ambulate 4 times • verbalize control of incisional pain • begin to verbalize feelings regarding change in body image and functions • exhibit effective coping • verbalize beginning understanding of home care instructions • begin to participate in care of ostomy
Assessments, tests, and treatments	CBC Electrolytes Chem profile Urinalysis Chest x-ray Baseline physical assessment with a focus on respiratory status and gastrointestinal function Assess and record the description, location, duration, and characteristics of client's pain	CBC Electrolytes Vital signs and O_2 saturation, neurovascular assessment, dressing and wound drainage assessment q15min × 4; q30min × 4; q1hr × 4 and then q4hr and prn Assess respiratory status and gastrointestinal function q4hr and prn	Vital signs, dressing, and wound drainage assessment q4hr and prn Assess respiratory status and gastrointestinal function q4hr Incentive spirometer q2hr until fully ambulatory Intake and output every shift Assess ostomy output q2–4hr and prn If still in place, assess patency and output of NG tube q4–8hr Assess urinary output q2–4hr

Total Proctocolectomy with Permanent Ileostomy *(continued)*

	Date _____ **Preoperative**	Date _____ **1st 24 Hours Postoperative**	Date _____ **2nd–3rd Days Postoperative**
Assessments, tests, and treatments (continued)	Reduce or eliminate pain-producing factors such as fear and anxiety Visit with enterostomal therapist for stoma location Consider visit with ostomate before surgery	Incentive spirometer q2hr Intake and output every shift Assess patency of NG tube q2hr, noting volume q4–8hr Assess urinary output q2hr and prn Assess and record the description, location, duration, and characteristics of client's pain q2–4hr and prn Encourage verbalization of pain and discomfort Reduce or eliminate pain-producing factors and employ distraction or relaxation techniques Provide back rubs Encourage client to request analgesic or use PCA (if in use) before pain becomes severe Assess effectiveness of pain relief measures Assess stoma for edema, cyanosis, and bleeding Assess peristomal skin for erythema, integrity, and irritation Assess appliance for proper fit	Using sterile asepsis, change dressing; assess wound healing and wound drainage Assess and record the description, location, duration, and characteristics of client's pain q4hr and prn Reduce or eliminate pain-producing factors, employ distraction or relaxation techniques, and offer back rubs Assess effectiveness of pain relief measures Assess stoma for edema, cyanosis, and bleeding Assess peristomal skin for erythema, integrity, or irritation Assess appliance for proper fit
Knowledge deficit	Orient to room and surroundings Provide simple, brief instructions Review preoperative preparation including hospital and surgical routines Include family in teaching Discuss surgery and specific postoperative care: turning, coughing, deep breathing, splinting incision, incentive spirometer, mobilization, possible tubes (nasogastric [NG] and intravenous [IV]), and pain management Instruct regarding distraction techniques, such as slow rhythmic breathing and guided imagery, to provide pain relief Instruct in relaxation techniques, such as tensing and relaxing muscle groups and rhythmic breathing Evaluate understanding of teaching	Reorient to room and postoperative routine Include family in teaching Review plan of care and importance of early mobilization Review importance of turning, coughing, deep breathing, splinting incision, incentive spirometer, mobilization, drainage and intravenous tubes, and pain management Evaluate understanding of teaching	Reinforce earlier teaching regarding ongoing care Include family in teaching Begin discharge teaching regarding wound care/dressing change and care of stoma and skin, including application of an appliance, and signs and symptoms of bowel obstruction Encourage and provide opportunities for self-care of ostomy Provide opportunity for client to meet with other ostomates if desired Evaluate understanding of teaching

	Date _____ **Preoperative**	Date _____ **1st 24 Hours Postoperative**	Date _____ **2nd–3rd Days Postoperative**
Psychosocial	Assess anxiety related to diagnosis and pending surgery Assess fears of the unknown related to surgery Encourage verbalization of concerns Minimize external stimuli (eg, noise, movement) Assess availability of support persons and resources for client Assess responses of support persons Allow for client's input regarding care Be supportive of client's effective coping behaviors	Assess level of anxiety Encourage verbalization of concerns Provide information and ongoing support and encouragement to client and family Encourage client and family to verbalize their feelings about the ostomy Listen to client and family and show interest and concern rather than giving advice Allow client to respond to loss of body function and changed body image with denial, shock, anger, depression, and other grieving behaviors	Encourage verbalization of concerns Provide ongoing support and encouragement Encourage client and family to verbalize their feelings about the ostomy Listen to client and family and show interest and concern rather than giving advice Allow client to respond to loss of body function and changed body image with denial, shock, anger, depression, and other grieving behaviors Be supportive of client's effective coping behaviors Support client's strengths and assist client to look at self in totality
Diet	NPO Baseline nutritional and hydration assessment	NG tube until return of bowel sounds NPO	When NG tube removed, begin clear liquids as tolerated
Activity	Assess safety needs and provide appropriate measures Activity as ordered	Maintain safety precautions Assist to chair 2 times	Maintain safety precautions Ambulate 4 times with assistance
Medications	Preoperative medications as ordered Oral antibiotics as ordered Enemas as ordered	IV fluids IV antibiotics Analgesics as ordered	IV fluids IV antibiotics When ordered, convert IV to intermittent IV device Analgesics as ordered
Transfer/ discharge plans	Assess potential discharge needs and support system Establish discharge goals with client and family	Review progress toward discharge goals with client and family Consult with social service regarding VNA and projected needs for home health care (if any)	Review progress toward discharge goals with client and family Make appropriate discharge referrals

➤

Total Proctocolectomy with Permanent Ileostomy *(continued)*

	Date _____ **4th Day Postoperative**	Date _____ **5th Day Postoperative**	Date _____ **6th–7th Days Postoperative**
Daily outcomes	Client will: • be afebrile and have stable vital signs • have a clean, dry wound with edges well-approximated, healing by first intention • have intact, non-reddened peristomal skin • tolerate ordered diet without nausea or vomiting • have a patent ostomy, active bowel sounds, and a soft non-distended abdomen • maintain urine output >30 mL/hr • ambulate 4–6 times • verbalize control of incisional pain • begin to verbalize feelings regarding change in body image and functions • exhibit effective coping • verbalize beginning understanding of home care instructions • participate in ostomy care	Client will: • be afebrile and have stable vital signs • have a clean, dry wound with edges well-approximated, healing by first intention • have intact, non-reddened peristomal skin • tolerate ordered diet without nausea or vomiting • maintain urine output >30 mL/hr • have a patent ostomy, active bowel sounds, and a soft non-distended abdomen • ambulate 4–6 times • verbalize control of incisional pain • begin to verbalize feelings regarding change in body image and functions • exhibit effective coping • verbalize understanding of home care instructions • participate actively in ostomy care	Client is afebrile and has stable vital signs Client has a clean, dry wound with edges well-approximated, healing by first intention Client's peristomal skin remains intact and without redness Client manages pain with non-pharmacologic measures and any ordered medications Client is independent in self-care, including ostomy care Client is fully ambulatory Client has resumed preadmission urine elimination pattern Client has a patent ostomy, active bowel sounds, and a soft non-distended abdomen Client verbalizes home care instructions Client tolerates usual diet Client verbalizes feelings regarding change in body image and function Client exhibits effective coping with ongoing stressors
Assessments, tests, and treatments	Vital signs, dressing, and wound drainage assessment q4hr Incentive spirometer q2hr until fully ambulatory Intake and output every shift Assess ostomy output q4hr and prn Assess respiratory status and gastrointestinal function q4–8hr Using sterile asepsis, change dressing; assess wound healing and wound drainage Assess and record description, location, duration, and characteristics of client's pain q4hr and prn Encourage client to employ distraction or relaxation techniques	Vital signs, dressing, and wound drainage assessment q4hr Assess respiratory status and gastrointestinal function q4–8hr Assess ostomy output q4hr and prn Remove dressing and assess wound healing and drainage Assess and record description, location, duration, and characteristics of client's pain q4hr and prn Encourage client to employ distraction or relaxation techniques	Vital signs, dressing, and wound drainage assessment q4–8hr Assess respiratory status and gastrointestinal function Assess wound healing Assess urine and ostomy output Assess and record description, location, duration, and characteristics of client's pain q4hr and prn Encourage client to employ distraction or relaxation techniques

	Date _____ **4th Day Postoperative**	Date _____ **5th Day Postoperative**	Date _____ **6th–7th Days Postoperative**
Knowledge deficit	Include family in teaching Initiate discharge teaching regarding wound care, diet, and activity Review teaching related to stoma care, including care of stoma, peristomal skin, and application of appliance Review written discharge instructions with client and family Evaluate understanding of teaching	Continue discharge teaching to client and family regarding wound care, diet, signs and symptoms to report, medications, and activity Reinforce teaching related to stoma care, including care of stoma, peristomal skin, and application of appliance Review written discharge instructions with client and family Evaluate understanding of teaching	Complete discharge teaching to include wound care, diet, follow-up care, signs and symptoms to report, activity, and medications: name, purpose, dose, frequency, route, dietary interactions, and side effects Refer any teaching needs related to stoma care, including care of stoma, peristomal skin, application of appliance, and so on, to visiting nurse Provide client with written discharge instructions Evaluate understanding of teaching
Psychosocial	Encourage verbalization of concerns Provide ongoing support and encouragement Encourage client and family to verbalize their feelings about the ostomy Use active listening skills Allow the client to respond to the loss of body function and changed body image with denial, shock, anger, depression, and other grieving behaviors Support client's strengths and assist client to look at self in totality	Encourage verbalization of concerns Provide ongoing support and encouragement Encourage client and family to verbalize their feelings about the ostomy Use active listening skills Allow the client to respond to the loss of body function and changed body image with denial, shock, anger, depression, and other grieving behaviors Support client's strengths and assist client to look at self in totality	Encourage verbalization of concerns Provide ongoing support and encouragement Encourage client and family to verbalize their feelings about the ostomy Use active listening skills Allow the client to respond to the loss of body function and changed body image with denial, shock, anger, depression, and other grieving behaviors Support client's strengths and assist client to look at self in totality
Diet	If tolerating clear liquids, advance to full liquids as tolerated	Advance diet to soft, regular diet as tolerated	Regular diet as tolerated
Activity	Ambulate independently at least 4 times Maintain safety precautions	Fully ambulatory Maintain safety precautions	Fully ambulatory
Medications	Offer oral analgesics Intermittent IV device for any IV medications; D/C when ordered	Offer oral analgesics	Offer oral analgesics
Transfer/ discharge plans	Continue to review progress toward discharge goals	Finalize discharge plans Continue to review progress toward discharge goals Finalize plans for home care if needed	Complete discharge instructions Refer to VNA for any identified knowledge deficits

Total Proctocolectomy with Permanent Ileostomy

Possible Complications

- Peritonitis
- Ileus
- Fluid and electrolyte disturbances

Health Conditions

- Undernutrition
- Pre-existing respiratory problems

Nursing Diagnoses

- Altered nutrition: less than body requirements
- Risk for infection
- Impaired skin integrity

Total Proctocolectomy with Permanent Ileostomy

Activity

- Gradually return to usual level of activity by increasing activity each day. Alternate activity with rest periods. Avoid fatigue and plan rest periods throughout the day.
- You may go up and down stairs.
- Avoid heavy housework, working, straining, heavy lifting, and driving for the period designated by your physician.
- You may shower with your pouch on.

Diet

- Eat a well-balanced diet, including all food groups.
- Drink 6–8 glasses of fluid each day.

Signs and Symptoms to Report

Notify physician if any of these symptoms occur:
- Increase in pain, or any redness or swelling in wound.
- Sudden increase in wound drainage, especially if drainage has pus or a foul odor.
- Nausea, vomiting, or change in bowel habits such as an increase or decrease in the amount, color, or consistency of stool.
- Redness or skin breakdown around stoma.
- Foul-smelling urine.
- Chills, or fever greater than 100F or 38C

Follow-Up Care and General Health Care

- Schedule follow-up appointment with physician as directed.
- Refer to local support group.
- Avoid wearing constrictive clothing over stoma.

Medications

- Review written list of medications, including dose, route, frequency, food interactions, and side effects.
- Discuss alcohol use with your physician.
- Avoid over-the-counter medications—especially those that will affect your bowel movements, such as laxatives or antidiarrheals.

Wound and Dressing Care

- Cleanse skin around incision daily with mild soap and water.
- If you are directed to use a dressing, change your dressing daily and as often as necessary to keep dressing dry and clean.
- Remove dressing prior to showering and replace with a clean dressing afterward.
- Drainage, if present, should gradually decrease.
- If there is a marked increase in drainage, swelling, tenderness, or fever, or if drainage is foul-smelling, notify physician.

Stoma Care

- Drain your drainage bag when it is one-half full, and then rinse your pouch with warm water.
- Plan to change your drainage system every 3–5 days. If there is evidence of leakage before this time, be sure to change the system.
- Before changing the system, gather your supplies and prepare the pouch.
- Remove the old bag from around the stoma and discard the old bag.
- Cleanse the skin around the stoma with warm water and skin cleanser. Rinse the skin well and pat it dry. Carefully inspect the skin around the stoma for any signs of irritation, chafing, or rash. Check the skin every time you change the bag. If there is redness or skin breakdown, notify your ostomy nurse or physician.
- Wipe the skin around the stoma with the skin gel protective wipe. Allow it to dry thoroughly.
- Apply the pouch over the stoma and press it firmly into place. Make sure the adhesive is sealed firmly around the stoma. Smooth the tape around the edges.
- Report any significant changes in the character, quality, or quantity of stool output.
- Your stoma may shrink after surgery as the edema subsides. If stool leaks onto the skin, you will need to use a pouch with a smaller opening.
- Consult with the stoma nurse if problems, questions, or needs arise.

Critical Pathway for Client Following

Splenectomy

Expected length of stay: 5 days

	Date _____ **Preoperative**	Date _____ **1st 24 Hours Postoperative**	Date _____ **2nd Day Postoperative**
Daily outcomes	Client verbalizes understanding of preoperative teaching, including: turning, coughing, deep breathing, incentive spirometer, mobilization, possible tubes, and pain management Client exhibits effective coping Client verbalizes understanding of procedure, indications for procedure and comparative risks, benefits and implications of treatment options Obtain informed consent	Client will: • be afebrile, free of signs of infection, and have stable vital signs • have a clean, dry wound with edges well-approximated, healing by first intention • recover from anesthesia, as evidenced by VS return to baseline and being awake, alert, and oriented • verbalize understanding and demonstrate cooperation with turning, coughing, deep breathing and splinting • verbalize control of incisional pain • transfer out of bed with assistance 2–3 times • exhibit effective coping	Client will: • be afebrile, free of signs of infection, and have stable vital signs • have a clean, dry wound with edges well-approximated, healing by first intention • have active bowel sounds • tolerate ordered diet without vomiting • demonstrate cooperation with turning, coughing, deep breathing and splinting • ambulate 4 times • verbalize control of incisional pain • exhibit effective coping • verbalize beginning understanding of home care instructions
Assessments, tests, and treatments	CBC Urinalysis Baseline physical assessment with a focus on respiratory, gastrointestinal, and nutritional status Minimize exposure to infections	CBC Vital signs and O_2 saturation, neurovascular assessment, dressing and wound drainage assessment q15min × 4; q30min × 4; q1hr × 4 and then q4hr and prn Assess respiratory status and gastrointestinal function q4hr and prn Incentive spirometer q2hr Intake and output every shift Assess voiding—if unable to void, try suggestive voiding techniques or, if still unable, catheterize q8hr or prn Assess and record the description, location, duration, and characteristics of client's pain q2–4hr and prn Encourage verbalization of pain and discomfort Reduce or eliminate pain-producing factors and employ distraction or relaxation techniques	Vital signs and dressing and wound drainage assessment q4hr and prn Assess respiratory status and gastrointestinal function q4hr Incentive spirometer q2hr until fully ambulatory Intake and output every shift Assess voiding pattern every shift Using sterile asepsis, change dressing; assess wound healing and wound drainage Assess and record the description, location, duration, and characteristics of client's pain q4hr and prn Reduce or eliminate pain-producing factors, employ distraction or relaxation techniques, and offer back rubs Minimize exposure to infection Monitor for signs of infection

Splenectomy *(continued)*

	Date _____ **Preoperative**	Date _____ **1st 24 Hours Postoperative**	Date _____ **2nd Day Postoperative**
Assessments, tests, and treatments (continued)		Provide back rubs Encourage client to request analgesic or use PCA before pain becomes severe Minimize exposure to infections Monitor for signs of infection	
Knowledge deficit	Orient to room and surroundings Provide simple, brief instructions Review preoperative preparation, including hospital and surgical routines Discuss surgery and specific postoperative care: turning, coughing, deep breathing, splinting incision, incentive spirometer, mobilization, possible tubes, and pain management (PCA or prn medications) Instruct regarding distraction techniques, such as slow rhythmic breathing and guided imagery, to produce pain relief Instruct in relaxation techniques, such as tensing and relaxing muscle groups and rhythmic breathing Evaluate understanding of teaching	Reorient to room and postoperative routine Review plan of care and importance of early mobilization Review importance of turning, coughing, deep breathing, splinting incision, incentive spirometer, mobilization, drainage and intravenous tubes, and pain management (PCA or prn medications) Evaluate understanding of teaching	Reinforce earlier teaching regarding ongoing care Begin discharge teaching regarding wound care/dressing change Evaluate understanding of teaching
Psychosocial	Assess anxiety related to diagnosis and pending surgery Assess fears of the unknown related to surgery Encourage verbalization of concerns Minimzie external stimuli (eg, noise, movement)	Assess level of anxiety Encourage verbalization of concerns Provide ongoing support and encouragement	Encourage verbalization of concerns Provide ongoing support and encouragement
Diet	NPO after 12 MN Baseline nutritional assessment	NPO until return of bowel sounds	If bowel sounds present, begin clear liquids as tolerated
Activity	Provide safety precautions Activity as ordered	Provide safety precautions Bathroom privileges with assistance Ambulate 2–3 times with assistance	Provide safety precautions Ambulate 4–6 times with assistance
Medications	Preoperative medications as ordered	IV fluids IV antibiotics if ordered Analgesics as ordered	IV fluids When ordered, convert IV to intermittent IV device Analgesics as ordered

➤

Splenectomy *(continued)*

	Date _____ **Preoperative**	Date _____ **1st 24 Hours Postoperative**	Date _____ **2nd Day Postoperative**
Transfer/ discharge plans	Assess potential discharge needs and support system Establish discharge goals with client and family	Review progress toward discharge goals with client and family Consult with social service regarding projected needs for home health care (if any)	Review progress toward discharge goals with client and family

	Date _____ **3rd Day Postoperative**	Date _____ **4th Day Postoperative**	Date _____ **5th Day Postoperative**
Daily outcomes	Client will: • be afebrile, free of signs of infection, and have stable vital signs • have a clean, dry wound with edges well-approximated, healing by first intention • tolerate ordered diet without nausea or vomiting • ambulate 4–6 times • verbalize control of incisional pain • exhibit effective coping • verbalize beginning understanding of home care instructions	Client will: • be afebrile, free of signs of infection, and have stable vital signs • have a clean, dry wound with edges well-approximated, healing by first intention • tolerate ordered diet without nausea or vomiting • ambulate 4–6 times • verbalize control of incisional pain • exhibit effective coping • verbalize beginning understanding of home care instructions	Client is afebrile, free of signs of infection, and has stable vital signs Client has a clean, dry wound with edges well-approximated, healing by first intention Client manages pain with non-pharmacologic measures Client is independent in self-care Client is fully ambulatory Client has resumed preadmission urine and bowel elimination pattern Client verbalizes home care instructions Client tolerates usual diet Client exhibits effective coping with ongoing stressors
Assessments, tests, and treatments	Vital signs, dressing, and wound drainage assessment q4hr Incentive spirometer q2hr until fully ambulatory Intake and output every shift Assess voiding pattern every shift Assess respiratory status and gastrointestinal function q4–8hr Using sterile asepsis, change dressing; assess wound healing and wound drainage Assess and record description, location, duration, and characteristics of client's pain q4hr and prn Encourage client to employ distraction or relaxation techniques Monitor for signs of infection	Vital signs, dressing, and wound drainage assessment q4hr Assess respiratory status and gastrointestinal function q4–8hr Remove dressing and assess wound healing and drainage Assess and record description, location, duration, and characteristics of client's pain q4hr and prn Encourage client to employ distraction or relaxation techniques Monitor for signs of infection	Vital signs, dressing, and wound drainage assessment q4–8hr Assess respiratory status and gastrointestinal function Assess wound healing Assess and record description, location, duration, and characteristics of client's pain q4hr and prn Encourage client to employ distraction or relaxation techniques Monitor for signs of infection

	Date _____ **3rd Day Postoperative**	Date _____ **4th Day Postoperative**	Date _____ **5th Day Postoperative**
Knowledge deficit	Initiate discharge teaching regarding wound care, diet, and activity Review written discharge instructions with client and family Evaluate understanding of teaching	Continue discharge teaching regarding wound care, diet, prevention of infection, signs and symptoms to report, medications, and activity Review written discharge instructions with client and family Evaluate understanding of teaching	Complete discharge teaching to include wound care, diet, prevention of infection, follow-up care, signs and symptoms to report, activity, and medications: dose, frequency, route, and side effects Provide client with written discharge instructions Evaluate understanding of teaching
Psychosocial	Encourage verbalization of concerns Provide ongoing support and encouragement	Encourage verbalization of concerns Provide ongoing support and encouragement	Encourage verbalization of concerns Provide ongoing support and encouragement
Diet	If tolerating clear liquids, advance to full liquids as tolerated	Advance diet to soft, regular diet as tolerated	Regular diet as tolerated
Activity	Ambulate independently at least 4 times	Fully ambulatory	Fully ambulatory
Medications	Provide oral analgesics	Provide oral analgesics	Provide oral analgesics
Transfer/ discharge plans	Continue to review progress toward discharge goals	Finalize discharge plans Continue to review progress toward discharge goals Finalize plans for home care if needed	Complete discharge instructions

Potential Client Variances
Splenectomy

Possible Complications
- Infection, sepsis
- Hemorrhage
- Thrombophlebitis
- Subphrenic abscess

Health Conditions
- Anemia
- Pre-existing infections
- Undernutrition

Nursing Diagnoses
- Risk for infection
- Altered nutrition: less than body requirements
- Fatigue

Discharge Teaching for Client Following
Splenectomy

Activity
- Gradually return to usual level of activity by increasing activity each day. Alternate activity with rest periods. Avoid fatigue.
- You may go up and down stairs.
- Avoid heavy housework, working, straining, heavy lifting, and driving for the period designated by your physician.

Diet
- Eat a well-balanced diet, including all food groups.
- Drink 6–8 glasses of fluid each day.

Signs and Symptoms to Report
Notify physician if any of these symptoms occur:
- Signs or symptoms of an infection
- Nausea, vomiting, or change in bowel habits.
- Increase in pain, redness, or swelling
- Sudden increase in wound drainage, especially if drainage has pus or a foul odor
- Chills, or fever greater than 100F or 38C

Follow-Up Care and General Health Care
- Schedule follow-up appointment with physician as directed.

Medications
- Review written list of medications, including dose, route, frequency, food interactions, and side effects.

Wound and Dressing Care
- Cleanse skin around incision daily with mild soap and water.
- If dressing present, change it daily and as often as necessary to keep dressing dry and clean.
- Remove dressing prior to showering and replace with a clean dressing afterward.
- Drainage, if present, should gradually decrease.
- If there is a marked increase in drainage, swelling, tenderness, or fever, or if drainage is foul-smelling, notify physician.

Thyroidectomy

Expected length of stay: 3 days

	Date _____ **1st Day Postoperative**	Date _____ **2nd Day Postoperative**	Date _____ **3rd Day Postoperative**
Daily outcomes	Client will: • be afebrile and have stable vital signs • have a clean, dry wound with edges well-approximated, healing by first intention • recover from anesthesia, as evidenced by VS return to baseline and being awake, alert, and oriented • verbalize understanding and demonstrate cooperation with turning, coughing, deep breathing, and splinting • demonstrate strategies to minimize stress on the suture line • tolerate ordered diet without nausea or vomiting • verbalize control of incisional pain • exhibit effective coping	Client will: • be afebrile and have stable vital signs • have a clean, dry wound with edges well-approximated, healing by first intention • demonstrate cooperation with turning, coughing, deep breathing, and splinting • tolerate ordered diet without nausea or vomiting • ambulate 4 times per day • verbalize control of incisional pain • exhibit effective coping • verbalize beginning understanding of home care instructions	Client is afebrile and has stable vital signs Client has a clean, dry wound with edges well-approximated, healing by first intention Client manages pain with non-pharmacologic measures Client is independent in self-care Client is fully ambulatory Client has resumed preadmission urine and bowel elimination pattern Client verbalizes/demonstrates home care instructions Client verbalizes understanding of neck range of motion exercises Client tolerates usual diet Client exhibits effective coping with ongoing stressors
Assessments, tests, and treatments	CBC Vital signs and O_2 saturation, neurovascular assessment, dressing and wound drainage assessment q15min × 4; q30min × 4; q1hr × 4 and then q4hr and prn Assess respiratory status and voice quality and tone q2–4hr and prn Incentive spirometer q2hr Intake and output every shift Assess voiding—if unable to void, try suggestive voiding techniques or, if still unable, catheterize q8hr or prn Keep HOB elevated 30 degrees Place a small pillow under the head Monitor for signs and symptoms of hypocalcemia, respiratory distress, hemorrhage, thyroid storm, or laryngeal nerve damage	Vital signs, dressing, and wound drainage assessment q4hr and prn Assess respiratory status and voice tone and quality q4hr and prn Incentive spirometer q2hr until fully ambulatory Intake and output every shift Assess voiding pattern every shift Keep HOB elevated 30 degrees Keep a small pillow under the head	Vital signs, dressing, and wound drainage assessment q4hr and prn Assess respiratory status and voice tone and quality q4hr and prn Keep HOB elevated 30 degrees Keep a small pillow under the head

	Date _____ **1st Day Postoperative**	Date _____ **2nd Day Postoperative**	Date _____ **3rd Day Postoperative**
Knowledge deficit	Reorient to room and postoperative routine Include family in teaching Review plan of care and importance of early mobilization Begin discharge teaching regarding wound care/dressing change Instruct regarding the importance of minimizing stress on the suture line, including avoiding quick movements and hyperextension of the neck, and supporting head and neck when moving Evaluate understanding of teaching	Initiate discharge teaching regarding wound care, diet, and activity Include family in teaching Review written discharge instructions Reinforce instructions regarding the importance of minimizing stress on the suture line Instruct client regarding the importance of neck range of motion exercises; demonstrate exercises, providing written copy Evaluate understanding of teaching	Complete discharge teaching to include wound care, diet, follow-up care, signs and symptoms to report, activity, and medications: name, purpose, dose, frequency, route, dietary interactions, and side effects Include family in teaching Provide client with written discharge instructions Evaluate understanding of teaching
Psychosocial	Assess level of anxiety Encourage verbalization of concerns Provide information and ongoing support and encouragement to client and family	Encourage verbalization of concerns Provide information and ongoing support and encouragement to client and family	Encourage verbalization of concerns Provide information and ongoing support and encouragement to client and family
Diet	Clear liquids to regular diet as tolerated	Regular diet as tolerated	Regular diet as tolerated
Activity	Provide safety precautions Bathroom privileges with assistance Ambulate 4 times with assistance	Provide safety precautions Ambulate independently at least 4 times	Fully ambulatory
Medications	Analgesics as ordered IV fluids or intermittent IV device	Analgesics as ordered Intermittent IV device	Analgesics as ordered D/C intermittent IV device
Transfer/ discharge plans	Assess discharge needs with client and family Establish discharge goals with client and family	Complete discharge plans Make any appropriate referrals Continue home care instructions	Complete discharge instructions

Potential Client Variances
Thyroidectomy

Possible Complications

- Hypocalcemia
- Hemorrhage
- Respiratory distress
- Laryngeal nerve damage
- Thyroid storm

Health Conditions

- Pre-existing respiratory problems
- Undernutrition

Nursing Diagnoses

- Ineffective airway clearance
- Acute pain
- Impaired verbal communication

Discharge Teaching for Client Following
Thyroidectomy

Activity

- Gradually return to usual level of activity by increasing activity each day. Alternate activity with rest periods. Avoid fatigue.
- No strenuous activity until okayed by physician.
- Avoid heavy housework, straining, and driving for the period designated by your physician.

Diet

- Eat a well-balanced diet, including all food groups.
- Drink 6–8 glasses of fluid each day.

Signs and Symptoms to Report

Notify physician if any of these symptoms occur:
- Chills, or fever greater than 100F or 38C
- Increasing difficulty breathing or shortness of breath

Follow-Up Care and General Health Care

- Schedule follow-up appointment with physician as directed.
- Avoid individuals with respiratory infections.

Wound and Dressing Care

- Cleanse skin around incision daily with mild soap and water.
- If dressing present, change it daily and as often as necessary to keep dressing dry and clean.
- Remove dressing prior to showering and replace with a clean dressing afterward.
- Drainage, if present, should gradually decrease.
- It there is a marked increase in drainage, swelling, tenderness, or fever, or if drainage is foul-smelling, notify physician.

Transurethral Resection of the Prostate

Expected length of stay: 3 days following surgery

	Date _____ **Preoperative**	Date _____ **1st 24 Hours Postoperative**
Daily outcomes	Client verbalizes understanding of preoperative teaching including: turning, coughing, deep breathing, incentive spirometer, mobilization, tubes (Foley catheter, continuous bladder irrigation, and intravenous), and pain management (prn medications) Client verbalizes understanding of procedures Client verbalizes ability to cope Obtain informed consent	Client will: • have stable vital signs • recover from anesthesia as evidenced by VS return to baseline, and being awake, alert, and oriented, with clear lungs • verbalize understanding and demonstrate cooperation with turning, coughing, and deep breathing • have a patent Foley catheter • tolerate ordered diet without nausea and vomiting • verbalize control of bladder spasms with ordered medications • demonstrate ability to cope If client received spinal anesthetic, client will have full return of preoperative neurologic function
Assessments, tests, and treatments	CBC PSA if ordered Urinalysis Baseline physical assessment with a focus on respiratory status and urinary elimation pattern Apply thigh-high anti-emboli stockings	Hct/Hgb Vital signs and O_2 saturation, and neurovascular assessment q15min × 4; q30min × 4; q1hr × 4 and then q4hr if stable Assess respiratory status, urinary, and gastrointestinal function q4hr and prn Incentive spirometer q2hr O_2 as indicated Remove and replace anti-emboli hose every shift
Knowledge deficit	Orient to room and surroundings Include family in teaching Provide simple, brief instructions Review preoperative preparation including hospital and surgical routines Discuss surgery and specific postoperative care: turning, coughing, deep breathing, incentive spirometer, mobilization, possible tubes (3-way catheter, continuous bladder irrigations, and intravenous), and pain management (prn medications) Evaluate understanding of teaching	Reorient to room and postoperative routine Include family in teaching Review plan of care and importance of early mobilization Begin discharge teaching Evaluate understanding of teaching

	Date _____ **Preoperative**	Date _____ **1st 24 Hours Postoperative**
Elimination	Observe amount, color, and character of urine output Maintain accurate intake and output If catheter present, maintain patency of retention catheter, provide catheter care, tape catheter to lower abdomen and maintain drainage receptacle below level of client's bladder Observe bowel elimination pattern Fleet enema if ordered	3-way Foley catheter: assess patency, color, and amount of urine, and presence of clots and character of urine output q15min × 4; q30min × 4; q1hr × 4 and then q2hr × 24 hr and prn Assess for spasms and meatal drainage q1hr Continuous bladder irrigation (CBI)—regulate flow so that urine is free flowing and pink in color for 12–24 hr Instruct client to avoid straining for BM Irrigate catheter prn Provide catheter care every shift and prn Explain the importance of reporting bladder spasms Maintain accurate intake and output Maintain drainage receptacle below level of client's bladder Notify MD with decreased or absent urine output or retention of CBI Assess bowel elimination pattern
Psychosocial	Assess anxiety related to diagnosis and pending surgery Assess fears of the unknown related to surgery Provide emotional support Encourage verbalization of concerns Minimize external stimuli (eg, noise, movement)	Assess level of anxiety Encourage verbalization of concerns Provide information Provide ongoing support and encouragement
Diet	Baseline nutritional assessment	Advance from clear liquids to regular diet as tolerated Encourage fluid intake as tolerated Encourage fluids that acidify urine such as cranberry juice
Activity	Assess safety needs and provide appropriate measures OOB ad lib until pre-medicated	Maintain appropriate safety precautions Reposition q2hr and prn Bed rest for 12–24 hr, then, if free of bleeding, up with assistance Avoid prolonged sitting
Medications	Laxatives if ordered	Analgesics and muscle relaxants as ordered IV antibiotics IV fluids or intermittent IV device Stool softener BID
Transfer/ discharge plans	Assess discharge needs and support system	Include family in discharge planning and teaching Assess potential discharge needs Begin home care teaching Assess need for appropriate referrals

	Date _____ **2nd Day Postoperative**	Date _____ **3rd Day Postoperative**
Daily outcomes	Client will: • be afebrile, have stable vital signs, and have clear lungs • demonstrate cooperation with turning, coughing, and deep breathing • tolerate ordered diet without nausea and vomiting • ambulate 4 times per day • verbalize control of bladder spasms • have a 3-way catheter • demonstrate ability to cope • verbalize beginning understanding of home care instructions	Client is afebrile, with stable vital signs and clear lungs Client manages pain with non-pharmacologic measures Client is independent in self-care Client is fully ambulatory Client has resumed preadmission bowel elimination pattern and is voiding in sufficient amounts and passing soft stools without straining Client verbalizes understanding of home care instructions Client tolerates usual diet Client demonstrates ability to cope with ongoing stressors
Assessments, tests, and treatments	Vital signs q4hr and prn Assess respiratory status and urinary function every shift and prn Incentive spirometer q2hr until fully ambulatory Intake and output every shift Remove and replace anti-emboli stockings every shift	Vital signs assessment q4hr Assess respiratory status and urinary function Monitor intake and output
Knowledge deficit	Include family in teaching Initiate discharge teaching regarding diet, bowel management, and activity Review written discharge instructions Evaluate understanding of teaching	When Foley catheter is removed, instruct client to void in urinal and notify nurse with each voiding Include family in teaching Complete discharge teaching to include diet, follow-up care and MD follow-up visit, signs and symptoms to report, activity, and medications: name, purpose, dose, frequency, route, and side effects Provide client with written discharge instructions that discuss: 1) no straining or lifting, 2) adequate fluid intake, 3) the importance of reporting heavy bleeding, 4) avoidance of aspirin, and 5) no prolonged sitting or car rides Evaluate understanding of teaching
Elimination	3-way Foley catheter: assess patency, color, and amount of urine, and presence of clots and character of urine q2–4 hr × 24 hr and prn Assess for spasms and meatal drainage q2–4hr D/C continuous bladder irrigation (CBI) Instruct client to avoid straining for BM Irrigate catheter prn Provide catheter care every shift and prn Explain the importance of reporting bladder spasms Maintain accurate intake and output Maintain drainage receptacle below level of client's bladder Notify MD with decreased or absent urine output Assess bowel elimination pattern	Remove 3-way catheter and monitor time and amount of voiding and record on intake and output Observe amount, color, and character of urine output Assess bowel elimination pattern

	Date _____ **2nd Day Postoperative**	Date _____ **3rd Day Postoperative**
Psychosocial	Encourage verbalization of concerns Provide ongoing support and encouragement	Encourage verbalization of concerns Provide ongoing support and encouragement
Diet	Regular diet as tolerated Encourage fluid intake of 2000 mL per day when IV fluids D/C Encourage fluids that acidify urine such as cranberry juice	Regular diet as tolerated Encourage fluids to 2000 mL per day Offer fluids that acidify urine such as cranberry juice
Activity	Maintain safety precautions Ambulate independently at least 4 times Avoid prolonged sitting	Fully ambulatory Avoid prolonged sitting
Medications	Analgesics and muscle relaxants as ordered IV or oral antibiotics Intermittent IV device Stool softener BID Laxative if no BM in 48 hr	Oral analgesics Stool softener BID D/C intermittent IV device
Transfer/ discharge plans	Complete discharge plans Continue home care instructions Make any referrals	Complete discharge instructions Discharge when voiding in sufficient amounts and without difficulty

Potential Client Variances
Transurethral Resection of the Prostate

Possible Complications
- Hemorrhage
- Infection
- Urinary incontinence

Health Conditions
- Pre-exisiting renal disease
- Diabetes

Nursing Diagnoses
- Urinary retention after catheter removal
- Altered sexuality patterns

Discharge Teaching for Client Following
Transurethral Resection of the Prostate

Activity

- Gradually return to usual level of activity by increasing activity each day. Alternate activity with rest periods. Avoid fatigue.
- You may go up and down stairs.
- Avoid heavy housework, straining, heavy lifting, and driving for the period designated by your physician.
- When sitting, keep legs elevated.

Diet

- Eat a well-balanced diet, including all food groups. Report nausea, vomiting, or change in bowel habits.
- Eat a diet high in fiber: fresh fruits, vegetables, and whole grain cereals and breads.
- Drink 1–2 quarts of liquids per day.

Signs and Symptoms to Report

Notify physician if any of these symptoms occur:
- Bright red urine or large clots
- Difficulty voiding, frequency, or urgency, or foul-smelling urine
- Chills, or fever greater than 100F or 38C

Follow-Up Care and General Health Care

- Schedule follow-up appointment with physician as directed.
- Intermittent small clots in the urine is normal for a period of 2–4 weeks.
- Avoid constipation or straining during bowel movement. Extra fiber and fluid will help prevent constipation.
- Check with your physician about taking laxatives.

Medications

- Review written list of medications, including dose, route, frequency, food interactions, and side effects.
- Discuss alcohol use with physician.

Obstetric Pathways

Labor and Delivery 237

Newborn 241

Postpartum Vaginal Delivery 245

Postpartum Cesarean Section 249

Labor and Delivery

	Date _____ **Stage I**	Date _____ **Stage II**
Outcomes	Woman effectively uses comfort measures during uterine contractions Woman discusses the labor and birth process Woman asks questions as needed Vital signs remain within expected normal parameters Fetal bradycardia absent Woman uses breathing techniques and relaxation measures as needed Woman voids spontaneously and evidences non-palpable bladder Woman's labor progresses within expected parameters of effacement, dilation, and fetal descent	Woman's vital signs remain within expected normal parameters Woman uses comfort techniques as desired Woman pushes effectively Fetal bradycardia absent Woman actively participates in the birth process Fetal descent progresses without impediment
Assessments, tests, and treatments	Assess uterine contractions, cervical effacement and dilation, fetal descent, status of membranes, comfort level, facial expressions, verbalizations, tone of voice, body movement, changes of behavior during contractions, degree of relaxation, and use of comfort measures; woman's B/P, pulse, respirations; and fetal status CBC Urinalysis Monitor woman's use of comfort measures and her ability to tolerate labor Provide support to woman and support person Utilize any of the following nursing comfort measures as needed: positioning, ambulation, showers, soothing cool cloth, warm blanket, back rub, effleurage, ice chips, sacral pressure Use aseptic technique during sterile vaginal exam and any invasive procedures Cleanse perineum frequently Note time of membrane rupture and character of fluid Assess fetal heart immediately after membrane rupture Assess voiding pattern and characteristics of urine, palpate bladder for distention Encourage voiding every 2–3 hours Monitor intake and output	Assess comfort level, effectiveness of pushing effort, ability to relax between contractions, woman's vital signs, fetal status, and bladder distention Provide ongoing support and encouragement to woman and support person Continue to monitor woman's ability to work with contraction Encourage relaxation between contractions Assist with positioning to push with each contraction Provide encouragement for specific pushing efforts Provide positive feedback for all efforts Keep woman and support person advised of progress Utilize nursing comfort measures Ensure aseptic technique during sterile vaginal exams and procedures Cleanse perineum frequently during pushing, and before and after birth Assess bladder distention and hydration status Encourage woman to empty bladder as needed Catheterize prn for distention

➤

	Date _____ **Stage I**	Date _____ **Stage II**
Knowledge deficit	Orient to room and unit Explain monitoring, labor and delivery care, and local and/or regional anesthesia to woman and support person Assess understanding of labor and birth process, breathing techniques, and comfort measures Validate woman's knowledge base and provide teaching to meet identified needs Provide opportunity for woman and support person to ask questions Review birth plan with couple	Review pushing techniques Have woman demonstrate understanding Provide ongoing teaching and explanation Assess need to reinforce teaching or to provide additional information Provide coaching or support the labor coach
Diet	Clear liquids as tolerated	Mouth care prn
Activity	Up ad lib	Position for pushing and delivery
Medications	Analgesics as ordered	Analgesics as ordered
Referral/ discharge plans	Assess discharge plans and adequacy of support system Establish discharge goals with woman and support person	Continue to assess support system

	Date _____ **Stage III**	Date _____ **Stage IV**
Daily outcomes	Woman's vital signs remain within expected normal parameters Woman uses comfort techniques as desired Woman pushes effectively Woman actively participates in the birth process Note: See also Newborn Critical Pathway	Woman's vital signs remain within expected parameters; fundus firm, midline, at umbilicus; moderate lochia rubra Woman exhibits no signs of discomfort Woman discusses labor, birth, and immediate fourth-stage changes Woman exhibits an absence of signs of infection Woman expresses satisfaction with her coping abilities during the labor and birth process Woman voids spontaneously in amounts >300 mL within 6–8 hours of delivery and exhibits non-palpable bladder Woman demonstrates accurate implementation of self-care and infant care procedures

	Date _____ **Stage III**	Date _____ **Stage IV**
Assessments, tests, and treatments	Assess comfort level, effectiveness of pushing effort, ability to relax between contractions, woman's vital signs, fetal status, and bladder distention Provide ongoing emotional support and encouragement Continue to monitor woman's ability to work with contractions Encourage relaxation between contractions Assist with positioning to push with each contraction Provide encouragement for specific pushing efforts Provide positive feedback for all efforts Keep woman and support person advised of progress Utilize nursing comfort measures Provide information regarding the status of the newborn Keep woman informed of process of placental expulsion Ensure aseptic technique during sterile vaginal exams and procedures Cleanse perineum frequently during pushing, and before and after birth Assess bladder distention and hydration status Encourage woman to empty bladder as needed Catheterize prn for distention Draw cord blood	Assess maternal vital signs, comfort level, perineum for redness, ecchymosis, edema, and discharge Assess woman's perception of her comfort, ability to rest, discomfort that interferes with interaction between herself and newborn and/or support person, and discomfort during fundal assessment Assess woman's vital signs, affect, and tenseness of body during assessment Assess interactions between parents and newborn Encourage opportunities for woman and newborn to bond Initiate breastfeeding if desired Monitor woman's ability to rest and relax between assessments Provide information regarding assessments needed and rationale for assessments Encourage woman to continue to use breathing and relaxation techniques during assessments Keep woman informed of her status Provide warmed blankets Provide fluids as desired Provide partial bath as desired Cleanse perineal area gently Change perineal pads and Chux as needed to maintain comfort Encourage position other than high Fowler's If fundal massage is necessary, complete with gentleness Arrange for desired support person(s) to be in attendance Ensure asepsis in placing perineal pads, cleansing perineum frequently Assess for bladder distention and hydration status Monitor voiding pattern Monitor intake and output Encourage woman to talk about birth experience Reinforce positive attachment behaviors Note: See also Vaginal Delivery Critical Pathway

	Date _____ **Stage III**	Date _____ **Stage IV**
Knowledge deficit	Provide ongoing teaching and explanation Assess need to reinforce teaching or to provide additional information Provide coaching or support the labor coach	Assess woman's expectations, cultural value system, ability to take in new information, and comfort level Assess knowledge regarding physiologic changes and psychologic changes common to postpartum period Assess knowledge of common postpartum self-care procedures Assess knowledge of and competence in providing basic infant care Provide information to meet identified needs Provide an environment conducive to asking questions Discuss and demonstrate or review self-care procedures, eg, perineal care, handwashing Demonstrate and discuss self-assessment Describe signs and symptoms to be reported to primary health care provider Evaluate understanding of postpartum teaching
Diet	Clear liquids as tolerated	Diet as tolerated
Activity	Position for expulsion of placenta	Encourage activity
Medications	Analgesics as ordered Pitocin as ordered	Analgesics as ordered Ice prn to perineum
Transfer/ discharge plans	Review progress toward discharge goals with woman and support person	Make appropriate discharge referrals Complete discharge instructions

Potential Client Variances
Labor and Delivery

Possible Complications

- Hemorrhage
- Hypertonic labor patterns
- Fetal distress
- Uterine rupture
- Precipitous labor

Health Conditions

- Pre-existing anemia
- Pre-existing diabetes
- Pregnancy-induced hypertension

Nursing Diagnoses

- Anxiety
- Ineffective individual coping
- Acute pain
- Risk for infection

Critical Pathway for

Newborn

	Date _____ **1–4 Hours Past Birth**	Date _____ **4–8 Hours Past Birth**	Date _____ **8–24 Hours Past Birth**
Outcomes	Newborn exhibits a clear airway Newborn's respiratory status is moving toward stabilization; assessments and interventions continue Newborn's temperature is maintained within normal limits (97.8 and 98.6 F) Newborn's trunk is pink, with slight acrocyanosis of hands and feet Newborn exhibits effective rooting, latch-on, sucking, and swallowing activities Newborn remains afebrile, no bleeding or discharge is present, and cord clamp is in place Mother and partner (if present) verbalize understanding of teaching Parents verbalize beginning understanding of normal newborn behavior and sleep and wake cycles Parents begin demonstrating attachment behaviors	Newborn exhibits a clear airway Newborn's respiratory status is moving toward stabilization; assessments and interventions continue Newborn's temperature is maintained within normal limits (97.8 and 98.6 F) Newborn's trunk is pink and acrocyanosis is absent from extremities Newborn tolerates first feedings and is satiated Signs of infection are absent at any areas where skin has been disturbed Mother and partner (if present) verbalize understanding of teaching Parents verbalize beginning understanding of newborn care needs	Newborn exhibits a clear airway Newborn's respiratory system has stabilized Newborn maintains own temperature within normal limits (97.8 and 98.6 F) Newborn's trunk is warm and acrocyanosis is absent from extremities Newborn's weight loss is within normal limits Feedings are taken without difficulty and retained Mother expresses satisfaction with the chosen feeding method Newborn remains free of infection, umbilical cord dries, and circumcision shows signs of healing Mother and partner (if present) verbalize/demonstrate understanding of teaching, including home care Parents exhibit attachment and caretaking behaviors Parents recognize newborn's interactive abilities, behavioral changes, and normal newborn characteristics Parents talk to newborn, use soothing techniques, and demonstrate willingness to complete caretaking activities such as diapering and feeding
Assessments, tests, and treatments	Assess respiratory rate and ease Assess for the presence of noisy respirations, nasal flaring, sternal retraction, snorting, or grunting Assess skin color Be alert for respiratory rate >60/min or cyanosis	Assess amount of mucus, respiratory ease, normal respiratory rate, the presence of noisy respirations, and skin color If respiratory difficulty: suction nares with bulb syringe and reassess need for further action Position newborn on side	Assess for stablization of respiration and for regurgitation of feeding Continue to assess respirations q2–4hr Continue side-lying position and keep bulb syringe within reach Continue to monitor and record axillary temperature q4hr

	Date _____ **1–4 Hours Past Birth**	Date _____ **4–8 Hours Past Birth**	Date _____ **8–24 Hours Past Birth**
Assessments, tests, and treatments (continued)	If respiratory difficulty occurs place in modified Trendelenburg position, suction nares with bulb syringe, and reassess need for further action Assess skin temperature and maintain temperature through use of skin probe Place hat on newborn Dry and cover infant with warmed blanket if given to parent, or place uncovered in radiant warmer Assess temperature q1hr Gestational exam Assess redness and discharge from umbilical cord and check that cord clamp is in place Maintain universal precautions Cord care per agency protocol Assess evidence of maternal attachment behaviors, including holding newborn *en face,* touching newborn, unwrapping newborn and examining physical characteristics, and accepting newborn's gender Assess parents' identification of newborn behaviors such as alertness, ability to see, vigorous suck, rooting behavior, and attention to human voice Delay eye prophylaxis to facilitate eye contact between newborn and parents Dim lights to help newborn keep eyes open Provide uninterrupted time for family during first hours of birth Assist parents in determining the personality and care needs of their newborn Cord blood per order Complete newborn identification procedures Record first void and/or meconium stool	Assess temperature q2–4hr and monitor temperature before and after first bath Dress newborn in hat, T-shirt, and diaper, and then wrap in 2 blankets and place in open crib Cord care per agency protocol Fold diaper below umbilical cord With plastic diapers, turn plastic layer away from the skin Report and document any redness or drainage from base of cord Monitor for first void and stool	Dress newborn in hat, T-shirt, diaper, and 1 or 2 blankets Assess signs of infection in umbilical cord area and at circumcision site: – Umbilical cord: check for discharge, or redness at base of cord. Check that cord is clean and dry, and cord clamp is in place – Circumcision: check for bleeding, discharge, or swelling. Check that Plastibell is in place and check voiding pattern Cord care per agency protocol Circumcision care: position newborn on side, change petroleum gauze when soiled, check incision site for redness or drainage Metabolic testing (PKU) (for accuracy PKU may be repeated at 72 hours post birth) Monitor voiding and stools

Newborn *(continued)*

	Date _____ **1–4 Hours Past Birth**	Date _____ **4–8 Hours Past Birth**	Date _____ **8–24 Hours Past Birth**
Knowledge deficit	Demonstrate use of bulb syringe if indicated Explain reasons for use of radiant warmer and need to keep newborn wrapped in warmed blankets when out of the radiant warmer	Reinforce teaching regarding need and use of bulb syringe Explain need to maintain newborn warmth through use of blankets and clothing Demonstrate how to take the newborn's axillary temperature, and read the thermometer, range of normal temperatures, and how to handle deviations. Also explain how to maintain newborn's normal temperature Discuss need to avoid tub baths until cord falls off Demonstrate cord care: wipe cord and base with rubbing alcohol, and allow to dry prior to diapering with diaper below cord Instruct parent to notify health care provider if discharge or redness appears or if cord remains moist	Reinforce previous teaching and discuss cleansing of bulb syringe Describe/identify to parents characteristics of normal respirations: rate, sneezing to clear airway, and no nasal flaring, retraction or grunting Demonstrate circumcision care: general cleaning, and position; report bleeding, redness, foul odor, swelling and/or decreased urine output Instruct parents about and demonstrate general newborn care, including bathing, feeding, suctioning, holding, and clothing Describe signs and symptoms of illness that need to be reported to health care providers, and explain importance of follow-up care
Nutrition	Assess level of alertness Assess rooting and sucking behaviors Assess for bowel sounds and abdominal distention Assist newborn to breastfeed in birthing area if mother desires Weigh newborn and measure length and head circumference Describe initial signs of feeding readiness and proper positioning for feeding	Assess for coordination of suck and swallow, choking, gagging, or pallor, patency of esophagus, and absence of respiratory difficulties with initial feeding Determine readiness to feed Provide initial feeding of 15–30 mL of sterile water or formula (per agency protocol) and observe newborn's response to the feeding Provide immediate support if signs of respiratory difficulties are present Assist with subsequent breast and/or bottle feedings Demonstrate proper positioning and burping, and discuss the signs of hunger and satiation	Weigh newborn prior to discharge Assess feeding patterns and voiding and stool patterns Monitor feedings Provide support and teaching as needed for chosen feeding method, the normal feeding requirements of newborns, how to handle feeding problems, and when to seek help
Medications	Within 1 hour of birth: – Vitamin K 1 mg IM as ordered – Erythromycin ophthalmic ointment in each eye	Medications as ordered	Hepatitis B vaccine as ordered
Referral/ discharge plans	Assess discharge plans and adequacy of support system Evaluate understanding of teaching	Review and reinforce teaching with mother and partner	Provide written copy of discharge instructions Make appropriate discharge referrals

Newborn

Possible Complications

- Infections
- Respiratory problems
- Cardiac defects
- Meconium aspiration
- Delivery trauma
- Prematurity

Health Conditions

- Congenital anomalies

Nursing Diagnoses

- Ineffective breathing pattern
- Decreased cardiac output
- Altered nutrition: less than body requirements

Vaginal Delivery

	Date _____ **1– 4 Hours Past Birth**	Date _____ **4–8 Hours Past Birth**	Date _____ **8–24 Hours Past Birth**
Outcomes	Mother exhibits normal physiologic responses to delivery: vital signs within expected parameters; fundus firm, midline, at level of umbilicus; moderate lochia rubra Mother uses comfort measures to enhance comfort during early postpartum period Mother rests and sleeps between assessments Mother exhibits no signs of infection Mother and partner (if present) begin to demonstrate appropriate attachment behaviors Mother verbalizes beginning understanding of knowledge about postpartum period and newborn care	Mother exhibits vital signs within expected normal parameters; fundus firm, midline, at level or umbilicus; moderate lochia rubra Mother exhibits no signs of developing infection Mother verbalizes increased comfort, and she employs comfort measures as indicated Mother discusses the importance of adequate rest and begin planning to ensure that she has opportunities to rest after discharge Parents verbalize their feelings about their birth experience and their newborn Mother begins to discuss postpartum changes, self-care measures, and newborn care	Mother exhibits vital signs within expected normal parameters; fundus firm, midline, at level or umbilicus; moderate lochia rubra Mother remains afebrile and exhibits an absence of infection Mother successfully employs appropriate comfort measures as needed Mother reports pain is 3 or less on a scale of 1 to 10 Mother has developed a plan for ensuring that she obtains adequate rest Mother rests and reports regaining energy Mother describes signs of infection and appropriate preventive measures Parents exhibit positive parenting and attachment behaviors, such as calling newborn by name; hugging, touching, smiling, and cuddling newborn; speaking to newborn in affectionate tones; and meeting newborn's physical needs promptly Mother (and partner) verbalize understanding essential information related to postpartum and newborn care, including self-care activities and changes in mother's condition that should be reported immediately Mother describes/identifies methods of coping with the stress of a newborn at home

	Date _____ **1– 4 Hours Past Birth**	Date _____ **4–8 Hours Past Birth**	Date _____ **8–24 Hours Past Birth**
Assessments, tests, and treatments	Assess history of factors predisposing to postpartal infection such as prolonged labor, hemorrhage, invasive procedures, and anemia Monitor pulse and B/P q15min × 6, q30min × 4 Assess temperature qlhr × 4 Assess firmness and position of fundus and character and amount of lochia q15min × 6, q30min × 4. Institute gentle fundal massage to maintain firmness as needed Assess perineum for redness, ecchymosis, edema, discharge and, where applicable, approximation of suture line. If signs of hematoma present, apply ice pack and notify primary health care provicer Assess for indications of bladder distention Encourage voiding q2–4hr Assess comfort level, facial expression, verbalizations of discomfort, ability to relax/rest, and use of comfort measures Assess level of fatigue, ability to relax/rest, factors that interfere with rest (eg, pain, visitors, newborn care needs, and environmental factors such as noise and temperature) Plan care activities to allow for uninterrupted periods If necessary, return newborn to central nursery for a time to allow mother to sleep Assess evidence of beginning maternal attachment behaviors such as calling newborn by name, touching newborn, holding newborn *en face*, accepting gender of newborn, speaking of newborn in affectionate terms Provide uninterrupted time for the family to become acquainted with new newborn during the first hour after birth	Monitor pulse and B/P q2hr Monitor temperature q2–4hr Assess firmness and position of fundus and lochia q2hr Assess perineum q2hr and prn Assess for indications of bladder distention Encourage voiding q2–4hr Assess comfort level, changes in types/sources of discomfort, ability to relax/rest, and use of comfort measures Assess level of fatigue. Provide opportunities for rest/sleep Assess breasts for signs of nipple redness or cracking Assess for signs of urinary tract infections such as dysuria Assess further development of attachment behaviors, such as kissing, hugging, cuddling, smiling at newborn, calling newborn by name in affectionate tones, or identifying positive family characteristics in newborn Support positive maternal behaviors, using praise and reinforcement Assist parents to discuss and understand their feelings, both positive and negative, about their birth experience and their newborn	Monitor vital signs q4hr and prn Assess firmness and position of fundus and character and amount of lochia q2–4hr and prn Assess perineum q4hr and prn Assess for indications of bladder distention Assess voiding q4hr Assess comfort level and sources of discomfort Assess mother's ability to successfully manage her discomfort Assess level of fatigue and factors that may interfere with rest/sleep Maintain a restful environment with periods of time for uninterrupted sleep Assess breasts for signs of nipple redness or cracking Assess for signs of developing infection Assess breastfeeding mother: cracked or bleeding nipples, areas of pain, tenderness, hardness or redness in the breasts Assess for ongoing developing of attachment behaviors such as holding the newborn close, expressing warm feelings about the newborn, and eagerness to care for newborn Ensure that a consistent, supportive nurse work with the mother as much as possible Reinforce positive parenting behaviors Provide appropriate opportunities for the new mother to express and work through her feelings about the newborn

	Date _____ **1– 4 Hours Past Birth**	Date _____ **4–8 Hours Past Birth**	Date _____ **8–24 Hours Past Birth**
Assessments, tests, and treatments (continued)	Delay eye prophylaxis to encourage eye contact between newborn and parents Explain factors (such as molding) that may affect the newborn's appearance Provide rooming-in so that parents have more time for interaction with the newborn		
Knowledge deficit	Provide information as to causes of discomfort and possible relief measures Perineal discomfort: explain perineal care, sitz baths, topical application of analgesics Hemorrhoidal discomfort: discuss sitz baths, topical ointments, digital replacement of external hemorrhoids in rectum, side-lying or prone position, stool softeners Afterpains: discuss lying prone with small pillow under abdomen, warm shower or sitz bath, ambulation, encourage voiding immediately before nursing Explain breast care and signs and symptoms to report Discuss with mother and family the importance of sufficient rest Elicit family's support in limiting phone calls and visitors	Reinforce teaching about possible comfort measures the mother can employ Assess mother's understanding of importance of adequate rest Begin discussing importance of adequate rest following discharge Discuss strategies for obtaining adequate rest, such as napping when the newborn naps, wearing a nightgown and robe for a few days, and accepting help from a family member or friend Explain to family members about the effects of fatigue and sleep deprivation Initiate teaching about child care as necessary to facilitate the development of maternal self-confidence and encourage return demonstrations Use positive reinforcement to support effective behaviors Evaluate understanding of teaching	Describe normal physiologic and psychologic changes during the postpartum period Demonstrate and discuss components of self-assessment of status and involution Assist with self-assessment Describe signs and symptoms to report promptly to primary health care provider Provide information on postpartum discomforts that may occur after the first day (such as breast engorgement, constipation) as well as postpartum complications (such as infected episiotomy, thrombophlebitis, mastitis, UTI) and the type of discomfort they may produce Describe signs of developing UTI or endometritis, which woman should be alert for following discharge Discuss self-care measures for discomforts Discuss the family's plan for ensuring that the new mother obtains adequate rest Reinforce teaching about self-care measures for preventing infection Discuss effective breastfeeding techniques to prevent engorgement, caked breasts, or nipple trauma if indicated Review printed teaching materials in the appropriate language Continue to provide opportunities for questions, discussion, and return demonstrations Evaluate knowledge of and competence in providing basic newborn care

Vaginal Delivery *(continued)*

	Date _____ **1– 4 Hours Past Birth**	Date _____ **4–8 Hours Past Birth**	Date _____ **8–24 Hours Past Birth**
Nutrition	Diet as tolerated Encourage fluids	Diet as tolerated Encourage fluids	Diet as tolerated Encourage fluids Encourage continuing prenatal vitamin and iron supplements for 6–8 weeks
Activity	Up and about with 2 assists Shower with assist	Up ad lib	Up ad lib
Medications	Medications as ordered Analgesics as ordered Colace 100 mg BID prn	Medications as ordered Analgesics as ordered Colace 100 mg BID prn	Medications as ordered Analgesics as ordered Colace 100 mg BID prn
Referral/ discharge plans	Assess discharge plans and adequacy of support system Evaluate understanding of teaching	Review and reinforce teaching with mother and partner	Provide written copy of discharge instructions Make appropriate discharge referrals for mother and family

Potential Client Variances
Vaginal Delivery

Possible Complications

- Uterine infections
- Urinary tract infection
- Mastitis
- Deep vein thrombosis
- Postpartum hemorrhage
- Fetal distress

Health Conditions

- Pre-existing anemia
- Pre-existing diabetes
- Pregnancy-induced hypertension (PIH)

Nursing Diagnoses

- Knowledge deficit
- Ineffective individual coping
- Altered patterns of urine elimination
- Acute pain
- Risk for infection

Cesarean Section

	Date _____ **Preoperative**	Date _____ **1st 24 Hours Postoperative**	Date _____ **24–48 Hours Postoperative**
Outcomes	Woman verbalizes understanding of and is able to demonstrate preoperative teaching, including: turning, coughing, deep breathing, incentive spirometer, mobilization, possible tubes (IV, Foley catheter), and pain management Woman demonstrates ability to cope Woman verbalizes understanding of procedure, indications for procedure, and comparative risks, benefits, and implications of all options Woman and family verbalize understanding of reason for cesarean, preoperative preparation, postoperative measures, and comfort measures after birth Woman and family have no further questions regarding the cesarean procedure Woman exhibits effective coping with preparations to cesarean birth	Mother exhibits anticipated physical status findings: skin warm and dry, vital signs are within normal limits; lungs clear; fundus firm, midline, at or below umbilicus; scant to moderate lochia rubra; pulse oximetry >90%; abdominal dressing dry and intact and without evidence of drainage; clear to amber drainage from indwelling catheter; intravenous fluids infusing at prescribed rate Mother uses comfort measures and verbalizes satisfaction with pain relief; describes pain as <5 on scale of 1 to 10 Mother coughs and deep breathes effectively; expectorates secretions efficiently Mother voices no complaints of nausea; displays absence of emesis Mother rests and sleeps between assessments Mother/couple exhibit appropriate attachment behaviours Mother verbalizes beginning understanding of knowledge about postpartum period and newborn care	Mother continues to exhibit normal findings for physical status indicators: vital signs within normal limits; lungs clear; fundus firm, 1 fingerbreadth below umbilicus; incision well-approximated, clean, and healing, active bowel sounds in all 4 abdominal quadrants; moderate lochia rubra Mother exhibits an absence of signs and symptoms of hemorrhage and infection Mother employs comfort measures as indicated and reports decreased discomfort Mother voids in amounts >300 mL within 6–8 hours of catheter removal and exhibits an absence of bladder distention Mother ambulates with minimal or no assistance; voices no complaints of vertigo or weakness Mother demonstrates implementation of self-care procedures to minimize potential for autoinfection Parents verbalize their feelings about the birth experience and their new infant; exhibit bonding behaviors Mother discusses the importance of adequate rest; begins planning to ensure opportunities for rest after discharge Mother describes common postpartum physiologic and psychologic changes

➤

	Date _____ **Preoperative**	Date _____ **1st 24 Hours Postoperative**	Date _____ **24–48 Hours Postoperative**
Assessments, tests, and treatments	CBC Type and cross-match 2 units packed cells Rh PTT RPR Urinalysis Assess for allergies and any sensitivities to medications or anesthetic agents in woman or immediate family Assess fetal size and status as evidenced by reactive non-stress test and fetal maturity tests Monitor fetal heart rate by external fetal monitor q15–30min per hospital policy Create a safe, nonthreatening environment for couple to work through unresolved negative feelings Encourage couple to identify events that would make the birth experience more positive Offer couple brief periods of privacy Determine client's knowledge regarding indications for procedure and comparative risks, benefits, and implications of all options to validate informed consent Assess fetal size and status Establish intravenous access and, if regional anesthesia is anticipated, infuse a minimum of 100 mL per hospital policy Insert indwelling catheter	Assess vital signs q15min × 4; q30min × 4; q1hr × 4; then q4hr Monitor patency and function of intravenous lines, indwelling catheter, pulse oximeter Assess dressing and wound q15min × 4, q30min × 4, q1hr × 4, then 4hr and prn Assess comfort level, facial expression, verbalizations of discomfort, ability to relax/rest, and use of comfort measures q2hr and prn Provide quiet, restful environment Assess firmness and position of fundus and amount and character of lochia q15min × 4; q30min × 4; then q4hr Assess Homan's sign, bowel sounds, and breasts BID Encourage change of position and support body parts Offer back rubs. Use therapeutic touch and music Assess for nausea and vomiting Provide information about newborn as soon as possible Provide opportunities for the parents to be with the newborn as soon as possible Provide opportunities to discuss feelings about the cesarean birth and woman's self-image as a mother Assess level of fatigue, ability to relax/rest, factors that interfere with rest (eg, pain, visitors, newborn care needs, and environmental factors such as noise and temperature) Plan care activities to allow for uninterrupted periods If necessary, return newborn to central nursery for a time to allow mother to sleep	Assess vital signs q4hr and prn Assess dressing/wound q1hr × 4, then q4hr × 24 hr Assess comfort level, changes in types/sources of discomfort, ability to relax/rest, and use of comfort measures Assess level of fatigue. Provide opportunities for rest/sleep Assess wound for approximation, redness, swelling, and drainage Assess dressing BID Assess firmness and position of fundus and lochia q8hr Assess Homan's sign, bowel sounds, and breasts BID Assess further development of attachment behaviors such as kissing, hugging, cuddling, smiling at newborn, calling newborn by name in affectionate tones, and identifying positive family characteristics in newborn Support positive maternal behaviors using praise and reinforcement Assist parents to discuss and understand their feelings, both positive and negative, about their birth experience and their newborn D/C IV per order D/C catheter per order and assess voiding

Cesarean Section *(continued)*

	Date _____ **Preoperative**	Date _____ **1st 24 Hours Postoperative**	Date _____ **24–48 Hours Postoperative**
Knowledge deficit	Assess reaction to and interpretation of past cesarean births or other surgical experiences Describe preoperative procedure: – abdominal prep – insertion of indwelling bladder catheter – insertion of IV – administration of preop medications Explain postoperative measures: turning, coughing, and deep breathing Discuss: – what is going to happen to woman's body and how it will feel – how to handle discomfort associated with procedures – what the woman will see and hear during the cesarean Demonstrate abdominal splinting	Provide information as to causes of discomfort and possible relief measures Reinforce earlier teaching Provide opportunities to ask questions Evaluate understanding of teaching	Reinforce teaching about possible comfort measures the mother can employ Assess mother's understanding of importance of adequate rest Begin discussing importance of adequate rest following discharge Discuss strategies for obtaining adequate rest such as napping when the newborn naps, wearing a nightgown and robe for a few days, and accepting help from a family member or friend Explain to family members about the effects of fatigue and sleep deprivation Discuss signs of developing UTI or endometritis, which mother should be alert for following discharge Initiate teaching about child care as necessary to facilitate the development of maternal self-confidence and encourage return demonstrations Use positive reinforcement to support effective behaviors
Nutrition	NPO	Diet as tolerated Encourage fluids	Progress diet based on bowel sounds Encourage fluids
Activity	Bathroom privileges with assistance	Up and about with 2 assists Shower with assist	Up ad lib with assistance as indicated
Medications	Preop medications as ordered Oral liquid antacid as ordered	Medications as ordered Antibiotics as ordered Analgesics as ordered Oxytocin as ordered Colace 100 mg BID prn	Medications as ordered Analgesics as ordered Colace 100 mg BID prn
Referral/ discharge plans		Assess discharge plans and adequacy of support system Evaluate understanding of teaching	Review and reinforce teaching with mother and partner

➤

	Date _____ **48–72 Hours Postoperative**	Date _____ **72 Hours Postoperative to Discharge**
Outcomes	Mother continues to exhibit normal findings for physical status indicators: vital signs within normal limits; evidences expected progression of normal involution; fundus firm, midline, 2 fingerbreadths below umbilicus; scant lochia rubra to serosa Mother exhibits an absence of signs and symptoms of hemorrhage, infection, and thrombophlebitis Mother employs appropriate comfort measures; describes pain as 3 or less on a scale of 1 to 10 Mother consistently implements self-care procedures accurately Mother reports obtaining adequate rest; naps periodically; reports feeling rested and regaining energy Mother has developed plans for ensuring adequate rest after discharge and coping with stress of a new infant Mother exhibits positive attachment behaviors such as calling infant by name; hugging, touching, smiling, and cuddling infant; speaking to infant in affectionate tones; meeting infant's physical needs promptly Parents exhibit positive parenting behaviors Client/couple verbalize understanding of essential information, including self-care activities and changes in mother's condition that should be reported immediately Mother accurately describes signs and symptoms to be reported promptly to the primary care provider including hemorrhage and infection Mother verbalizes satisfaction with childbearing experience and care	Mother continues to exhibit normal findings for physical status indicators: vital signs within normal limits; evidences expected progression of normal involution; fundus firm, midline, 2 fingerbreadths below umbilicus; scant lochia rubra to serosa Mother exhibits an absence of signs and symptoms of hemorrhage, infection, and thrombophlebitis Mother employs appropriate comfort measures; describes pain as 3 or less on a scale of 1 to 10 Mother consistently implements self-care procedures accurately Mother reports obtaining adequate rest; naps periodically; reports feeling rested and regaining energy Mother has developed plans for ensuring adequate rest after discharge and coping with the stress of a newborn Parents exhibit positive parenting behaviors Client/couple verbalize understanding of self-care activities and normal changes occurring during the postpartum period Mother accurately describes signs and symptoms to be reported promptly to the primary care provider including hemorrhage and infection Mother verbalizes satisfaction with childbearing experience care

	Date _____ **48–72 Hours Postoperative**	Date _____ **72 Hours Postoperative to Discharge**
Assessments, tests, and treatments	Assess comfort level and sources of discomfort Assess mother's ability to successfully manage her discomfort Assess level of fatigue and factors that may interfere with rest/sleep Maintain a restful environment with periods of time for uninterrupted sleep Assess vital signs q4hr Assess wound BID Assess fundus and lochia BID and prn Assess Homan's sign and breasts BID Assess for signs of developing infection Assess redness, edema, ecchymosis, or drainage from any incisions, including episiotomy Assess breastfeeding mother for cracked or bleeding nipples, areas of pain, tenderness, hardness or redness in the breasts Assess for signs of developing endometritis such as changes in lochia (eg, profuse, scant, or foul-smelling), pronounced uterine tenderness, malaise, chills, tachycardia Assess for ongoing development of attachment behaviors such as holding newborn close, expressing warm feelings about newborn, eagerness to care for newborn Ensure that a consistent, supportive nurse works with mother as much as possible Reinforce positive parenting behaviors Provide appropriate opportunities for the new mother to express and work through her feelings about her newborn Assess voiding and monitor for signs and symptoms of infection	Assess comfort level and sources of discomfort Assess mother's ability to successfully manage her discomfort Assess level of fatigue and factors that may interfere with rest/sleep Maintain a restful environment with periods of time for uninterrupted sleep Assess vital signs q4hr Assess wound BID Assess fundus and lochia BID and prn Assess Homan's sign and breasts BID Assess for signs of developing infection Assess redness, edema, ecchymosis, or drainage from any incisions, including episiotomy Assess breastfeeding mother for cracked or bleeding nipples, areas of pain, tenderness, hardness or redness in the breasts Assess for signs of developing endometritis such as changes in lochia (eg, profuse, scant, or foul-smelling), pronounced uterine tenderness, malaise, chills, tachycardia Assess for ongoing development of attachment behaviors such as holding newborn close, expressing warm feelings about newborn, eagerness to care for newborn Ensure that a consistent, supportive nurse works with mother as much as possible Reinforce positive parenting behaviors Provide appropriate opportunities for the new mother to express and work through her feelings about her newborn Assess voiding and monitor for signs and symptoms of infection

➤

	Date _____ **48–72 Hours Postoperative**	Date _____ **72 Hours Postoperative to Discharge**
Knowledge deficit	Describe signs and symptoms to report promptly to primary health care provider Provide information on postpartum discomforts that may occur (eg, breast engorgement, constipation) as well as postpartum complications (eg, infected episiotomy, mastitis, UTI) and the type of discomfort they may produce Discuss self-care measures for these discomforts Discuss the family's plan for ensuring that the new mother obtains adequate rest Reinforce teaching about self-care measures for preventing infection Describe effective breastfeeding techniques to prevent engorgement, caked breasts, or nipple trauma Review printed teaching materials in the appropriate language Continue to provide opportunities for questions, discussion, and return demonstrations Assess knowledge of and competence in providing basic infant care	Describe normal physiologic and psychologic changes during the postpartum period Demonstrate and discuss components of self-assessment of status and involution Assist with self-assessment Review strategies to manage postpartum discomforts Reivew signs and symptoms of complications and importance of reporting them to primary health care provider Review teaching about self-care measures for preventing infection Continue to provide opportunities for questions and discussion
Nutrition	Diet as tolerated Encourage fluids	Diet as tolerated Encourage fluids Encourage continuing prenatal vitamin and iron supplements for 6–8 weeks
Activity	Up ad lib	Up ad lib
Medications	Medications as ordered Analgesics as ordered Colace 100 mg BID prn	Medications as ordered Prescriptions for home as needed
Referral/ discharge plans	Review and reinforce teaching with mother and partner	Provide written copy of discharge instructions Make appropriate discharge referrals for mother and partner

Teaching new parents about the postpartum period and newborn care presents many challenges to caregivers in these practice areas. With shorter hospital stays and the varied needs of parents, it is imperative to develop systems that focus teaching and meet the specific needs of clients. One such model is a "Postpartum and Family Needs Assessment" which assists clients to identify learning needs and facilitates nursing staff efforts to provide the appropriate teaching. Once learner needs have been identified, the nurse can plan teaching that is directed to the learner's needs. Hospitals that have developed assessment tools such as this one have also organized education materials geared to the populations they serve.

POSTPARTUM AND FAMILY NEEDS ASSESSMENT

This sheet is designed to help you select the areas of teaching needs and assist the nurse to choose with you the most desired method of teaching and learning.

Please place a ✔ to indicate what you would like information on. What is your best way of learning?

☐ Audiovisual ☐ Hands-on demonstration ☐ Reading materials ☐ Any combination of same

MOTHER	BABY	FAMILY
☐ Hemorrhoids	☐ Feeding	☐ New roles for mother, father, other family members
☐ Breast and nipple care	☐ Growth and development	☐ Helping other children adjust
☐ Activity	☐ Circumcision	☐ Pets
☐ Nutrition	☐ Bathing	Are you concerned about:
☐ Need for exercise and rest	☐ Diapering	☐ Child care
☐ Sexuality and contraception	☐ Clothing	☐ Paying bills
☐ Emotions/feelings	☐ Taking temperature	☐ Having enough food/supplies/clothing
☐ Signs and symptoms to report	☐ Safety	☐ Other: _____
	☐ Normal newborn appearance and behavior	☐ Domestic violence/child abuse
	☐ Signs and symptoms to report	

☐ Would you like a home visit by a registered nurse to provide further information and assessment for you and your baby on any of the above topics?

My nurse and I have discussed the topics which I selected from these lists. I have received instruction and understand the instructions given to me.

Client: _____
Signature/Date

Nurse: _____
Signature/Date

POSTPARTUM AND FAMILY NEEDS ASSESSMENT (continued)

☐ List additional pamphlets given to client:

☐ Postpartum teaching and exercises

☐ Routine care of newborn teaching aid

☐ Newborn screening

☐ Breastfeeding

☐ Bottlefeeding teaching aid

☐ _____	☐ _____
☐ _____	☐ _____
☐ _____	☐ _____

INITIALS	TEACHER'S NAME AND TITLE
_____	_____
_____	_____
_____	_____

CODE: TEACHING METHOD

C = Class	H = Handout
A = Audiovisual	N = See notes
E = Explanation	N/A = Not Applicable
D = Demonstration	

SOURCE: Lakes Region General Hospital—Family Birthplace, Laconia, NH, 1994

Pediatric Pathways

Asthma 259

Diabetes (Type I) 263

Myringotomy and Insertion of Pressure-Equalizer Tubes 266

Pyloric Stenosis (Surgical Repair) 269

Respiratory Infection (Acute) 272

Tonsillectomy and Adenoidectomy 276

Asthma

Expected length of stay: 3 days

	Date _____ **Admission Day**	Date _____ **Day 2**	Date _____ **Day 3**
Daily outcomes	Client will: • evidence stabilization of vital signs • exhibit a patent airway; experience resolution of acute respiratory distress • verbalize understanding and demonstrate cooperation with respiratory therapy Family verbalizes feelings regarding illness Family displays effective coping Family verbalizes beginning understanding of asthma and ongoing care and treatments	Client will: • evidence stable vital signs and be afebrile • exhibit absence of respiratory infection • exhibit unlabored respirations and patent airway • tolerate ordered activity without evidence of respiratory distress, weakness, or exhaustion • have moist mucous membranes and have urine specific gravity = 1.005–1.020 • verbalize understanding and demonstrate cooperation with respiratory therapy Family exhibits effective coping mechanisms Family verbalizes beginning understanding of home care instructions including trigger agents, signs and symptoms of impending attack and appropriate actions	Client is afebrile with stable vital signs Client exhibits a patent airway and unlabored respirations with activity Client's respiratory rate and status has returned to baseline Client tolerates ordered activity without evidence of respiratory distress, weakness, or exhaustion Client's mucous membranes are moist Client's urine specific gravity = 1.005–1.020 Client tolerates usual diet Family verbalizes/demonstrates home care instructions, including strategies to reduce exposure to infectious illnesses and respiratory irritants Family exhibits ability to cope with lifestyle changes and effects of chronic illness Family demonstrates/verbalizes ability to cope with ongoing stressors Family verbalizes understanding of need to identify and avoid trigger agents and situations Family provides a home environment that enables normal growth and development

➤

	Date _____ **Admission Day**	Date _____ **Day 2**	Date _____ **Day 3**
Assessments, tests, and treatments	CBC ABGs Electrolytes Urinalysis Theophylline level Chest x–ray Skin tests as ordered Urine specific gravity q8hr Sputum for C and S Vital signs and O_2 saturation, q1–2hr and prn Assess respiratory status q1–2hr and prn Monitor carefully for changes in respiratory rate, skin color, retractions, and/or flaring Strict intake and output Respiratory therapy as ordered Humidification as ordered Position client in semi–Fowler's or high Fowler's position Oxygen as ordered Provide quiet, restful environment Assess cognitive/developmental level Reassure client and family of ongoing surveillance of client status and responses to therapy	CBC Theophylline level Urine specific gravity q8hr Note results of cultures Vital signs and O_2 saturation q4hr and prn Assess respiratory status q4hr and prn. Monitor carefully for changes in respiratory rate, skin color, retractions, and/or flaring Strict intake and output Respiratory therapy as ordered Humidification as ordered Position client in semi–Fowler's or high Fowler's position Oxygen as ordered D/C oxygen if O_2 saturation over 96% on room air Provide quiet, restful environment Reassure client and family of ongoing surveillance of client status and responses to therapy	Theophylline level Urine specific gravity q8hr Read and record results of skin tests Vital signs and O_2 saturation q4hr and prn Assess respiratory status q4hr and prn. Monitor carefully for changes in respiratory rate, skin color, retractions, and/or flaring Respiratory therapy as ordered Provide quiet, restful environment
Knowledge deficit	Initiate teaching regarding ongoing care including procedures, treatments, and medications Initiate teaching about asthma, its treatments, trigger agents, avoidance of respiratory infections and irritants, early signs and symptoms of infections Include family in teaching Evaluate understanding of teaching Provide information at developmental/cognitive level	Reinforce earlier teaching regarding ongoing care Reinforce teaching about asthma and treatments Renew detailed teaching with family/client regarding home care including medications, respiratory therapy, activity, trigger agents, avoidance of respiratory infections and irritants, early signs and symptoms of an impending attack, and follow-up care Include family in teaching Evaluate understanding of teaching	Reinforce earlier teaching regarding ongoing care Complete discharge teaching to include diet, follow-up care, signs and symptoms to report, follow-up MD visit, activity, and medications: name, purpose, dose, frequency, route, dietary interactions, and side effects Provide family/client with written discharge instructions Refer unmet teaching needs to outpatient services Include family in teaching Evaluate understanding of teaching Refer knowledge deficits to community resources

	Date _____ **Admission Day**	Date _____ **Day 2**	Date _____ **Day 3**
Psychosocial	Encourage verbalization of concerns Encourage family to participate in care Provide ongoing support and encouragement to client and family	Encourage verbalization of concerns Encourage family to participate in care Provide ongoing support and encouragement to client and family	Encourage verbalization of concerns Provide ongoing support and encouragement to client and family
Diet	Based on respiratory status NPO or advance from clear liquids to diet as tolerated, providing small, frequent, nutritious feedings Avoid cold fluids Encourage fluid intake	Diet as tolerated, providing small, frequent, nutritious feedings Avoid cold fluids Encourage fluid intake	Diet as tolerated, providing small, frequent, nutritious feedings Avoid cold fluids Encourage fluid intake
Activity	Assess safety needs and provide adequate precautions Balance activity with planned rest periods Side-lying or semiprone position Encourage age- and status-appropriate diversional activities	Maintain safety precautions Balance activity with planned rest periods Side-lying or semiprone position Increase activity as ordered Encourage age- and status-appropriate diversional activities	Maintain safety precautions Balance activity with planned rest periods Encourage age- and status-appropriate diversional activities
Medications	IV fluids as ordered IV aminophyllin Bronchodilators as ordered Steroids as ordered Oral antibiotics Inhalers as ordered Tylenol as ordered for temp over 101F	IV fluids as ordered/IV intermittent device Wean from IV aminophyllin to oral meds Bronchodilators as ordered Steroids as ordered Oral antibiotics Inhalers as ordered Tylenol as ordered for temp over 101F	D/C IV or intermittent IV device Oral theophylline as ordered Bronchodilators as ordered Oral steroids as ordered Inhalers as ordered Oral antibiotics
Transfer/ discharge plans	Continue to review progress toward discharge goals Review discharge plans	Continue to review progress toward discharge goals Determine need for home respiratory therapy and outpatient teaching for breathing exercises Finalize discharge plans Make appropriate referrals	Finalize plans for home care if needed Make any appropriate referrals Complete discharge teaching

Potential Client Variances
Asthma

Possible Complications
- Status asthmaticus
- Respiratory arrest

Health Conditions
- Pneumonia
- Respiratory acidosis
- Pneumothorax

Nursing Diagnoses
- Ineffective individual or family coping
- Fluid volume deficit
- Ineffective management of therapeutic regimen

Discharge Teaching for Pediatric Client with
Asthma

Activity
- Gradually return to usual level of activity by increasing activity each day. Alternate activity with rest periods. Avoid fatigue.
- Gradually increase activities. Monitor response to activity and stop activity if shortness of breath or wheezing occur. Avoid overexertion.
- Practice breathing exercises on a regular basis.

Diet
- Eat a well-balanced diet, including fruits, meat, vegetables, breads and starches, and milk products. Avoid any foods that cause symptoms.
- Plan rest periods after meals whenever possible.

Signs and Symptoms to Report
Notify physician if any of these symptoms occur:
- Shortness of breath, wheezing, or difficulty breathing
- Early signs and symptoms of an asthma attack

Follow-up Care and General Health Care
- Schedule follow-up appointment with physician as directed.
- Notify physician if activity intolerance occurs.
- Avoid others with respiratory infections.
- Establish a dust-free environment and stay away from respiratory irritants or allergy-producing substances.
- Avoid circumstances that precipitate symptoms of allergy or asthma.
- Consider support groups.

Medications
- Review written list of medications including dose, frequency, food interactions, and side effects.
- Carry a list of medications with listed doses.
- Avoid over-the-counter medications unless recommended by physician.

Diabetes (Type I)

Expected length of stay: 3 days

	Date _____ **Day 1**	Date _____ **Day 2**	Date _____ **Day 3**
Daily outcomes	Client will: • exhibit stable vital signs. • have hyperglycemia treated and blood sugar within expected therapeutic range • verbalize beginning understanding of diabetes and importance of diet compliance and regular blood sugar testing • verbalize beginning understanding of the purpose of insulin • experience early identification of impending hypoglycemia or hyperglycemia Family/client verbalize feelings regarding diagnosis Family/client exhibit effective coping	Client will: • exhibit stable vital signs • have blood sugar within therapeutic range • verbalize beginning understanding of diabetes and the importance of insulin therapy • verbalize understanding and importance of diet compliance and regular blood sugar testing • demonstrate beginning ability to prepare and administer insulin accurately • perform blood glucose monitoring accurately • begin to demonstrate ability to safely and correctly perform self-monitoring of blood glucose • verbalize beginning understanding of home care instructions Client/family evidence beginning acceptance of and effective coping with diagnosis	Client is afebrile, with stable vital signs Client has blood sugar within normal limits Client/family verbalizes/demonstrates home care instructions including aspects of diabetic care: 1) diet control, 2) SMBG, 3) insulin administration, 4) foot care, 5) general health care rules, and 6) signs, symptoms, and management of hypo- and hyperglycemia Client/family verbalizes importance of ongoing nursing and medical care Client tolerates ordered diet Client/family verbalizes understanding of the importance of health maintenance activities including regular dental care, physical exams, and care of cuts and scratches Family encourages planning and adhering to recommended exercise regimen Client/family displays effective coping with ongoing stressors
Assessments, tests, and treatments	CBC Fasting blood sugar Fingerstick blood sugar ac, hs, and prn; if blood glucose over 240 mg then obtain serum glucose Urine ketones if BS >250 mg Glycosylated hemoglobin Baseline laboratory work Vital signs q4hr and prn Weight Monitor for signs and symptoms of hypo- and hyperglycemia; follow appropriate protocol if symptoms occur Intake and output q8hr	Fasting blood sugar Fingerstick blood sugar ac, hs, and prn; if blood glucose over 240 mg then obtain serum glucose Urine ketones if BS >250 mg Vital signs q4hr if stable Weight Monitor for signs and symptoms of hypo- and hyperglycemia; follow appropriate protocol if symptoms occur Intake and output q8hr	Fasting blood sugar Fingerstick blood sugar ac, hs, and prn; if blood glucose over 240 mg then obtain serum glucose Urine ketones if BS >250 mg Vital signs q4hr if stable Weight Monitor for signs and symptoms of hypo- and hyperglycemia; follow appropriate protocol if symptoms occur

Diabetes (Type I) *(continued)*

	Date _____ **Day 1**	Date _____ **Day 2**	Date _____ **Day 3**
Knowledge deficit	Orient to room and hospital routine Review plan of care Assess readiness for teaching Assess current knowledge of and explain pathophysiology of diabetes Include client and family in teaching program Review steps of insulin administration and provide written instruction sheets Describe and explain factors that influence blood glucose levels including exercise, illness, and stress Review steps of SMBG Consult with diabetic nurse educator and registered dietitian and develop age-appropriate plan for care and instruction Evaluate understanding of teaching Keep teaching sessions short and priority-focused	Reinforce prior teaching Review steps of insulin administration and SMBG Review plan of care Include client and family in teaching Reinforce accurate performance of SMBG and preparation and administration of insulin Review site rotation Discuss hypo- and hyperglycemia and home management Provide client and family with teaching materials that reinforce teaching and meet specific learning needs and styles Allow client to practice with related equipment Show client and family videotapes related to Type I diabetes and self-care practices Evaluate understanding of teaching	Review plan of care Include family in teaching Supervise client/family in self-administration of insulin and performing SMBG and reinforce accurate performance Client and family attend classes on general health care practices and foot care and watch video related to identifying and managing hypo-and hyperglycemia and sick day management Refer knowledge deficits to outpatient diabetes program Evaluate understanding of teaching
Psychosocial	Assess level of anxiety Encourage verbalization of concerns Assess cognitive and developmental levels Provide ongoing support and encouragement	Assess level of anxiety Encourage verbalization of concerns Provide ongoing support and encouragement	Encourage verbalization of concerns Provide ongoing support and encouragement
Diet	Dietary consult ADA diet as ordered Encourage fluid intake	Diet teaching per dietitian ADA diet as ordered Encourage fluid intake	ADA diet as ordered Encourage fluid intake
Activity	Assess safety needs and provide appropriate precautions Activity as ordered Provide rest periods	Maintain safety precautions Activity as ordered Encourage rest periods Discuss the relationship of exercise to blood glucose control Identify usual form of exercise Collaboratively plan for regular exercise after discharge	Maintain safety precautions Activity as ordered Encourage rest periods Review the relationship of exercise to blood glucose control
Medications	Regular insulin to scale ac and hs	Regular insulin to scale ac and hs NPH insulin per order	Regular insulin to scale ac and hs NPH insulin per order

Diabetes (Type I) *(continued)*

	Date _____ **Day 1**	Date _____ **Day 2**	Date _____ **Day 3**
Transfer/ discharge plans	Establish discharge goals with client and family Consult with outpatient diabetes teaching program	Review progress towards discharge goals with client and family Refer to outpatient teaching program	Review progress toward discharge goals with client and family Refer to diabetic support group Refer to outpatient teaching program for continued teaching after discharge Make any appropriate referrals

Potential Client Variances
Diabetes (Type I)

Possible Complications
- Diabetic ketoacidosis
- Hypoglycemia
- Hyperglycemia
- Infection

Health Conditions
- Pre-existing illness or infection
- Surgery

Nursing Diagnoses
- Risk for infection
- Ineffective management of therapeutic regimen
- Ineffective individual or family coping

Discharge Teaching for Pediatric Client with
Diabetes (Type I)

Activity
- Continue exercise program as recommended by physician

Diet
- Follow prescribed diabetic diet as instructed. (Diet plan and exchange lists provided.)
- Increase fiber as instructed.

Signs and Symptoms to Report
Notify physician if any of these symptoms occur:
- Episodes of hypoglycemia or hyperglycemia
- Blood sugar over 240 mg
- Ketones in the urine
- Evidence of complications such as infections

Follow-Up Care and General Health Care
- Schedule follow-up appointment with physician as directed
- Continue blood sugar testing as recommended and maintain record
- Continue outpatient diabetic teaching as directed
- Consider attending a support group or summer camp for diabetics
- Wear a MedicAlert tag or bracelet

Medications
- Review written list of medications, including dose, route, frequency, food interactions, and side effects
- Administer insulin as directed. Rotate sites as directed.

Myringotomy and Insertion of Pressure-Equalizer Tubes

Expected length of stay: less than 6 hours

	Date _____ **Preoperative**	Date _____ **Postoperative**
Daily outcomes	Parent/client verbalizes understanding of preoperative teaching including IV fluids, antiemetics, activity, and pain management Parent/client exhibits effective coping Validate informed consent	Client evidences stable vital signs and is alert and responsive Client recovers from anesthesia Client indicates relief of pain from oral analgesics Client is independent in self–care Client is ambulatory Parent verbalizes/demonstrates home care instructions Client tolerates ordered diet without vomiting
Assessments, tests, and treatments	CBC Urinalysis Baseline physical assessment with a focus on respiratory status Anesthesia consult Assess developmental/cognitive level	Position on side until fully awake Vital signs and O_2 saturation, and neurovascular assessment q15min × 4; q30min × 4; q1hr × 4 and then q4hr and prn Assess lung sounds q1–2hr and prn Monitor intake and output Encourage voiding prior to discharge Assess pain and evaluate effectiveness of pain medications
Knowledge deficit	Orient to room and surroundings Include family in teaching Provide simple, brief instructions Review preoperative preparation including hospital and surgical routines Reinforce preoperative teaching Evaluate understanding of teaching Provide information at cognitive /developmental level	Reorient to room and postoperative routine Include family in teaching Review plan of care and importance of early mobilization, as well as any activity restrictions Complete discharge teaching regarding postoperative assessments, follow-up care, signs and symptoms to report, medications, diet, avoidance of infection and possible temporary hearing loss Explain to parent that myringotomy tubes will eventually be rejected and that a small plastic tube may fall from the ear Discuss the hazards of contaminated water entering the ear canal. Instruct the parent/client to use ear plugs or equivalent for showering, shampooing, or swimming Review the hazards of diving Evaluate understanding of teaching
Psychosocial	Assess anxiety related to pending surgery Assess fears of the unknown related to surgery Encourage verbalization of concerns Provide emotional support to client and family Provide information regarding surgical experience Minimize external stimuli (eg, noise, movement)	Assess level of anxiety Encourage verbalization of concerns Provide emotional support to client and family Provide information and ongoing support and encouragement

	Date _____ **Preoperative**	Date _____ **Postoperative**
Diet	NPO Baseline nutritional assessment	Advance diet from clear to full liquids following surgery Encourage fluids
Activity	OOB ad lib until premedicated for surgery	Provide safety precautions Bathroom privileges with assistance after surgery and begin progressive ambulation as tolerated
Medications	NPO except ordered medications	Analgesics as ordered Antibiotics if ordered IV fluids until adequate oral intake then D/C intermittent IV device
Transfer/ discharge plans	Assess discharge plans and support system	Probable discharge within 6 hours of surgery Complete discharge home care teaching when fully awake and oriented and before discharge Provide a written copy of discharge instructions

Potential Client Variances
Myringotomy and Insertion of Pressure-Equalizer Tubes

Possible Complications
- Infection
- Tube occlusion

Health Conditions
- Acute otitis media
- Acute respiratory infection

Nursing Diagnoses
- Fluid volume deficit
- Ineffective management of therapeutic regimen
- Risk for infection

Discharge Teaching for Pediatric Client Undergoing
Myringotomy and Insertion of Pressure-Equalizer Tubes

Activity
- Rest when you return home. Gradually return to usual level of activity by increasing activity each day.
- Avoid strenuous exercise or activity for the first few days following surgery.

Diet
- Advance diet from liquids to usual diet as tolerated.
- Drink 2 liters of fluid each day.

Signs and Symptoms to Report
Notify physician if any of these symptoms occur:
- Chills, or fever greater than 100F or 38C
- Worsening ear pain or discomfort
- Purulent drainage from either ear
- Nausea or vomiting
- Crying or irritability
- Lack of appetite

Follow-Up Care and General Health Care
- Schedule follow-up appointment with physician as directed.
- The ear tubes will eventually be rejected and you may find them as they fall out of the ear canal.
- Avoid others with respiratory infections.
- Avoid getting contaminated water in the ear canal. Use ear plugs when showering, shampooing, or swimming. No diving until the ear tubes are rejected.
- Avoid allergens and respiratory irritants
- If you fly, swallow frequently during take-off, so as to equalize pressure.

Medications
- Review written list of medications, including dose, route, frequency, food interactions, and side effects.

Surgical Repair of Pyloric Stenosis

Expected length of stay: 3 days

	Date _____ **1st 24 Hours Postoperative**	Date _____ **24–48 Hours Postoperative**	Date _____ **3 Days Postoperative**
Daily outcomes	Client will: • have stable vital signs and be alert and responsive • have lungs clear to auscultation • have unlabored respirations and maintain oxygen saturation above 95% • have a clean, dry dressing • recover from anesthesia • tolerate ordered diet without vomiting • have moist mucous membranes • have a urine specific gravity = 1.005–1.020 • demonstrate pain control Family displays effective coping with ongoing stressors	Client will: • have stable vital signs and be alert and responsive • have lungs clear to auscultation • have unlabored respirations and maintain oxygen saturation above 95% • have a clean, dry wound with edges well–approximated, healing by first intention • tolerate ordered diet without vomiting • have moist mucous membranes • have a urine specific gravity = 1.005–1.020 Family will demonstrate beginning understanding of home care instructions Family displays effective coping with ongoing stressors	Client is afebrile, has stable vital signs, and is alert and oriented Client has lungs clear to auscultation and unlabored respirations with an O_2 saturation >95% Client has clean, dry wound with edges well–approximated, healing by first intention Client has moist mucous membranes and urine specific gravity = 1.005–1.020 Family verbalizes/demonstrates home care instructions Client tolerates ordered diet without vomiting Family exhibits ability to cope with ongoing stressors
Assessments, tests, and treatments	Electrolytes Urine specific gravity q8hr Weight Vital signs and O_2 saturation and wound drainage assessment q15min × 4; q30min × 4; q1hr × 24 and prn Assess respiratory status q2–4hr and prn Change position frequently Assess abdomen and bowel sounds q8hr and prn Oxygen as ordered Observe responses to feeding and feeding technique Strict intake and output Record and report vomiting Monitor temperature and provide warming measures as indicated Provide ongoing emotional support to family	Weight Urine specific gravity q8hr Vital signs, O_2 saturation, and dressing and wound drainage assessment q2–4hr and prn Assess respiratory status q4hr and prn Change position frequently Assess abdomen and bowel sounds q8hr and prn Dressing change and wound assessment BID and prn Strict intake and output Observe responses to feeding and feeding technique Record and report vomiting Monitor temperature and provide warming measures as indicated	Weight Urine specific gravity q8hr Vital signs, O_2 saturation, and dressing and wound drainage assessment q4–8hr and prn Assess respiratory status q4–8hr Change position frequently Assess wound and apply dry sterile dressing every day and prn Assess abdomen and bowel sounds q8hr and prn Observe responses to feeding and feeding technique Record and report vomiting Monitor temperature and provide warming measures as indicated

➤

	Date _____ **1st 24 Hours Postoperative**	Date _____ **24–48 Hours Postoperative**	Date _____ **3 Days Postoperative**
Knowledge deficit	Orient family to room and surroundings Provide simple, brief instructions Encourage family involvement in care Review specific postoperative care: turning, intravenous, pain management Provide family instructions regarding feeding Evaluate understanding of teaching	Review plan of care Begin discharge teaching regarding wound care/dressing change and diet Review written discharge instructions with family Continue to encourage family participation in care Observe and coach family members regarding feeding Evaluate understanding of teaching	Complete discharge teaching to include wound care, diet, follow-up care and appointment, signs and symptoms to report, activity, and medication: name, purpose, dose, frequency, route, food interactions, and side effects Provide family with written discharge instructions regarding home care Evaluate understanding of teaching
Psychosocial	Assess anxiety related to surgery Encourage verbalization of concerns Assess coping status of family Provide emotional support to client and family Cuddle prn and encourage parents to cuddle child	Assess level of anxiety Encourage verbalization of concerns Assess coping status of family Provide emotional support to client and family Provide information and ongoing encouragement	Assess level of anxiety Encourage verbalization of concerns Assess coping status of family Provide emotional support to client and family Provide information and ongoing encouragement
Diet	When fully awake, begin progressive diet as ordered Position on right side with head up after feedings Burp before feedings and frequently during feedings Pacifier between meals	Continue progressing diet as ordered Position on right side with head up after feedings Burp before feedings and frequently during feedings Pacifier between meals	Diet as ordered Position on right side with head up after feedings Burp before feedings and frequently during feedings Pacifier between meals
Activity	Assess safety needs and provide adequate precautions	Maintain safety precautions	Maintain safety precautions
Medications	IV fluids Analgesics as ordered	Intermittent IV device Analgesics as ordered	Analgesics as ordered D/C IV device
Transfer/discharge plans	Establish discharge objectives with family Determine discharge needs Assess support system Begin home care instructions	Review progress toward discharge goals Make appropriate referrals Finalize discharge plans	Finalize any home care arrangements Complete discharge instructions

Potential Client Variances
Surgical Repair of Pyloric Stenosis

Possible Complications

- Infection
- Dehydration
- Metabolic alkalosis
- Peritonitis

Health Conditions

- Acute respiratory infection

Nursing Diagnoses

- Fluid volume deficit
- Ineffective management of therapeutic regimen
- Ineffective family coping

Discharge Teaching for Infant Following
Surgical Repair of Pyloric Stenosis

Activity

- Provide calm, restful environment
- Provide adequate rest

Diet

- Burp before feedings and frequently during feedings.
- Advance diet as directed.
- Position with head up and on right side after meals.

Signs and Symptoms to Report

Notify physician if any of these symptoms occur:
- Chills, or fever greater than 100F or 38C
- Vomiting
- Excessive crying or irritability

Follow-Up Care and General Health Care

- Schedule follow-up appointment with physician as directed.

Medications

- Review written list of medications, including dose, route, frequency, food interactions, and side effects.

Wound Care

- Keep incision clean and dry.
- Report any increasing redness, swelling, tenderness, or drainage.

Acute Respiratory Infection

Expected length of stay: 3 days

	Date _____ **Admission Day**	Date _____ **Day 2**	Date _____ **Day 3**
Daily outcomes	Client will: • experience stabilization of vital signs • experience fever reduction in response to antipyretics and cooling measures • evidence a patent airway and an absence of respiratory distress • exhibit a respiratory rate within 10 of baseline • verbalize understanding of and demonstrate cooperation with respiratory therapy • remain calm and be comforted by nursing measures and family presence Family verbalizes feelings regarding illness Family demonstrates ability to cope Family verbalizes beginning understanding of ongoing care and treatments	Client will: • exhibit stable vital signs • evidence effective control of fever with antipyretics and cooling measures • exhibit unlabored respirations with activity • maintain a patent airway and tolerate activity without evidence of weakness, exhaustion, or labored respirations • have moist mucous membranes • have urine specific gravity between 1.005–1.020 • verbalize understanding of and demonstrate cooperation with respiratory therapy • remain calm and be comforted by nursing measures and family presence • have an oral intake of 2000 mL/day Family exhibits effective coping Family verbalizes beginning understanding of home care instructions	Client is afebrile with stable vital signs Client has a patent airway, unlabored respirations with activity, and clear lungs Client's respiratory rate and status have returned to baseline Client tolerates ordered activity without evidence of weakness, exhaustion, or labored respirations Client's mucous membranes are moist Client's urine specific gravity is between 1.005–1.020 Client tolerates usual diet Family verbalizes/demonstrates home care instructions, including strategies to reduce exposure to infectious illnesses Family exhibits effective coping Family demonstrates/verbalizes ability to cope with ongoing stressors
Assessments, tests, and treatments	CBC ABGs Urinalysis Chest x–ray Skin tests as ordered Urine specific gravity q8hr Sputum for C and S Vital signs and O_2 saturation q1–2hr and prn Assess respiratory status q1–2hr and prn Monitor carefully for changes in respiratory rate, skin color, retractions, and/or flaring Strict intake and output Respiratory therapy as ordered	CBC Urine specific gravity q8hr Note results of cultures Vital signs and O_2 saturation, q4hr and prn Assess respiratory status q4hr and prn Monitor carefully for changes in respiratory rate, skin color, retractions, and/or flaring Strict intake and output Respiratory therapy as ordered Suction as indicated Humidification as ordered Position client in semi–Fowler's or high Fowler's position	Urine specific gravity q8hr Read and record results of skin tests Vital signs and O_2 saturation q4hr if stable Assess respiratory status q4hr and prn Monitor carefully for changes in respiratory rate, skin color, retractions, and/or flaring Respiratory therapy as ordered Provide quiet, restful environment

Acute Respiratory Infection (continued)

	Date _____ **Admission Day**	Date _____ **Day 2**	Date _____ **Day 3**
Assessments, tests, and treatments (continued)	Humidification as ordered Suction as indicated Position client in semi–Fowler's or high Fowler's position Administer oxygen per order Provide quiet, restful environment Plan nursing activities to minimize energy expenditures Assess developmental/cognitive level	Administer oxygen to maintain saturation at 92% D/C oxygen if O_2 saturation over 96% on room air Provide quiet, restful environment Plan nursing activities to minimize energy expenditures	
Knowledge deficit	Initiate teaching regarding ongoing care, including explaining procedures, treatments, and medications; reinforce prn Include family in teaching Present information at developmental/cognitive level Evaluate understanding of teaching	Reinforce earlier teaching regarding ongoing care Initiate detailed teaching with family/client regarding home care including medications, activity, the avoidance of respiratory infections, and follow–up care Include family in teaching Evaluate understanding of teaching	Reinforce earlier teaching regarding ongoing care Complete discharge teaching to include diet, follow–up care, signs and symptoms to report, follow–up MD visit, activity, and medications: name, purpose, dose, frequency, route, dietary interactions, and side effects Provide family/client with written discharge instructions Refer unmet teaching needs to outpatient services Include family in teaching Evaluate understanding of teaching
Psychosocial	Encourage verbalization of concerns Encourage family to participate in care Provide ongoing support and encouragement to client and family Cuddle young clients and encourage parents to cuddle with child	Encourage verbalization of concerns Encourage family to participate in care Provide ongoing support and encouragement to client and family	Encourage verbalization of concerns Provide ongoing support and encouragement to client and family
Diet	Based on respiratory status: NPO or advance from clear liquids to diet as tolerated, providing age-appropriate diet as ordered Offer fluids slowly and carefully monitor response	Diet as tolerated, providing age-appropriate diet as ordered	Age-appropriate diet as tolerated

➤

	Date _____ **Admission Day**	Date _____ **Day 2**	Date _____ **Day 3**
Activity	Assess safety needs and provide adequate precautions Balance activity with planned rest periods Position of comfort with HOB up; turn q2hr and prn Provide age-appropriate diversions	Maintain safety precautions Balance activity with planned rest periods Position of comfort with HOB up; turn q2hr and prn Provide age-appropriate diversions	Maintain safety precautions Balance activity with planned rest periods Position of comfort with HOB up; turn q2hr and prn Provide age-appropriate diversions
Medications	IV fluids as ordered IV aminophyllin if ordered Bronchodilators as ordered Antibiotics as ordered Inhalers as ordered Tylenol as ordered for temp over 101F	IV fluids as ordered/IV intermittent device Wean from IV aminophyllin to oral meds as directed Bronchodilators as ordered Antibiotics as ordered Inhalers as ordered Tylenol as ordered for temp over 101F	D/C IV or intermittent IV device Bronchodilators as ordered Inhalers as ordered Antibiotics as ordered
Transfer/ discharge plans	Continue to review progress toward discharge goals Review discharge plans	Continue to review progress toward discharge goals Finalize discharge plans Make appropriate referrals	Finalize plans for home care if needed Make any appropriate referrals Complete discharge teaching

Potential Client Variances
Acute Respiratory Infection

Possible Complications

- Empyema
- Pneumothorax
- Laryngeal obstruction
- Respiratory arrest

Health Conditions

- Pre-existing respiratory conditions
- Acute epiglottitis
- Immunosuppression

Nursing Diagnoses

- Ineffective individual or family coping
- Fluid volume deficit
- Ineffective management of therapeutic regimen

Discharge Teaching for Pediatric Client with
Acute Respiratory Infection

Activity

- Gradually return to usual level of activity by increasing activity each day. Alternate activity with rest periods. Avoid fatigue.
- Gradually increase activities. Monitor response to activity and stop activity if shortness of breath occurs. Avoid overexertion.

Diet

- Eat a well-balanced diet, including fruits, meat, vegetables, breads and starches, and milk products.
- Plan rest periods after meals whenever possible.

Signs and Symptoms to Report

Notify physician if any of these symptoms occur:
- Shortness of breath, wheezing, and difficulty breathing
- Chills, or fever greater than 100F or 38C

Follow-up Care and General Health Care

- Schedule follow-up appointment with physician as directed.
- Notify physician if activity intolerance occurs.
- Avoid others with respiratory infections.

Medications

- Review written list of medications including dose, frequency, food interactions, and side effects.
- Carry a list of medications, with listed doses.
- Avoid over-the-counter medications unless recommended by physician.

Tonsillectomy and Adenoidectomy

Expected length of stay: less than 6 hours

	Date _____ **Day 1**	Date _____ **Day 2**
Daily outcomes	Parent/client verbalizes understanding of preoperative teaching including IV fluids, antiemetics, ice pack to neck, activity, and pain management Parent/client displays effective coping Validate informed consent	Client has a patent airway and has minimal drainage in the throat Client has stable vital signs and is alert and responsive Client remains free of signs/symptoms of hemorrhage and hemoglobin and hematocrit remains within normal limits Client manages pain with ordered medications Parent/client verbalizes/demonstrates home care instructions Client tolerates liquids without complaints of severe pain or vomiting
Assessments, tests, and treatments	CBC Urinalysis PTT Baseline physical assessment with a focus on respiratory status Anesthesia consult Assess cognitive/developmental level	Position on side until fully awake; then Fowler's position Vital signs and O_2 saturation, neurovascular assessment, and bleeding assessment q15min × 4; q30min × 4; q1hr × 4 and then q4hr and prn Assess lung sounds q1–2hr and prn Discourage coughing or clearing of throat Monitor for frequent swallowing Ice pack to neck Monitor intake and output; encourage voiding prior to discharge Offer/administer analgesics on schedule as ordered for 24 hours Assess pain and effectiveness of pain medications
Knowledge deficit	Orient to room and surroundings Include family in teaching Provide simple, brief instructions Review preoperative preparation, including hospital and surgical routines Emphasize probability of the presence of old blood in the nose, between the teeth, and in emesis Reinforce preoperative teaching Evaluate understanding of teaching Provide information at developmental/cognitive level	Reorient to room and postoperative routine Include family in teaching Review plan of care and importance of early mobilization, as well as diet and activity restrictions Complete discharge teaching regarding postoperative assessments, follow-up care, signs and symptoms to report, medications, and diet Explain to client to avoid coughing or clearing throat and to avoid gargling Review the importance of reporting any signs or symptoms of bleeding during the postoperative period up to 10 days following surgery Evaluate understanding of teaching

	Date _____ **Day 1**	Date _____ **Day 2**
Psychosocial	Assess anxiety related to pending surgery Assess fears of the unknown related to surgery Encourage verbalization of concerns Provide emotional support to client and family Minimize external stimuli (eg, noise, movement) Reassure child that he/she will be able to talk	Assess level of anxiety Encourage verbalization of concerns Provide emotional support to client and family Provide information and encouragement to client and family
Diet	NPO Baseline nutritional assessment	Advance to clear liquid to full liquid following surgery; offer cool fluids Encourage large sips of fluids No straws No citrus juices
Activity	OOB ad lib until premedicated for surgery	Provide safety precautions Encourage bed rest for first 24 hours, then bathroom privileges with assistance after surgery
Medications	NPO except ordered medications	Analgesics as ordered Antibiotics if ordered IV fluids until adequate oral intake; then D/C NO ASPIRIN
Transfer/ discharge plans	Assess discharge plans and support system	Probable discharge within 6 hours of surgery Complete discharge home care teaching when fully awake and oriented and before discharge Provide a written copy of discharge instructions

Potential Client Variances
Tonsillectomy and Adenoidectomy

Possible Complications

- Hemorrhage
- Infection

Health Conditions

- Pre-existing cardiac or respiratory disease
- Upper respiratory infection
- Developmental delays

Nursing Diagnoses

- Pain
- Fluid volume deficit
- Ineffective management of therapeutic regimen

Discharge Teaching for Pediatric Client Undergoing
Tonsillectomy and Adenoidectomy

Activity

- Rest in bed when you return home. Gradually return to usual level of activity by increasing activity each day. Alternate activity with rest periods.
- Avoid strenuous exercise or activity for the first few days following surgery.

Diet

- Start with clear and full liquids. Cold fluids are best tolerated. Take large sips as they are easier to swallow. Gradually begin to introduce soft, bland foods such as jello, cooked fruits, soup, and mashed potatoes. Avoid citrus fruits or juices.
- Do not use straws.
- Drink 2 –3 liters of fluid each day.

Signs and Symptoms to Report

Notify physician if any of these symptoms occur:
- Bleeding of any type
- Chills, or fever greater than 100F or 38C
- Inability to drink fluids
- Nausea or vomiting

Follow–Up Care and General Health Care

- Schedule follow–up appointment with physician as directed.
- Avoid people with respiratory infections.
- Avoid coughing or clearing the throat.
- Avoid gargling or vigorous tooth brushing.

Medications

- Review written list of medications, including dose, route, frequency, food interactions, and side effects.
- NO ASPIRIN or aspirin-containing medications.

Psychiatric Pathways

Alcohol Withdrawal 281

Anorexia Nervosa 287

Bipolar Disorder: Manic Phase 292

Dementia 299

Depression Without Psychotic Features or Agitation 304

Panic Disorder: Outpatient Treatment 310

Alcohol Withdrawal

Expected length of stay: 6 days

	Date _____ **Day 1**	Date _____ **Day 2**	Date _____ **Day 3**
Daily outcomes	Client will: • evidence stable vital signs • remain oriented to time, place, and person • withdraw from alcohol without injury • consume 1500 kcal and 2000 mL of fluid each day unless contraindicated • verbalize thoughts and feelings • verbalize commitment to detox program • maintain a stable weight • exhibit effective coping	Client will: • evidence stable vital signs • remain oriented to time, place, and person • withdraw from alcohol without injury • consume 2000 kcal and 3000 mL of fluid each day unless contraindicated • verbalize thoughts and feelings • verbalize commitment to detox program • attend AA and/or scheduled groups daily • maintain a stable weight • identify strategies to promote sleep/rest • exhibit alternate coping mechanisms	Client will: • be afebrile, with stable vital signs • remain oriented to time, place, and person • withdraw from alcohol without injury • remain free of signs and symptoms of delirium tremens • consume 2000 kcal and 3000 mL of fluid each day unless contraindicated • verbalize thoughts and feelings • begin to verbalize alcohol's negative effects on significant others and lifestyle • verbalize commitment to detox program • attend AA and/or scheduled groups daily • maintain a stable weight • identify strategies to promote sleep/rest • exhibit alternate coping mechanisms

	Date _____ **Day 1**	Date _____ **Day 2**	Date _____ **Day 3**
Assessments, tests, and treatments	CBC Urinalysis Chemistry profile Electrolytes Serum magnesium Chest x-ray EKG PPD Assess need for HIV testing Vital signs q4hr and prn Intake and output Blood alcohol level Weight Assess q1–2hr for signs and symptoms of withdrawal, including anxiety, agitation, irritability, tremors, tachycardia, hypertension, diaphoresis, and hallucinations Assess drinking history and patterns Establish the date and time of last drink	Vital signs q4hr and prn Intake and output Assess q1–2hr for signs and symptoms of withdrawal, including anxiety, agitation, irritability, tremors, tachycardia, hypertension, diaphoresis, and hallucinations	Repeat laboratory studies as indicated Vital signs every shift and prn D/C intake and output if stable Assess q1–2hr for signs and symptoms of withdrawal, including anxiety, agitation, irritability, tremors, tachycardia, hypertension, diaphoresis, and hallucinations Monitor for delirium tremens Read PPD Weight
Knowledge deficit	Orient client and family to room and routine Include family in teaching Review plan of care Evaluate understanding of teaching	Review plan of care with client and family Include family in teaching Evaluate understanding of teaching	Review plan of care with client and family Include family in teaching Initiate discharge teaching regarding the need for ongoing outpatient therapy and attending a self-help group Evaluate understanding of teaching
Diet	Encourage up to 3000 mL of fluids each day (unless contraindicated) Limit caffeine intake Provide frequent, small, nutritious feedings, inclusive of all food groups Nutritional assessment	Encourage up to 3000 mL of fluids each day (unless contraindicated) Limit caffeine Provide frequent, small, nutritious feedings, inclusive of all food groups	Encourage up to 3000 mL of fluids each day (unless contraindicated) Limit caffeine Provide frequent, small, nutritious feedings, inclusive of all food groups
Activity	Assess safety needs and maintain appropriate precautions Activity as tolerated Assist with hygiene as needed	Maintain safety precautions Activity as tolerated Prompt and assist with hygiene as needed	Maintain safety precautions Self-care/shower

	Date _____ **Day 1**	Date _____ **Day 2**	Date _____ **Day 3**
Psychosocial	Approach in non-judgmental manner Assess level of anxiety Assess sleep patterns and provide measures that promote rest and sleep Encourage expression of thoughts and feelings Explore availability of support system Encourage regular aerobic exercise Explore interests and potential hobbies Explore attending an AA meeting Use gentle confrontation strategies Provide education and set limits Explore lifestyle changes Provide information and ongoing support and encouragement to client and family	Approach in non-judgmental manner Assess level of anxiety Encourage verbalization of concerns Provide measures that promote rest and sleep Encourage expression of thoughts and feelings Explore availability of support system Explore interests and potential hobbies Prompt to attend an AA meeting Use gentle confrontation strategies Provide education and set limits Explore lifestyle changes Provide information and ongoing support and encouragement to client and family	Approach in non-judgmental manner Assess level of anxiety Encourage verbalization of concerns Provide measures that promote rest and sleep Encourage expression of thoughts and feelings Explore availability of support system Prompt to choose and begin regular aerobic exercise Explore interests and potential hobbies Prompt to attend an AA meeting Use gentle confrontation strategies Provide education and set limits Explore lifestyle changes Provide information and ongoing support and encouragement to client and family
Medications	Thiamine 100 mg IM or po Routine meds as ordered Librium as ordered	Thiamine 100 mg po Folic acid 1 mg po Multivitamin po Routine meds as ordered Librium as ordered	Thiamine 100 mg po Folic acid 1 mg po Multivitamin po Routine meds as ordered Librium as ordered
Transfer/ discharge plans	Family assessment if not previously completed Consult with internist if indicated Refer to neurologist if indicated Discuss self-help groups Establish discharge objectives with client and family	Review discharge objectives and anticipated discharge care with client and family Refer to self-help groups Refer family to self-help groups Complete discharge planning	Review progress toward discharge objectives with client and family Make appropriate referrals

Alcohol Withdrawal *(continued)*

	Date _____ **Day 4**	Date _____ **Day 5**	Date _____ **Day 6–Discharge Day**
Daily outcomes	Client will: • be afebrile, with stable vital signs • remain oriented to time, place, and person • withdraw from alcohol without injury • remain free of signs and symptoms of delirium tremens • consume 2000 kcal and 3000 mL of fluid each day unless contraindicated • verbalize thoughts and feelings • begin to verbalize alcohol's negative effects on lifestyle • verbalize commitment to detox program • attend AA or scheduled groups daily • maintain a stable weight • establish sleep/rest routine to promote sleep • exhibit effective coping	Client will: • be afebrile, with stable vital signs • remain oriented to time, place, and person • withdraw from alcohol without injury • remain free of signs and symptoms of delirium tremens • consume 2000 kcal and 3000 mL of fluid each day unless contraindicated • verbalize thoughts and feelings • begin to verbalize alcohol's negative effects on lifestyle • verbalize commitment to detox program • attend AA or scheduled groups daily • maintain a stable weight • establish sleep/rest routine to promote sleep • exhibit effective coping • discuss alternate coping strategies	Client is afebrile, with stable vital signs Client is alert and oriented Client has withdrawn from alcohol safely and without injury Client maintains adequate nutrition and fluid intake Client's weight remains stable Client verbalizes understanding of hazards of alcohol Client is independent in self-care Cleint verbalizes times and places for AA meetings Client verbalizes commitment to detox program and regular attendance at AA meetings or scheduled groups Client verbalizes home care instructions, including the importance of ongoing counseling Client has established a sleep/rest pattern and verbalizes understanding of sleep-promoting measures Client exhibits effective coping with ongoing stressors
Assessments, tests, and treatments	Vital signs BID and prn Assess for signs and symptoms of withdrawal, including anxiety, agitation, irritability, tremor, tachycardia, hypertension, diaphoresis, and hallucinations Monitor for delirium tremens Weight	Vital signs BID and prn Assess for signs and symptoms of withdrawal, including anxiety, agitation, irritability, tremor, tachycardia, hypertension, diaphoresis, and hallucinations Monitor for delirium tremens Weight	Vital signs BID and prn Assess for signs and symptoms of withdrawal, including anxiety, agitation, irritability, tremor, tachycardia, hypertension, diaphoresis, and hallucinations Monitor for delirium tremens Weight
Knowledge deficit	Review plan of care Include family in teaching Continue discharge teaching regarding the need for ongoing care and self-help groups Evaluate understanding of teaching	Review plan of care with client and family Continue discharge teaching regarding detox program and need for ongoing counseling Evaluate understanding of teaching	Client and/or family verbalizes understanding of discharge teaching, including exercise program, strategies to prevent relapse, diet, signs and symptoms to report, follow-up care and MD appointment, and medications: name, purpose, dose, frequency, route, dietary interactions, and side effects Evaluate understanding of teaching

Alcohol Withdrawal *(continued)*

	Date _____ **Day 4**	Date _____ **Day 5**	Date _____ **Day 6–Discharge Day**
Diet	Encourage up to 3000 mL of fluids each day (unless contraindicated) Limit caffeine intake Provide frequent, small, nutritious feedings, inclusive of all food groups	Encourage up to 3000 mL of fluids each day (unless contraindicated) Limit caffeine intake Provide frequent, small, nutritious feedings, inclusive of all food groups	Encourage up to 3000 mL of fluids each day (unless contraindicated) Limit caffeine intake Provide frequent, small, nutritious feedings, inclusive of all food groups
Activity	Maintain safety precautions Self-care/shower	Maintain safety precautions Self-care/shower	Maintain safety precautions Self-care/shower
Psychosocial	Approach in non-judgmental manner Assess level of anxiety Encourage verbalization of concerns Provide measures that promote rest and sleep Encourage expression of thoughts and feelings Explore availability of support system Prompt to continue regular aerobic exercise Explore interests and potential hobbies Prompt to attend an AA meeting Use gentle confrontation strategies Provide education and set limits Explore lifestyle changes Encourage verbalization of concerns Provide information and ongoing support and encouragement to client and family	Approach in non-judgmental manner Assess level of anxiety Encourage verbalization of concerns Provide measures that promote rest and sleep Encourage expression of thoughts and feelings Explore availability of support system Prompt to continue regular aerobic exercise Explore interests and potential hobbies Prompt to attend an AA meeting Use gentle confrontation strategies Provide education and set limits Explore lifestyle changes Encourage verbalization of concerns Provide information and ongoing support and encouragement to client and family	Approach in non-judgmental manner Assess level of anxiety Encourage verbalization of concerns Provide measures that promote rest and sleep Encourage expression of thoughts and feelings Explore availability of support system Prompt to continue regular aerobic exercise Explore interests and potential hobbies Prompt to attend an AA meeting Use gentle confrontation strategies Provide education and set limits Explore lifestyle changes Encourage verbalization of concerns Provide information and ongoing support and encouragement to client and family
Medications	Thiamine 100 mg po Folic acid 1 mg po Multivitamin po Librium as ordered Routine meds as ordered	Thiamine 100 mg po Folic acid 1 mg po Multivitamin po Librium as ordered Routine meds as ordered	Thiamine 100 mg po Folic acid 1 mg po Multivitamin po Librium as ordered Routine meds as ordered
Transfer/ discharge plans	Review with client and family discharge objectives regarding home care	Review with client and family discharge objectives regarding home care Complete referrals for outpatient care/therapy	Discharge with referrals for outpatient care/therapy

Alcohol Withdrawal

Possible Complications

- Alcohol intoxication
- Nutritional deficits
- Pancreatitis
- Ulcer disease
- Liver disease
- Delirium tremens

Health Conditions

- Pre-existing respiratory or cardiac problems
- Liver disease
- Clotting disorders
- Seizure disorders

Nursing Diagnoses

- Risk for injury
- Risk for violence
- Self-care deficits
- Sleep pattern disturbance
- Ineffective management of therapeutic regimen

Anorexia Nervosa

Expected length of stay: 24–32 days

	Date _____ **Days 1–3**	Date _____ **Days 3–7**	Date _____ **Days 7–14**
Daily outcomes	Client will: • remain free of malnutrition, infection, and electrolyte and cardiac abnormalities • identify initial goals for hospitalization • remain oriented to time, place, and person • participate in assessment • identify current dietary pattern and food preferences • identify current elimination pattern • identify current self-care patterns, including sleep, physical activity, and hygiene • remain free of dehydration • maintain oral intake per contract • ingest food provided as per contract • remain free of self-induced vomiting	Client will: • remain free of malnutrition, infection, and electrolyte and cardiac abnormalities • participate in development of transdisciplinary treatment plan • remain oriented to time, place, and person • participate in menu plan for balanced meal • remain free of dehydration evidenced by moist mucous membranes and urine output >30 mL/hr • maintain oral intake of 1000 mL/day • ingest food provided per contract • gain 1/2 lb each day • remain free of self-induced vomiting	Client will: • remain free of malnutrition, infection, and electrolyte and cardiac abnormalities • identify two positive attributes of self • participate in transdisciplinary treatment plan • remain oriented to time, place, and person • consume diet as per menu plan • remain free of dehydration, evidenced by moist mucous membranes and urine output >30 mL/hr • maintain oral intake per contract • ingest food provided per contract • make dietary choices consistent with a well-balanced diet • gain 1/2 lb each day • remain free of self-induced vomiting
Assessments, tests, and treatments	CBC Urinalysis Chemistry profile Thyroid profile EKG Other laboratory tests as ordered Complete psychosocial assessment to include mental status, mood, affect, behavior, and communication every shift and prn Contract for safety Negotiate contract regarding food/fluid intake with client Observe for safety per protocol Complete nursing database assessment Weight Vital signs BID	Psychosocial assessment every shift and prn Observe for safety per protocol Monitor dietary intake, sleep pattern, and bowel elimination pattern Monitor effects of and compliance with medications Routine vital signs Weight	Daily psychosocial assessment Observe for safety per protocol Monitor dietary intake, sleep pattern, and bowel elimination pattern Monitor effects of and compliance with medications Routine vital signs Repeat laboratory studies if indicated Weight

➤

Anorexia Nervosa (continued)

	Date _____ **Days 1–3**	Date _____ **Days 3–7**	Date _____ **Days 7–14**
Knowledge deficit	Orient client and family to patients, staff, and program Review initial plan of care Assess learning needs of client and family Instruct client and family regarding behavior modification program Evaluate understanding of teaching	Review unit orientation with emphasis on program Reinforce behavior modification program Evaluate understanding of teaching	Review plan of care Include family in teaching Continue behavior modification program Evaluate understanding of teaching
Psychosocial	Observe behavior Assess level of anxiety Encourage verbalization of feelings and thoughts Listen attentively, giving adequate time to respond Approach with non-judgmental, accepting, matter-of-fact attitude and positive expectations Formulate initial plan of care with client and family Identify current support system Provide information regarding illness and treatment Provide ongoing support and encouragement to client and family Avoid discussion of food and eating habits Meet with client 4 times each shift for 5–10 minute periods focused on establishing relationship	Observe behavior Assess level of anxiety Encourage verbalization of concerns and feelings Approach with non-judgmental, accepting, matter-of-fact attitude and positive expectations Provide information and ongoing support and encouragement to client and family Provide simple, structured activities Identify potential support system and strategies to access additional supports Prompt to attend group therapy Acknowledge accomplishments Meet with client 10–15 minutes every shift during waking hours to focus on initial goals Avoid discussion of food and eating habits Discuss problem-solving strategies	Observe behavior Assess level of anxiety Approach with non-judgmental, accepting, matter-of-fact attitude and positive expectations Encourage verbalization of concerns and feelings Provide information and ongoing support and encouragement to client and family Review strategies to access support system using problem-solving strategies Acknowledge accomplishments Meet with client 15 minutes twice every shift during waking hours to work on therapeutic goals Explore effective coping strategies Explore fears related to sexuality and weight gain Client attends group therapy independently with spontaneous involvement × 1 Client practices problem-solving strategies
Diet	Nutritional assessment Dietary consultation Monitor dietary intake Diet as tolerated: encourage small, frequent feedings from all food groups Provide preferred snacks and foods Encourage fluids Provide pleasant mealtime environment	Monitor dietary intake Diet per menu plan: encourage small, frequent feedings from all food groups Encourage fluids Provide preferred snacks and foods Provide pleasant mealtime environment	Monitor dietary intake Diet per menu plan: encourage small, frequent feedings from all food groups Encourage fluids Provide preferred snacks and foods Provide pleasant mealtime environment

Anorexia Nervosa *(continued)*

	Date ____ **Days 1–3**	Date ____ **Days 3–7**	Date ____ **Days 7–14**
Activity	Assess safety needs and maintain appropriate precautions Encourage brief periods of activity and interaction Engage client in identifying reasonable activity/exercise plan	Maintain safety precautions Encourage activities during the day Client participates in exercise program of moderate intensity and duration	Maintain safety precautions Encourage involvement in 50–75% of activities Client participates in exercise program of moderate intensity and duration
Medications	Routine meds as ordered	Routine meds as ordered	Routine meds as ordered
Transfer/ discharge plans	Family assessment Establish discharge objectives with client and family	Review discharge objectives with client and family Initiate referrals for discharge care	Review progress toward discharge objectives with client and family Make appropriate referrals to support groups

	Date ____ **Days 15–21**	Date ____ **Days 22–26**	Date ____ **Day 26–Discharge Day**
Daily outcomes	Client will: • remain free of malnutrition, infection, and electrolyte and cardiac abnormalities • communicate feelings spontaneously and appropriately in 1:1 and group activities • identify method in which strengths can be used to improve coping skills • participate in transdisciplinary plan • begin to explore issues of body image and self-esteem • maintain oral intake per contract • ingest food provided per contract • make dietary choices consistent with a well-balanced diet • gain 1/2 lb each day • begin to verbalize accurate assessment of body size and nutritional needs	Client will: • remain free of malnutrition, infection, and electrolyte and cardiac abnormalities • communicate feelings spontaneously and appropriately in 1:1 and group activities • identify methods in which strengths can be used to improve coping skills • verbalize plan to use strengths to enhance coping skills • participate in transdisciplinary plan • realistically discuss issues related to body image and self-esteem • maintain oral intake per contract • ingest food provided per contract • make dietary choices consistent with a well-balanced diet • gain 1/2 lb each day • continue to verbalize accurate assessment of body size and nutritional needs • participate in discharge planning	Client is free of malnutrition, infection, and electrolyte and cardiac abnormalities Client expresses positive self-perception and self-esteem Client expresses reduced anxiety about weight gain Client verbalizes accurate assessment of body size and nutritional needs Client communicates feelings honestly and openly Client participates in activities that promote physical health Client develops sustaining relationships with friends and family members Client verbalizes/demonstrates home care instructions including the importance of ongoing mental health care Client demonstrates ability to adaptively cope with ongoing stressors Client verbalizes positive attributes regarding self Client accepts positive feedback

	Date _____ **Days 15–21**	Date _____ **Days 22–26**	Date _____ **Days 26–Discharge Day**
Assessments, tests, and treatments	Daily psychosocial assessment Observe for safety Monitor dietary intake, sleep pattern, and bowel elimination pattern Weight Monitor effects of and compliance with medications Routine vital signs	Daily psychosocial assessment Observe for safety Monitor dietary intake, sleep pattern, and bowel elimination pattern Monitor effects of and compliance with medications Weight	Psychosocial assessment Monitor dietary intake, sleep pattern, and bowel elimination pattern Monitor effects of and compliance with medications Weight
Knowledge deficit	Review current level of knowledge regarding medications, treatments, symptom management and follow-up care Review plan of care Include family in teaching Initiate teaching regarding coping strategies, utilizing client strengths Evaluate understanding of teaching	Review plan of care with client and family Reinforce current level of knowledge regarding medications, treatments, symptom management and follow-up care Evaluate understanding of teaching	Client and/or family verbalizes understanding of discharge teaching including activity and exercise program, diet, signs and symptoms to report, follow-up care arrangements and MD appointment, medications: name, purpose, dose, frequency, route, dietary interactions, and side effects Evaluate understanding of teaching Make referrals to community caregivers for any knowledge deficits regarding medications, treatments, symptoms management, and follow-up care
Psychosocial	Assess level of anxiety Support client in implementing stress-and anxiety-reduction strategies Client independently attends scheduled group therapy sessions Reinforce skills learned in group therapy Identify progress with cognitive restructuring and reinforce learning Acknowledge accomplishments Encourage verbalization of feelings and concerns Meet with client 15 minutes twice every shift during waking hours to discuss progress toward therapeutic goals Encourage client to discuss body image and self-esteem as well as role in family Encourage client to acknowledge accomplishments	Assess level of anxiety Reinforce stress- and anxiety-reduction strategies Encourage verbalization of concerns and feelings Client independently attends group therapy Provide specific, realistic feedback Encourage constructive expression of feelings Meet with client 15 minutes twice every shift during waking hours to discuss progress toward therapeutic goals Encourage client to discuss relationship to others in family Encourage realistic discussion of body image Encourage client to acknowledge accomplishments Provide information and ongoing support and encouragement to client and family	Assess level of anxiety Reinforce stress- and anxiety-reduction strategies Encourage verbalization of concerns and feelings Client independently attends group therapy Meet with client 15 minutes every shift during waking hours to discuss progress towards therapeutic goals Acknowledge accomplishments Provide information and ongoing support and encouragement to client and family

	Date _____ **Days 15–21**	Date _____ **Days 22–26**	Date _____ **Day 26–Discharge Day**
Psychosocial (continued)	Provide information and ongoing support and encouragement to client and family		
Diet	Diet as tolerated: encourage small, frequent feedings from all food groups Encourage fluids Provide preferred snacks and foods Monitor dietary intake Provide pleasant mealtime environment	Diet as tolerated: encourage small, frequent feedings from all food groups Encourage fluids Provide preferred snacks and foods Monitor dietary intake Provide pleasant mealtime environment	Diet as tolerated: encourage small, frequent feedings from all food groups Encourage fluids Provide preferred snacks and foods Monitor dietary intake Provide pleasant mealtime environment
Activity	Maintain safety precautions Encourage involvement in 75–100% of activities Engage client and family in identifying reasonable activity plan following discharge Client participates in exercise program of moderate intensity and duration	Maintain safety precautions Encourage involvement in 100% of activities Client participates in exercise program of moderate intensity and duration	Maintain safety precautions Client is independently involved in 100% of activities Client participates in exercise program of moderate intensity and duration
Medications	Routine meds as ordered	Routine meds as ordered	Routine meds as ordered
Transfer/ discharge plans	Review discharge objectives with client and family	Review discharge objectives with client and family Complete referrals for discharge care	Refer to support group and ongoing mental health care Review need for any discharge referrals Discharge with referrals

Potential Client Variances
Anorexia Nervosa

Possible Complications

- Electrolyte disturbances
- Dysrhythmias
- Cardiac arrest

Health Conditions

- Suicide attempt or ideation
- Metabolic disorders

Nursing Diagnoses

- Self-esteem disturbances
- Ineffective management of therapeutic regimen
- Ineffective individual/family coping

Bipolar Disorder: Manic Phase

Expected length of stay: 10–14 days

	Date _____ **Day 1**	Date _____ **Days 2–4**	Date _____ **Days 5–7**

Daily outcomes	Client will:
	• remain free of injury to self or others
	• identify initial goals for hospitalization
	• contract for management of intrusive behaviors
	• participate in transdisciplinary treatment plan:
	  – participate in assessment
	  – identify most recent medication regimen
	  – drink 2000 mL of fluids each day
	  – identify current dietary pattern and food preferences
	• remain oriented to time, place, and person
		Client will:
		• remain free of injury to self or others
		• identify initial goals for hospitalization
		• maintain contract for management of intrusive behaviors
		• participate in transdisciplinary treatment plan:
		  – participate in assessment
		  – begin to verbalize need for medications
		  – participate in menu planning
		  – drink 2000 mL of fluids each day
		  – participate in physical activity groups as scheduled
		  – respond to redirection while participating in physical activity groups
		  – establish rest/sleep promoting environment
		  – increase sleep period by 5% if sleep period less than 4 hr
		• remain oriented to time, place, and person
			Client will:
			• remain free of injury to self or others
			• identify initial goals for hospitalization
			• maintain contract for management of intrusive behaviors
			• participate in transdisciplinary treatment plan:
			  – verbalize reasons for medications
			  – consume diet per menu plan
			  – drink 2000 mL of fluids each day
			  – listen and respond to topic for a few minutes
			  – increase sleep period by 5%
			  – participate in physical activity groups as scheduled
			  – respond to redirection while participating in physical activity groups
			  – perform self-care activities independently 50% of time
			  – establish rest/sleep-promoting environment
			  – stay focused on simple task for a few minutes
			• remain oriented to time, place, and person

Bipolar Disorder: Manic Phase *(continued)*

	Date _____ **Day 1**	Date _____ **Days 2–4**	Date _____ **Days 5–7**
Assessments, tests, and treatments	CBC Urinalysis Thyroid profile Chemistry profile Drug screen RPR Electrolytes Lithium level Other laboratory tests as ordered Psychosocial assessment every shift and prn: mental status, mood, affect, behavior, and communication Complete nursing database assessment Observe behavior and activity level Weight Monitor fluid intake Vital signs BID and prn	Lithium level Day 3 Psychosocial assessment every shift and prn Observe for safety per protocol Monitor behavior and activity level Monitor effects and compliance with medication Monitor fluid intake Assess sleep pattern Lithium level Day 3 Routine vital signs	Lithium level Day 7 Psychosocial assessment every shift and prn Observe for safety per protocol Monitor behavior and activity level Monitor effects and compliance with medication Monitor fluid intake Assess sleep pattern Lithium level Day 7 Routine vital signs
Knowledge deficit	Orient client/family to unit and program Assess learning needs of client and family Review initial plan of care Initiate medication teaching Evaluate understanding of teaching	Review unit orientation with emphasis on program Continue medication teaching Evaluate understanding of teaching	Review plan of care Include family in teaching Initiate teaching regarding treatment modalities and preventive techniques Assess medication teaching response and need for additional teaching Evaluate understanding of teaching
Psychosocial	Approach with non-judgmental and accepting manner Observe and monitor behavior Direct to structured activities as per contract Minimize environmental stimuli and provide a safe environment Redirect intrusive behaviors: sexual, aggressive, and/or manipulative Provide information regarding illness and treatment to client and family Avoid power struggles by maintaining a kind but consistent approach Redirect frequent requests and attempt to meet demands in effective manner Maintain scheduled contacts	Approach with non-judgmental and accepting manner Observe and monitor behavior Direct to structured activities as per contract Minimize environmental stimuli and provide a safe environment Redirect intrusive behaviors: sexual, aggressive, and/or manipulative Provide information regarding illness and treatment to client and family Avoid power struggles by maintaining a kind but consistent approach Redirect frequent requests and attempt to meet demands in effective manner Maintain scheduled contacts	Approach with non-judgmental and accepting manner Observe and monitor behavior Direct to structured activities as per contract Minimize environmental stimuli and provide a safe environment Redirect intrusive behaviors: sexual, aggressive, and/or manipulative Provide information regarding illness and treatment to client and family Avoid power struggles by maintaining a kind but consistent approach Redirect frequent requests and attempt to meet demands in effective manner Maintain scheduled contacts

➤

	Date _____ **Day 1**	Date _____ **Days 2–4**	Date _____ **Days 5–7**
Diet	Monitor dietary intake Diet as tolerated: encourage small, frequent feedings from all food groups Provide preferred snacks and foods Encourage fluids and finger foods, making them accessible throughout the day	Monitor dietary intake Diet as tolerated: encourage small, frequent feedings from all food groups Provide preferred snacks and foods Encourage fluids and finger foods, making them accessible throughout the day	Monitor dietary intake Diet as tolerated: encourage small, frequent feedings from all food groups Provide preferred snacks and foods Encourage fluids and finger foods, making them accessible throughout the day
Activity	Assess safety needs and maintain appropriate precautions Observe activity level Develop schedule for stimulus titration (ie, quiet time) Manage agitation with periods of physical activity Provide sleep-enhancing atmosphere for 45 minutes prior to sleep	Maintain safety precautions Observe activity level Maintain schedule for stimulus titration Manage agitation with periods of physical activity Prompt to attend physical activity groups Prompt and assist with hygiene as necessary Provide sleep-enhancing atmosphere for 45 minutes prior to sleep	Maintain safety precautions Observe activity level Maintain schedule for stimulus titration Manage agitation with periods of physical activity Prompt to attend physical activity groups Encourage to attend small group activities Prompt with hygiene as necessary Provide sleep-enhancing atmosphere for 45 minutes prior to sleep
Medications	Identify target symptoms Lithium as ordered Tegretol, depakoate, or valproic acid as ordered Antipsychotics as ordered Routine meds as ordered	Assess target symptoms Lithium as ordered Tegretol, depakoate, or valproic acid as ordered Antipsychotics as ordered Routine meds as ordered	Assess target symptoms Lithium as ordered Tegretol, depakoate, or valproic acid as ordered Antipsychotics as ordered Routine meds as ordered
Transfer/ discharge plans	Family assessment Consult with internist if ordered Consult with occupational and recreational therapist Establish discharge objectives with client and family	Review discharge objectives with client and family Complete discharge planning	Review progress toward discharge objectives with client and family Make appropriate referrals to support groups

	Date _____ **Days 8–9**	Date _____ **Days 10–12**	Date _____ **Days 13–14—Discharge Day**
Daily outcomes	Client will: • remain free of injury to self or others • discuss goals for hospitalization • contract for management of intrusive behaviors • participate in transdisciplinary treatment plan • verbalize reasons for medications and understanding of side effects of medications • consume diet per menu plan • participate in physical activity groups as scheduled • listen and respond to topic for increasing periods of time • increase sleep period by 5% • begin to identify consequences of manic behavior • respond to redirection when participating in physical activity groups • perform self-care activities independently 75% of time • establish sleep/rest-promoting environment • stay focused on simple task for 10 minute period • maintain usual elimination patterns • remain oriented to time, place, and person	Client will: • remain free of injury to self or others • discuss goals for hospitalization • contract for management of intrusive behaviors • participate in transdisciplinary treatment plan • verbalize reasons for medications and need for long term therapy • consume diet per menu plan • participate in physical activity groups as scheduled • adaptively use listening skills • respond to redirection when participating in physical activity groups • perform self-care activities independently 100% of time • establish sleep/rest-promoting environment • stay focused on simple task for 15 minute period • maintain usual elimination patterns • remain oriented to time, place, and person	Client is free of injury to self or others Client is alert and oriented Client communicates feelings of self-worth Client's weight is stable Client achieves maximum independence in self-care Client adaptively uses listening skills Client enjoys 6 hours of uninterrupted sleep Client identifies plan if symptoms recur Client eats a well balanced diet inclusive of all food groups Client drinks 2000 mL of fluids each day Client has resumed preadmission urine and bowel elimination pattern Client verbalizes/demonstrates home care instructions including the importance of ongoing mental health care Client participates in regular exercise program Client demonstrates ability to adaptively cope with ongoing stressors
Assessments, tests, and treatments	Psychosocial assessment BID and prn Observe for safety per protocol Monitor behavior and activity pattern Monitor effects and compliance with medication Monitor fluid intake Assess sleep pattern	Lithium level Day 12 Psychosocial assessment BID prn Observe for safety per protocol Monitor behavior and activity pattern Monitor effects and compliance with medication Monitor fluid intake Assess sleep pattern	Psychosocial assessment Observe for safety per protocol Monitor behavior and activity pattern Monitor effects and compliance with medication Monitor fluid intake Assess sleep pattern

➤

Bipolar Disorder: Manic Phase (continued)

	Date _____ **Days 8–9**	Date _____ **Days 10–12**	Date _____ **Days 13–14—Discharge Day**
Knowledge deficit	Review plan of care Include family in teaching Review current level of knowledge regarding medications, treatments, symptom management, and follow-up care Evaluate understanding of teaching	Review plan of care with client and family Reinforce current level of knowledge regarding medications, treatments, symptom management, and follow-up care Evaluate understanding of teaching	Patient and/or significant other verbalizes understanding of discharge teaching including activity level and exercise program, diet, signs and symptoms to report, follow-up care arrangements and MD appointment, and medications: name, purpose, dose, frequency, route, dietary interactions, and side effects Evaluate understanding of teaching Make referrals to community caregivers for any knowledge deficits regarding medications, treatments, symptoms management, and follow-up care
Psychosocial	Approach with non-judgmental and accepting manner Observe and monitor behavior Direct to structured activities as per contract Minimize environmental stimuli and provide a safe environment Redirect intrusive behaviors: sexual, aggressive, and/or manipulative Provide information regarding illness and treatment to client and family Avoid power struggles by maintaining a kind but consistent approach Redirect frequent requests and attempt to meet needs in effective manner Prompt to attend physical activity groups Independently attends short, small group activities Prompt to start attending group therapy as tolerated Meet with client 2 times each shift for 5 minute periods focused on activities of daily living and behavior Maintain scheduled contacts	Approach with non-judgmental and accepting manner Observe and monitor behavior Direct to structured activities as per contract Minimize environmental stimuli and provide a safe environment Redirect intrusive behaviors: sexual, aggressive, and/or manipulative Provide information regarding illness and treatment to client and family Avoid power struggles by maintaining a kind but consistent approach Redirect frequent requests and attempt to meet needs in effective manner Eats meals in dining room without prompting Independently attends group therapy for increasingly longer periods Independently attends short small-group activities Attends discharge planning group Meet with client 2 times each shift for 5 minute periods to work on discharge goals Maintain scheduled contacts	Approach with non-judgmental and accepting manner Observe and monitor behavior Direct to structured activities as per contract Minimize environmental stimuli and provide a safe environment Redirect intrusive behaviors: sexual, aggressive, and/or manipulative Provide information regarding illness and treatment to client and family Avoid power struggles by maintaining a kind but consistent approach Redirect frequent requests and attempt to meet needs in effective manner Meet with client 2 times each shift for 5 minute periods to discuss after discharge care and management Maintain scheduled contacts

	Date _____ **Days 8–9**	Date _____ **Days 10–12**	Date _____ **Days 13–14—Discharge Day**
Diet	Monitor dietary intake Diet as tolerated: encourage small, frequent feedings from all food groups Provide preferred snacks and foods Encourage fluids and finger foods, making them accessible throughout the day	Monitor dietary intake Diet as tolerated: encourage small, frequent feedings from all food groups Provide preferred snacks and foods Encourage fluids and finger foods, making them accessible throughout the day	Monitor dietary intake Diet as tolerated: encourage small, frequent feedings from all food groups Provide preferred snacks and foods Encourage fluids and finger foods, making them accessible throughout the day
Activity	Maintain safety precautions Observe activity level Maintain schedule for stimulus titration Encourage to work at activities until completion Manage agitation with periods of physical activity Encourage to eat meals in dining room Prompt with hygiene as necessary Provide sleep-enhancing atmosphere for 45 minutes prior to sleep	Maintain safety precautions Observe activity level Maintain schedule for stimulus titration Manage agitation with periods of physical activity Independently attends physical activity groups Independent in self-care Provide sleep-enhancing atmosphere for 45 minutes prior to sleep	Maintain safety precautions Observe activity level Maintain schedule for stimulus titration Manage agitation with periods of physical activity Prompt to attend physical activity groups Independent in self-care Provide sleep-enhancing atmosphere for 45 minutes prior to sleep
Medications	Monitor target symptoms Lithium as ordered Tegretol, depakoate, or valproic acid as ordered Antipsychotics as ordered Routine meds as ordered	Monitor target symptoms Lithium as ordered Tegretol, depakoate, or valproic acid as ordered Antipsychotics as ordered Routine meds as ordered	Monitor target symptoms Lithium as ordered Tegretol, depakoate, or valproic acid as ordered Antipsychotics as ordered Routine meds as ordered
Transfer/ discharge plans	Review discharge objectives with client and family	Review progress toward discharge objectives with client and family Complete referrals for discharge care	Discharge with referrals

Bipolar Disorder: Manic Phase

Possible Complications

- Violence toward self or others
- Physical exhaustion

Health Conditions

- Other psychiatric illness
- Pre-existing renal or metabolic disease

Nursing Diagnoses

- Risk for injury
- Risk for violence toward self or others
- Ineffective individual coping
- Ineffective management of therapeutic regimen
- Altered nutrition: less than body requirements

Dementia

Expected length of stay: 6–10 days

	Date _____ **Day 1**	Date _____ **Days 2–3**	Date _____ **Days 4–5**
Daily outcomes	Client will: • evidence stable vital signs • remain free of injury • consume 1500 kcal and 2000 mL of fluid each day • verbalize thoughts and feelings • sleep 6–8 hr/night • participate in self-care to ability • demonstrate trust with caregivers and family	Client will: • evidence stable vital signs • remain free of injury • consume 1500 kcal and 2000 mL of fluid each day • verbalize thoughts and feelings • maintain a stable weight • sleep 6–8 hr/night • participate in self-care to ability • demonstrate trust with caregivers and family • establish a regular urine and bowel elimination pattern • spend short intervals with diversional activity • demonstrate increasing attention span	Client will: • evidence stable vital signs • remain free of injury • consume 1500 kcal and 2000 mL of fluid each day • verbalize thoughts and feelings • maintain a stable weight • sleep 6–8 hr/night • participate in self-care to ability • demonstrate trust with caregivers and family • establish a regular urine and bowel elimination pattern • spend short intervals with diversional activity • stay focused on a simple task for 10 minutes • demonstrate increasing attention span
Assessments, tests, and treatments	CBC Urinalysis Chemistry profile Electrolytes Folate level Chest x-ray EKG PPD Other diagnostic tests as indicated Assess need for HIV testing Mental status exam on admission and every 8 hr and prn Vital signs q4hr and prn Intake and output Weight Assess mood, affect, and behavior q1–2hr Assess urine and bowel elimination pattern Initiate bowel protocol	Mental status exam q12hr and prn Vital signs q4hr and prn Intake and output Assess mood, affect, and behavior q1–2hr Monitor urine and bowel elimination and sleep patterns Continue bowel protocol	Repeat laboratory studies as indicated Mental status exam q12hr and prn Vital signs every shift and prn D/C intake and output if balanced Assess mood, affect, and behavior q1–2hr Read PPD Weight on Day 4 Monitor urine and bowel elimination and sleep patterns

Dementia *(continued)*

	Date _____ **Day 1**	Date _____ **Days 2–3**	Date _____ **Days 4–5**
Knowledge deficit	Orient client and family to room and routine Use simple words and phrases Include family in teaching Review plan of care Evaluate understanding of teaching	Review plan of care with client and family Use simple words and phrases Include family in teaching Evaluate understanding of teaching	Review plan of care with client and family Use simple words and phrases Include family in teaching Initiate discharge teaching regarding the need for ongoing outpatient care and medications Evaluate understanding of teaching
Psychosocial	Approach in calm, quiet, non-judgmental manner Assess level of anxiety Provide information and ongoing support and encouragement to client and family Use simple commands Assess sleep patterns and provide measures that promote rest and sleep Encourage expression of thoughts and feelings Explore availability of support system Explore interests	Approach in calm, quiet, non-judgmental manner Assess level of anxiety Encourage verbalization of concerns Provide information and ongoing support and encouragement to client and family Use simple commands Provide measures that promote rest and sleep Encourage expression of thoughts and feelings Explore availability of support system	Approach in calm, quiet, non-judgmental manner Assess level of anxiety Encourage verbalization of concerns Provide information and ongoing support and encouragement to client and family Use simple commands Provide measures that promote rest and sleep Encourage expression of thoughts and feelings
Diet	Encourage up to 2000 mL of fluids each day (unless contraindicated) Limit caffeine intake Provide frequent, small, nutritious feedings inclusive of all food groups Nutritional assessment, including calorie count if indicated	Encourage up to 2000 mL of fluids each day (unless contraindicated) Limit caffeine Provide frequent, small, nutritious feedings inclusive of all food groups	Encourage up to 2000 mL of fluids each day (unless contraindicated) Limit caffeine Provide frequent, small, nutritious feedings inclusive of all food groups
Activity	Assess safety needs and maintain appropriate precautions Frequent observation Activity as tolerated Physical therapy evaluation if indicated Toilet q2–3hr while awake and prn Assist with hygiene	Maintain safety precautions Frequent observation Activity as tolerated Prompt and assist with hygiene as needed Occupational therapy evaluation Toilet q2–3hr while awake and prn	Maintain safety precautions Frequent observations Activity as tolerated Prompt and assist with hygiene as needed Toilet q2–3hr while awake and prn
Medications	Routine meds as ordered Meds for agitation prn	Routine meds as ordered Meds for agitation prn	Routine meds as ordered Meds for agitation prn

Dementia *(continued)*

	Date _____ **Day 1**	Date _____ **Days 2–3**	Date _____ **Days 4–5**
Referral/ discharge plans	Family assessment if not previously complete Refer to neurologist and/or psychiatrist if indicated Establish discharge objectives with client and family	Review discharge objectives and anticipated discharge care with client and family Refer to social service for discharge planning	Review progress toward discharge objectives with client and family Make appropriate referrals

	Date _____ **Day 6**	Date _____ **Day 7**	Date _____ **Day 8—Discharge Day**
Daily outcomes	Client will: • have stable vital signs • remain free of injury • consume 1500 kcal and 2000 mL of fluid each day • verbalize thoughts and feelings • maintain a stable weight • establish sleep/rest routine to promote sleep • sleep 6-8 hr/night • participate in self-care to ability • demonstrate trust with caregiver and family • maintain a regular urine and bowel elimination pattern • spend increasing periods of time with diversional activities • stay focused on a simple task for 15 minutes • demonstrate increasing attention span	Client will: • have stable vital signs • remain free of injury • consume 1500 kcal and 2000 mL of fluid each day • verbalize thoughts and feelings • maintain a stable weight • establish sleep/rest routine to promote sleep • sleep 6–8 hr/night • participate in self-care to ability • demonstrate trust with caregiver and family • maintain a regular urine and bowel elimination pattern • spend increasing periods of time with diversional activities • stay focused on a simple task for 15 minutes • demonstrate increasing attention span	Client is afebrile with stable vital signs Client remains free of injury Client maintains adequate nutrition and fluid intake Client's weight remains stable Client/family verbalizes discharge plans Client has established a sleep/rest pattern and sleeps 6–8 hr/night Client participates in self-care to ability Client demonstrates trust with caregiver and family Client maintains a regular urine and bowel elimination pattern Client spends increasing periods of time with diversional activities Client stays focused on a simple task for 15 minutes Client demonstrates increasing attention span
Assessments, tests, and treatments	Mental status q12hr and prn Assess mood, affect, and behavior q1–2hr Weight Vital signs BID and prn Monitor urine and bowel elimination and sleep pattern Continue bowel protocol	Mental status q12hr and prn Assess mood, affect, and behavior q1–2hr Vital signs BID and prn Monitor urine and bowel elimination and sleep patterns Continue bowel protocol Weight	Mental status q12hr Assess mood, affect, and behavior q1–2hr Vital signs BID and prn Monitor urine and bowel elimination and sleep patterns Continue bowel protocol

►

Dementia *(continued)*

	Date _____ **Day 6**	Date _____ **Day 7**	Date _____ **Day 8—Discharge Day**
Knowledge deficit	Review plan of care Use simple words and phrases Include family in teaching Continue discharge teaching regarding medications and activity Evaluate understanding of teaching	Review plan of care with client and family Use simple words and phrases Continue discharge teaching medications, activity, and managing agitation Evaluate understanding of teaching	Client and/or family verbalizes understanding of discharge teaching, including exercise, diet, signs and symptoms to report, follow-up care and MD appointment, home care arrangements, and medications: name, purpose, dose, frequency, route, dietary interactions, and side effects Evaluate understanding of teaching
Diet	Encourage up to 2000 mL of fluids per day (unless contraindicated) Provide frequent, small, nutritious feedings inclusive of all food groups	Encourage up to 2000 mL of fluids per day (unless contraindicated) Provide frequent, small, nutritious feedings inclusive of all food groups	Encourage up to 2000 mL of fluids per day (unless contraindicated) Provide frequent, small, nutritious feedings inclusive of all food groups
Activity	Maintain safety precautions Frequent observation Activity as tolerated Prompt with self-care and hygiene	Maintain safety precautions Frequent observation Activity as tolerated Prompt with self-care and hygiene	Maintain safety precautions Frequent observation Activity as tolerated Prompt with self-care and hygiene
Psychosocial	Approach in calm, quiet, nonjudgmental manner Assess level of anxiety Provide information and ongoing support and encouragement to client and family Use simple commands Provide measures that promote rest and sleep Encourage expression of thoughts and feelings Encourage verbalization of concerns	Approach in calm, quiet, nonjudgmental manner Assess level of anxiety Provide information and ongoing support and encouragement to client and family Use simple commands Provide measures that promote rest and sleep Encourage expression of thoughts and feelings Encourage verbalization of concerns	Approach in calm, quiet, nonjudgmental manner Assess level of anxiety Provide information and ongoing support and encouragement to client and family Use simple commands Provide measures that promote rest and sleep Encourage expression of thoughts and feelings Encourage verbalization of concerns
Medications	Routine meds as ordered Meds for agitation prn	Routine meds as ordered Meds for agitation prn	Routine meds as ordered Meds for agitation prn
Referral/ discharge plans	Review discharge objectives with client and family	Review discharge objectives with client and family Complete referrals for discharge	Discharge with completed referrals

Dementia

Possible Complications

- Injuries, including fractures
- Aphasia
- Depression

Health Conditions

- HIV/AIDS
- Arteriosclerosis
- Depression
- Other psychiatric diagnoses

Nursing Diagnoses

- Risk for injury
- Ineffective family coping
- Altered thought process
- Altered role performance

Depression Without Psychotic Features or Agitation

Expected length of stay: 7–8 days

	Date _____ **Day 1**	Date _____ **Days 2–3**	Date _____ **Day 4**

Daily outcomes	Client will:
	• remain free of self-inflicted injury
	• communicate suicide ideation
	• contract for safety
	• identify initial goals for hospitalization
	• verbalize need for medications
	• remain oriented to time, place, and person with prompting
	• participate in assessment:
	  – identify current dietary pattern and food preferences
	  – identify current elimination pattern
	  – identify recreation and leisure interest and capabilities
	  – identify current self-care patterns—including sleep, physical activity, and hygiene
		Client will:
		• remain free of self-inflicted injury
		• communicate feelings related to depressed mood
		• maintain contract for safety
		• participate in development of transdisciplinary treatment plan:
		  – identify name, dose, and major side effects of medications
		  – demonstrate orientation to time, place, and person
		  – participate in menu plan for balanced meals
		  – identify need for laxative if no BM in 3 days
		  – attend 25% of leisure activities as scheduled, with prompting and support
			Client will:
			• remain free of self-inflicted injury
			• identify at least one reason for living
			• identify three positive attributes of self
			• identify one misperception or misbelief
			• communicate feelings related to managing loss and stress
			• participate in transdisciplinary treatment plan:
			  – identify changes in symptoms as a result of medications
			  – remain oriented to time, place, and person
			  – consume diet as per menu plan
			  – attend 50% of scheduled activities independently
			  – identify need for laxative
			  – perform self-care activities independently 50% of time

Assessments, tests, and treatments	CBC Urinalysis Chemistry profile Thyroid profile RPR Other laboratory tests as ordered Complete psychosocial assessment to include mental status, mood, affect, behavior, and communication every shift and prn Assess suicidal ideation, gestures, threats, plans, and means Contract for safety Observe for safety per protocol Complete nursing database assessment Weight Initiate suicide precautions as indicated Vital signs BID	Psychosocial assessment every shift and prn Observe for safety per protocol Monitor dietary intake, sleep pattern, and bowel elimination pattern Continue suicide assessment Reinforce safety contract Suicide precautions as indicated Monitor effects of and compliance with medications Routine vital signs	Daily psychosocial assessment and prn Observe for safety per protocol Monitor dietary intake, sleep pattern, and bowel elimination pattern Continue suicide assessment Reinforce safety contract Suicide precautions as indicated Monitor effects of and compliance with medications Routine vital signs

Depression Without Psychotic Features or Agitation *(continued)*

	Date _____ **Day 1**	Date _____ **Days 2–3**	Date _____ **Day 4**
Knowledge deficit	Orient client and family to patients, staff, and program Review initial plan of care Assess learning needs of client and family Initiate medication teaching Evaluate understanding of teaching	Review unit orientation with emphasis on program Continue medication teaching Evaluate understanding of teaching	Review plan of care Include family in teaching Initiate teaching regarding anxiety, depression, treatment modalities, and preventive techniques Evaluate medication teaching response and need for additional teaching Evaluate understanding of teaching
Psychosocial	Observe behavior Assess level of anxiety Encourage verbalization of feelings and thoughts Listen attentively, giving adequate time to respond Approach with non-judgmental and accepting manner Formulate initial plan of care with client and family Offer realistic hope to client and family Identify current support system Engage in structured activities Provide information regarding illness and treatment Provide ongoing support and encouragement to client and family Meet with client 4 times each shift for 5-minute periods focused on establishing relationship	Observe behavior Assess level of anxiety Encourage verbalization of concerns and feelings Provide information and ongoing support and encouragement to client and family Provide simple structured activities Identify potential support system and strategies to access additional supports Prompt to attend group therapy Acknowledge accomplishments Meet with client 10–15 minutes twice a shift during waking hours and focus on working on initial goals	Observe behavior Assess level of anxiety Encourage verbalization of concerns and feelings Provide information and ongoing support and encouragement to client and family Provide increasingly complex structured activities Initiate cognitive restructuring Review strategies to access support system using problem-solving strategies Client attends group therapy independently with spontaneous involvement × 1 Acknowledge accomplishments Meet with client 15 minutes every shift waking hours to work on therapeutic goals
Diet	Monitor dietary intake Diet as tolerated: encourage small, frequent feedings from all food groups Provide preferred snacks and foods Provide adequate time for meals and snacks Encourage fluids Low tyramine diet if taking MAO inhibitors	Monitor dietary intake Diet per menu plan: encourage small, frequent feedings from all food groups Provide preferred snacks and foods Provide adequate time for meals and snacks Encourage fluids Low tyramine diet if taking MAO inhibitors	Monitor dietary intake Diet per menu plan: encourage small, frequent feedings from all food groups Provide preferred snacks and foods Provide adequate time for meals and snacks Encourage fluids Low tyramine diet if taking MAO inhibitors

➤

Depression Without Psychotic Features or Agitation *(continued)*

	Date _____ **Day 1**	Date _____ **Days 2–3**	Date _____ **Day 4**
Activity	Assess safety needs and maintain appropriate precautions Encourage client to be in milieu 10 hours/day Encourage brief periods of activity and interaction Provide sleep-enhancing atmosphere for 45 minutes prior to sleep	Maintain safety precautions Encourage activities during the day—prompt client to attend 25% of activities Prompt and assist with hygiene as necessary Encourage to participate in simple exercise Prompt to engage in simple structured activities Provide sleep-enhancing atmosphere 45 minutes prior to sleep	Maintain safety precautions Encourage involvement in 50–75% of activities Prompt with hygiene as necessary Prompt to participate in exercise
Medications	Identify target symptoms Antidepressants as ordered Routine meds as ordered	Assess target symptoms Antidepressants as ordered Routine meds as ordered Colace/metamucil if indicated Laxative prn if no BM in 3 days	Assess target symptoms Antidepressants as ordered Routine meds as ordered Colace/metamucil if indicated Laxative prn if no BM in 3 days
Referral/ discharge plans	Family assessment Establish discharge objectives with client and family Occupational and recreational therapist	Review discharge objectives with client and family Initiate referrals for discharge care	Review progress toward discharge objectives with client and family Make appropriate referrals to support groups

	Date _____ **Day 5**	Date _____ **Day 6**	Date _____ **Days 7–8—Discharge Day**
Daily outcomes	Client will: • remain free of self-inflicted injury • verbalize at least one reason for living • communicate feelings spontaneously and appropriately in 1:1 and group activities • identify method in which strengths can be used to improve coping skills • describe how distorted perceptions affect coping • begin to reframe false beliefs	Client will: • remain free of self-inflicted injury • verbalize at least one reason for living • communicate feelings spontaneously and appropriately in 1:1 and group activities • identify methods in which strengths can be used to improve coping skills • describe how distorted perceptions affect coping • reframe distorted beliefs • verbalize plan to use strengths to enhance coping skills	Client is free of self-inflicted injury and verbalizes reasons for living Client is alert and oriented Client expresses a positive self-perception and self-esteem Client communicates feelings honestly and openly Client participates in activities that promote physical health Client identifies cues to increasing depression Client develops sustaining relationships with friends and family members Client utilizes strengths and skills in managing current and ongoing stressors

Depression Without Psychotic Features or Agitation *(continued)*

	Date _____ **Day 5**	Date _____ **Day 6**	Date _____ **Days 7–8—Discharge Day**

Daily outcomes
(continued)
	• participate in transdisciplinary plan:
	  – consume diet as per menu plan
	  – perform self–care independently 75% of time
	  – attend 75% of scheduled activities independently
	  – identify need for laxative
	  – identify changes in symptoms as a result of medications
	  – verbalize awareness of long-term medication needs for depression
	  – identify discharge activity pattern
	• remain oriented to time, place, and person
		• participate in transdisciplinary plan:
		  – consume diet as per menu plan
		  – perform self-care independently 75% of time
		  – attend 75% of scheduled activities independently
		  – identify need for laxative
		  – identify changes in symptoms as a result of medications
		  – demonstrate self-administration of medication safely and correctly
		  – verbalize awareness of and committment to long-term medication therapy for depression
		• remain oriented to time, place, and person
			Client verbalizes/demonstrates home care instructions including the importance of ongoing mental health care
			Client attains maximum independence in self-care
			Client demonstrates ability to adaptively cope with ongoing stressors

Assessments, tests, and treatments	Daily psychosocial assessment and prn Observe for safety Monitor dietary intake, sleep pattern, and bowel elimination pattern Weight Continue suicide assessment Reinforce safety contract Suicide precautions if indicated Monitor effects of and compliance with medications Routine vital signs	Daily psychosocial assessment and prn Observe for safety Monitor dietary intake, sleep pattern, and bowel elimination pattern Continue suicide assessment Reinforce safety contract Suicide precautions if indicated Monitor effects of and compliance with medications Routine vital signs	Psychosocial assessment Observe for safety Monitor dietary intake, sleep pattern, and bowel elimination pattern Suicide assessment Monitor effects of and compliance with medications
Knowledge deficit	Review plan of care Include family in teaching Review teaching regarding anxiety Initiate teaching of coping strategies utilizing client strengths Review current level of knowledge regarding medications, treatments, symptom management, and follow-up care Evaluate understanding of teaching	Review plan of care with client and family Reinforce current level of knowledge regarding medications, treatments, symptom management and follow-up care Evaluate understanding of teaching	Client and/or significant other verbalizes understanding of discharge teaching including activity level and exercise program, safety measures, diet, signs and symptoms to report, follow-up care arrangements and MD appointment, medications: name, purpose, dose, frequency, route, dietary interactions, and side effects Evaluate understanding of teaching Make referrals to community resources for any knowledge deficits regarding medications, treatments, symptoms management, and follow-up care

	Date _____ **Day 5**	Date _____ **Day 6**	Date _____ **Days 7–8—Discharge Day**
Psychosocial	Assess level of anxiety Support client in implementing stress and anxiety-reduction strategies Provide information and ongoing support and encouragement to client and family Reinforce and utilize role-playing strategies as an approach to developing support system Client attends scheduled group therapy sessions independently Reinforce skills learned in group therapy Identify progress with cognitive restructuring and reinforce learning Acknowledge accomplishments Encourage verbalization of feelings and concerns Meet with client 15 minutes every shift during waking hours to discuss progress in terms of therapeutic goals Encourage client to acknowledge accomplishments Provide information and ongoing support and encouragement to client and family	Assess level of anxiety Reinforce stress and anxiety-reduction strategies Encourage verbalization of concerns and feelings Client attends group therapy independently Provide specific, realistic feedback Encourage constructive expression of feelings Meet with client 15 minutes every shift during waking hours to discuss progress in terms of therapeutic goals Reinforce strategies for cognitive restructuring and reinforce learning Encourage client to acknowledge accomplishments Provide information and ongoing support and encouragement to client and family	Assess level of anxiety Reinforce stress and anxiety-reduction strategies Encourage verbalization of concerns and feelings Client attends group therapy independently Meet with client 15 minutes every shift during waking hours to discuss progress in terms of therapeutic goals Acknowledge accomplishments Reinforce progress with and strategies for cognitive restructuring and reinforce learning Provide information and ongoing support and encouragement to client and family
Diet	Diet as tolerated: encourage small, frequent feedings from all food groups Encourage fluids Provide preferred snacks and foods Provide adequate time for meals and snacks Monitor dietary intake Low tyramine diet if taking MAO inhibitors	Diet as tolerated: encourage small, frequent feedings from all food groups Encourage fluids Provide preferred snacks and foods Provide adequate time for meals and snacks Monitor dietary intake Low tyramine diet if taking MAO inhibitors	Diet as tolerated: encourage small, frequent feedings from all food groups Encourage fluids Provide preferred snacks and foods Provide adequate time for meals and snacks Monitor dietary intake Low tyramine diet if taking MAO inhibitors
Activity	Maintain safety precautions Encourage involvement in 75–100% of activities Prompt with self-care Provide sleep-enhancing atmosphere for 45 minutes prior to sleep Engage client and family in identifying reasonable activity plan following discharge	Maintain safety precautions Encourage involvement in 100% of activities Client is independent in self-care Provide sleep-enhancing atmosphere for 45 minutes prior to sleep Identify plan to create sleep-enhancing environment after discharge	Maintain safety precautions Client is independently involved in 100% of activities Client is independent in self-care Provide sleep-enhancing atmosphere for 45 minutes prior to sleep

	Date _____ **Day 5**	Date _____ **Day 6**	Date _____ **Days 7–8—Discharge Day**
Medications	Assess target symptoms Antidepressants as ordered Routine meds as ordered Colace/Metamucil as indicated Laxative prn if no BM in 3 days	Assess target symptoms Antidepressants as ordered Routine meds as ordered Colace/Metamucil as indicated Laxative prn if no BM in 3 days	Assess target symptoms Antidepressants as ordered Routine meds as ordered Colace/Metamucil as indicated Laxative prn if no BM in 3 days

*Transfer/
discharge plans*
	Review discharge objectives with
	  client and family
	Discuss options for ongoing care
	  following discharge
		Review discharge objectives with
		  client and family
		Complete referrals for discharge
		  care
			Review progress toward discharge
			  objectives
			Review need for any discharge
			  referrals
			Discharge with referrals

Potential Client Variances
Depression Without Psychotic Features or Agitation

Possible Complications
- Suicide attempt
- Malnutrition
- Sleep pattern disturbances

Health Conditions
- History of depression or suicide attempt
- Other psychiatric diagnoses

Nursing Diagnoses
- Ineffective individual coping
- Hopelessness
- Social isolation
- Low self-esteem

Panic Disorder: Outpatient Treatment

Expected length of stay: 8 weeks

	Date _____ **Weeks 1–2**	Date _____ **Weeks 3–6**	Date _____ **Weeks 7–8**
Weekly outcomes	Client will: • identify initial goals for therapy • contract for ongoing treatment • participate in treatment plan • begin to identify sources of anxiety/panic	Client will: • identify ongoing goals for therapy • maintain contract for ongoing therapy • participate in treatment plan • identify strategies to manage anxiety and panic	Client describes ongoing strategies to manage panic disorder Client demonstrates ability to cope with ongoing feelings of panic Client describes strategies to cope with stressors
Assessments, tests, and treatments	Psychosocial assessment to include mental status, mood, affect, behavior, and communication Assist client to explore factors that precipitate panic attacks	Psychosocial assessment Assess recent history of anxiety and panic attacks Explore contributing factors Discuss effectiveness of cognitive restructuring strategies	Psychosocial assessment Assess recent history of anxiety and panic attacks Explore contributing factors Discuss effectiveness of cognitive restructuring strategies
Knowledge deficit	Orient client to therapy program Assess learning needs of client Review initial plan of care Evaluate understanding of teaching Discuss the etiology and management of anxiety and panic disorders Discuss the physical symptoms of panic and the importance of understanding the meaning of anxiety and panic disorders Instruct client to maintain journal of anxiety and panic attacks	Review therapy program and treatment objectives Review journal of recent panic attacks Assist client to identify the early signs of anxiety and panic attacks Discuss strategies to cope with early signs and symptoms of panic attacks, including talking or activity Discuss additional strategies to cope with panic attacks, including expressing anger, positive self-talk, and guided imagery Instruct regarding principles of cognitive restructuring; practice during session Instruct regarding relaxation techniques; practice during session Discuss use of exercise to alleviate anxiety/panic Assist client to explore problem-solving strategies Evaluate understanding of teaching	Review plan of care Review principles of cognitive restructuring Evaluate understanding of teaching

	Date _____ **Weeks 1–2**	Date _____ **Weeks 3–6**	Date _____ **Weeks 7–8**
Psychosocial	Approach with non-judgmental and accepting manner Observe and monitor behavior Assist client to understand relationship of unexpressed feelings to anxiety and panic experience Encourage client to express feelings, thoughts, ideas and beliefs	Approach with non-judgmental and accepting manner Encourage client to express feelings, thoughts, ideas, and beliefs Observe and monitor behavior Provide positive feedback for efforts to incorporate coping strategies into daily life Assist client to understand relationship of feelings to panic Assist client to realistically identify strengths and limitations Explore ways of re-framing limitations in a positive manner Assist client to practice and implement effective coping strategies Assist client to identify potentially stressful situations and role-play coping strategies	Approach with non-judgmental and accepting manner Encourage client to review strategies to manage anxiety and panic
Diet	Nutritional assessment Encourage well-balanced diet, including all food groups Contract with client to avoid stimulants	Encourage well-balanced diet from all food groups Encourage avoidance of stimulants	Encourage well-balanced diet, including all food groups Encourage avoidance of stimulants
Activity	Discuss the importance of regular aerobic exercise Contract for regular exercise program Sleep pattern assessment Discuss strategies to provide sleep-enhancing atmosphere for 45 minutes prior to sleep	Review ability to begin and continue exercise program Maintain contract for regular exercise program Encourage client to practice relaxation response Discuss effectiveness of sleep-enhancing strategies	Review ability to continue exercise program Maintain contract for regular exercise program Encourage client to practice relaxation response Discuss effectiveness of sleep-enhancing strategies
Medications	Identify target symptoms Routine meds as ordered	Assess target symptoms Assess need for medications and refer as indicated Routine meds as ordered	Assess target symptoms Routine meds as ordered
Transfer/ discharge plans	Family assessment Establish objectives of therapy with client	Review with client progress toward therapy objectives	Review with client progress toward therapy objectives Make appropriate referrals to support groups

Panic Disorder: Outpatient Treatment

Possible Complications

- Extreme restlessness or agitation
- Physical exhaustion

Health Conditions

- Any health problems
- Any psychiatric diagnoses

Nursing Diagnoses

- Ineffective individual coping
- Ineffective management of therapeutic regimen
- Anxiety/fear

The diverse needs of the psychiatric population and the great variations in symptoms and treatment approaches to psychiatric illnesses make it somewhat challenging to develop standardized teaching protocols. One approach to teaching individuals with mental health problems is to use a generic teaching protocol that can include client-specific information and can also document teaching efforts.

TEACHING PROTOCOL

TITLE: <u>DISCHARGE</u>

<table>
<tr><td align="center">PHASE OF LEARNING</td><td align="center">LEARNER</td></tr>
</table>

KEY: I = Initial Instruction   C or R = Client or Resident

       II = Repeated Instruction   F = Family

       III = Demonstrates Learning

Name: _____

RP = Responsible Party

Name: _____

PHASE OF LEARNING	I		II			III		LEARNER'S RESPONSE
LEARNER								
DATE								
OBJECTIVES	ENTER INSTRUCTOR'S INITIALS IN BOX:							LEARNER'S RESPONSE
<u>Knowledge Deficit</u> related to mental health problems and/or chemical dependency problems								
· Knows and can explain diagnosis in simple terms								
· Can name target symptoms								
· Verbalizes understanding of treatment plan post-discharge								
· Can describe self-care measures to stabilize symptoms								
Medication Teaching Protocol Completed								
<u>Knowledge Deficit</u> related to Health Maintenance Patterns								
· Can describe plan for maintaining own health in the following areas:								
· Diet – Nutrition								

Hospital Teaching Protocol	Client/Resident Identification

313

PHASE OF LEARNING		I	II	III	
LEARNER					
DATE					
OBJECTIVES		ENTER INSTRUCTOR'S INITIALS IN BOX:			LEARNER'S RESPONSE
· Sleep pattern					
· Exercise pattern/plan					
· Leisure activities					
· Verbalizes knowledge regarding interrelation of Health Maintenance Patterns					
· Arrangement for medical follow-up					
· Other (pre-existing medical problems, non-psych meds, etc.)					
Knowledge deficit related to transition/aftercare issues					
· Verbalizes plan for living arrangements					
· Verbalizes plan for vocational issues/money management					
· Verbalizes plan for sharing information related to hospitalization					
· Verbalizes plan for follow-up: when, with whom, etc. (Include review of substance abuse follow-up if applicable)					
· Verbalizes crisis plan in case of symptom recurrence/relapse/ impulse to self-harm/ etc.					
· Other					

Developed by N. Tisdale, MS, RN, C, CNA — Assistant Director of Nursing Standards, Education and Research, New Hampshire Hospital, Concord, NH 03301

Index

Accountability in critical pathways, 6
Abdominal aortic aneurysm repair
    critical pathway, 89–93
    discharge teaching form, 94
    potential client variances, 93
Alcohol withdrawal
    critical pathway, 281–285
    potential client variances, 286
Anorexia nervosa
    critical pathway, 287–291
    potential client variances, 291
Appendectomy
    critical pathway, 95–97
    discharge teaching form, 98
    potential client variances, 97
Arm fracture (upper) with open reduction
    critical pathway, 99–101
    discharge teaching form, 102
    potential client variances, 102
Asthma
    critical pathway, 259–261
    discharge teaching form, 262
    potential client variances, 262

Bipolar disorder: manic phase
    critical pathway, 292–297
    potential client variances, 298
Burns, severe thermal
    critical pathway, 19–20
    potential client variances, 21

Carotid endarterectomy
    critical pathway, 103–106
    discharge teaching form, 107
    potential client variances, 106
Case management, 6.
        See also Nurse case managers.
Cataract surgery
    critical pathway, 108–109
    discharge teaching form, 110
    potential client variances, 109
Cerebral vascular accident (CVA)
    critical pathway, 22–26
    discharge teaching form, 27
    potential client variances, 26
Cholecystectomy (laparoscopic)
    critical pathway, 111–112
    discharge teaching form, 113
    potential client variances, 112
Chronic obstructive pulmonary disease
        (COPD)
    critical pathway, 33–36
    discharge teaching form, 37
    potential client variances, 37

Clinical applications, 10
Colon resection
    critical pathway, 114–118
    discharge teaching form, 119
    potential client variances, 118
Computer models in documentation, 10–11
Congestive heart failure (CHF)
    critical pathway, 28–31
    discharge teaching form, 32
    potential client variances, 31
Coronary angioplasty, percutaneous
        transluminal (PTCA)
    critical pathway, 120–121
    discharge teaching form, 122
    potential client variances, 122
Coronary artery bypass surgery
    critical pathway, 123–129
    discharge teaching form, 130
    potential client variances, 129
Craniotomy for brain tumor
    critical pathway, 131–133
    discharge teaching form, 134
    potential client variances, 133
Critical pathways
    accountability of the health care team, 6
    case management by nurses, 3–4
    client involvement in care, 7
    clinical applications of, 10
    communication of care, 10
    computers in documentation of, 10–11
    defined, 3
    development process of, 3
    development strategies for, 6–7
    discharge outcomes, 9
    evaluation of, 10
    goals of, 3
    historical background of, 3
    home health care setting, use in, 10
    implementation strategies, 9–10
    influences in development of, 7
    information analysis, 7
    interdisciplinary classifications, 7–8
    interventions, planning of, 9
    nursing interventions, 4
    outcome-driven practice models, 4
    quality management, 4
    staff education and involvement, 9
    time line determination, 9
Cystectomy with ileal conduit
    critical pathway, 135–139
    discharge teaching form, 140
    potential client variances, 139

Deep vein thrombosis
    critical pathway, 38–41
    discharge teaching form, 42
    potential client variances, 42
Dementia
    critical pathway, 299–302
    potential client variances, 303
Depression without psychotic features or
        agitation
    critical pathway, 304–309
    potential client variances, 309
Diabetes (type I)
    critical pathway, 263–265
    discharge teaching form, 265
    potential client variances, 265
Diabetes, new onset (type II)
    critical pathway, 43–47
    discharge teaching form, 47
    potential client variances, 47
Diarrhea and dehydration
    critical pathway, 48–51
    discharge teaching form, 52
    potential client variances, 51
Discharge teaching form, sample of, 8
Diverticulitis and constipation
    critical pathway, 53–57
    discharge teaching form, 57
    potential client variances, 57

Femoral popliteal bypass graft
    critical pathway, 141–144
    discharge teaching form, 145
    potential client variances, 144

Gastrectomy, partial
    critical pathway, 146–150
    discharge teaching form, 151
    potential client variances, 150
Gastrointestinal bleeding (upper)
    critical pathway, 58–61
    discharge teaching form, 62
    potential client variances, 62

Hernia repair (laparoscopic)
    critical pathway, 152–153
    discharge teaching form, 154
    potential client variances, 153
Hip pinning (fractured hip with prosthesis
        or internal fixation)
    critical pathway, 155–161
    discharge teaching form, 162
    potential client variances, 162

Hip replacement (total)
    critical pathway, 163–166
    discharge teaching form, 167
    potential client variances, 167
Home health care, critical pathways in, 10
Hysterectomy (abdominal)
    critical pathway, 168–170
    discharge teaching form, 171
    potential client variances, 170
Hysterectomy (vaginal)
    critical pathway, 172–174
    discharge teaching form, 175
    potential client variances, 174

Implementation of critical pathway, 9–10
Interdisciplinary client care plan,
        example of, 5
Interdisciplinary interventions, 7
Interventions
    determination of, 9
    validation of, 11

Knee replacement (total)
    critical pathway, 176–180
    discharge teaching form, 181
    potential client variances, 181

Labor and delivery
    critical pathway, 237–240
    potential client variances, 240
Laminectomy (lumbar)
    critical pathway, 182–184
    discharge teaching form, 185
    potential client variances, 185
Laryngectomy
    critical pathway, 186–192
    discharge teaching form, 193
    potential client variances, 192
Lower leg fracture (open reduction and
        internal fixation)
    critical pathway, 194–196
    discharge teaching form, 197
    potential client variances, 197

Mastectomy
    critical pathway, 198–200
    discharge teaching form, 201
    potential client variances, 200
Microdiskectomy
    critical pathway, 202–203
    discharge teaching form, 204
    potential client variances, 204

Myocardial infarction (uncomplicated)
    critical pathway, 63–66
    discharge teaching form, 67
    potential client variances, 66
Myringotomy and insertion of
        pressure-equalizer tubes
    critical pathway, 266–267
    discharge teaching form, 268
    potential client variances, 267

Nephrectomy
    critical pathway, 205–209
    discharge teaching form, 210
    potential client variances, 209
Newborn
    critical pathway, 241–243
    potential client variances, 244
Nurse case managers
    information review by, 7
    responsibilities of, 3–4, 6
    validation of time line and
        interventions by, 11

Osteomyelitis
    critical pathway, 68–71
    discharge teaching form, 72
    potential client variances, 71
Outcome-driven management, 4
Outcomes, establishment of, 9

Pacemaker insertion (permanent)
    critical pathway, 211–213
    discharge teaching form, 214
    potential client variances, 213
Panic disorder: outpatient treatment
    critical pathway, 310–311
    discharge teaching form, 313–314
    potential client variances, 312
Pneumonia
    critical pathway, 73–76
    discharge teaching form, 77
    potential client variances, 76
Postpartum cesarean section
    critical pathway, 249–254
    discharge teaching form, 255–256
Postpartum vaginal delivery
    critical pathway, 245–248
    potential client variances, 248
Proctocolectomy with permanent
        ileostomy (total)
    critical pathway, 215–219
    discharge teaching form, 221
    potential client variances, 220

Pyloric stenosis (surgical repair)
    critical pathway, 269–270
    discharge teaching form, 271
    potential client variances, 271

Quality assurance improvement, 4

Respiratory infection (acute)
    critical pathway, 272–274
    discharge teaching form, 275
    potential client variances, 274

Sickle cell crisis
    critical pathway, 78–81
    discharge teaching form, 82
    potential client variances, 82
Splenectomy
    critical pathway, 222–225
    discharge teaching form, 226
    potential client variances, 225

Thyroidectomy
    critical pathway, 227–228
    discharge teaching form, 229
    potential client variances, 229
Time line
    determination of, 9
    validation of, 11
Tonsillectomy and adenoidectomy
    critical pathway, 276–277
    discharge teaching form, 278
    potential client variances, 277
Transurethral resection of the prostate
    critical pathway, 230–233
    discharge teaching form, 234
    potential client variances, 233

Variances in critical pathways
    computers used to analyze, 11
    defined, 10
    recording sheet, sample, 12–13

Weight loss program
    critical pathway, 83–84
    discharge teaching form, 84
    potential client variances, 84
Wound management at home
    critical pathway, 85
    discharge teaching form, 86
    potential client variances, 85